35.00

Cardiovascular Emergencies

This book is due for return on or before the last date shown below.

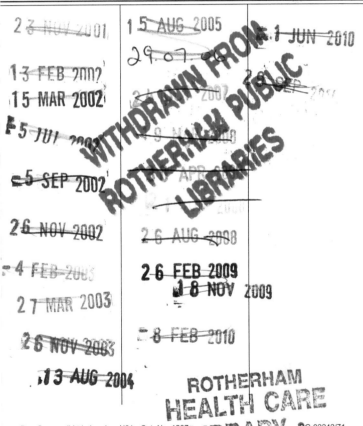

Don Gresswell Ltd., London, N21   Cat. No. 1207   DG 02242/71

Cardiovascular Emergencies

Edited by

Crispin Davies

Assistant Professor/Attending Cardiologist, Oregon Health Sciences University, Portland, USA

and

Yaver Bashir

Consultant Cardiologist, John Radcliffe Hospital, Oxford, UK

© BMJ Books 2001
BMJ Books is an imprint of the BMJ Publishing Group

First published in 2001
by BMJ Books, BMA House, Tavistock Square,
London WC1H 9JR

www.bmjbooks.com

British Library Cataloguing in Publication Data

A catalogue record for this book is available from the British Library

ISBN 0-7279-1484-7

Typeset by FiSH Books
Printed and bound by in Spain by GraphyCems, Navarra

Contents

Contributors

Yaver Bashir
Consultant Cardiologist
Department of Cardiology,
John Radcliffe Hospital, Oxford, UK

Keith Channon
BHF Reader in Cardiovascular Medicine
Honorary Consultant Cardiologist
Department of Cardiovascular Medicine, John Radcliffe
Hospital, Oxford, UK

Crispin Davies
Assistant Professor/Attending Cardiologist
Oregon Health Sciences University, Portland, USA

John Ferguson
Specialist Registrar (Cardiology)
John Radcliffe Hospital, Oxford, UK

M Hunt
Consultant in Emergency Medicine
Whipps Cross Hospital, Leytonstone, London, UK

Nigel Lever
Consultant Cardiologist
Wellington Hospital, Wellington, New Zealand

Intisor Mirza
Specialist Registrar (Cardiology)
John Radcliffe Hospital, Oxford, UK

Bruce Shively
Associate Professor/Attending Cardiologist
Oregon Health Science University, Portland, USA

David Sprigings
Consultant Cardiologist
Northampton General Hospital, Northampton, UK

Nick West
Research Fellow
Department of Cardiovascular Medicine, John Radcliffe
Hospital, Oxford, UK

Preface

Cardiovascular emergencies account for 30–40% of an acute medical workload that has grown inexorably over the last two decades. The same period has also witnessed unprecedented changes in the classification, investigation and treatment of acute cardiac problems, driven by advances in basic sciences, pharmacology and technology, but above all by a proliferating body of evidence from controlled trials. Nowhere has the shift from the traditional *laissez-faire* philosophy towards increasingly aggressive, interventionist approaches been more apparent than in the field of acute coronary syndromes. In 1980, the management of myocardial infarction consisted of little more than bed rest, analgesia and monitoring, while many physicians did not even recognise unstable angina as a distinct entity. Today, the same patients have to be guided through diverse and complex care pathways involving the use of potent but potentially hazardous drugs, and with much greater emphasis on invasive investigation and percutaneous revascularisation. For clinicians in the front line, the price of this progress has been that the management of common cardiovascular emergencies is now more complex and pressurised than in the past, requiring complex clinical judgements and frequent liaison with tertiary cardiac centres about the transfer of critically ill patients. Bed shortages, performance targets (for example, 'door-to-needle' times) and the growing threat of litigation have further compounded their anxieties. It is therefore hardly surprising that most junior doctors and general physicians from non-cardiac specialities regard this as perhaps the most stressful and demanding area of emergency medicine.

In producing 'Cardiovascular Emergencies' we have sought to fill a perceived gap in the literature. Standard internal medicine and cardiology textbooks have often failed to reflect the pace of change in this field and are too cumbersome for general reading. At the other end of the spectrum, emergency medicine pocket handbooks cater to the most junior medical staff, providing guidance on immediate management – of necessity, their format tends to be relatively didactic and does not allow more detailed consideration of the often complex issues surrounding management of these conditions. This book is intended to provide such essential background reading primarily for junior medical staff involved in acute general medical takes and specialist registrars in cardiology, intensive care or accident/emergency medicine. However, the subject matter may also be of interest to trainees in cardiothoracic surgery and anaesthesia, medical students and nurses working in cardiology wards, CCU or acute medical admissions units. Wherever possible, we have adopted a problem-orientated, stepwise approach to more closely reflect the way in which disorders present to clinicians in real-life, rather than the systematic layout of traditional textbooks. Mindful of modern bed pressures, due emphasis has been given to avoiding or shortening hospital admissions. No textbook can obviate the need for hard clinical experience or keeping abreast of the literature but our aim is to provide junior doctors with a basic framework for continuing professional development in this crucial area of acute medicine.

Crispin Davies
Yaver Bashir

1: Diagnosis of acute chest pain

DC SPRIGINGS, Y BASHIR, CH DAVIES

1.1 Introduction

Chest pain is the most common reason for referral of patients for acute medical admission. Prompt and accurate diagnosis is very important but our ability to differentiate between the patient with a life-threatening cardiac condition and someone with self-limiting musculoskeletal discomfort still depends primarily on clinical acumen plus interpretation of the ECG and (to a lesser extent) the chest radiograph. Unfortunately, such assessments have to be carried out against a background of conflicting priorities. Clinicians are encouraged to rapidly identify and offer fast-track thrombolysis to patients with acute myocardial infarction and ST elevation (shortening "door-to-needle time") while at the same time avoiding inappropriate, potentially hazardous treatment of those with conditions such as aortic dissection or pericarditis. Similarly, there is increasing pressure to reduce unnecessary admissions and minimise the length of hospital stay, but also a growing threat of litigation if a patient is sent home from the emergency department with a missed diagnosis of acute coronary syndrome and subsequently dies. These factors, combined with the fact that we often delegate responsibility for such decisions to relatively inexperienced doctors, may have contributed on the one hand to a steady growth in medico-legal actions, and on the other hand to an overcautious approach towards admitting patients with acute chest pain.

Another problem is that the traditional clinical approach to acute chest pain has relied on making a specific diagnosis in every patient either by pattern recognition or deductive analysis from a list of differential diagnoses. However, this "black or white" philosophy is unsuitable for many cases of suspected acute coronary syndrome in which key management decisions, particularly whether or not to admit, have to be made before a definite diagnosis can be reached. It is increasingly accepted that such decisions can be facilitated by risk-stratification algorithms which estimate the individual patient's short-term susceptibility to major cardiac events by integrating data from clinical assessment, ECG interpretation and biochemical markers such as troponins. The current chapter deals with the overall diagnostic approach to acute chest pain syndromes from this perspective. Discussion of the diagnosis of individual conditions is addressed in subsequent chapters.

1.2 Causes of acute chest pain

The causes of chest pain, grouped anatomically, are shown in Table 1.1. The relative frequency of the different diagnoses in clinical practice is shown in Figure 1.1. Ischaemic heart disease accounts for approximately 30% of cases of chest pain presenting to emergency departments, of whom 20% will have some form of acute coronary syndrome, but perhaps only 5% will exhibit acute ST elevation and be candidates for fast-track thrombolysis. It is important to note that acute coronary syndromes are far more common than other life-threatening conditions such as pulmonary embolism or aortic dissection (Figure 1.2). Among patients presenting with suspected acute coronary syndromes, but in whom ischaemic heart disease is not confirmed, oesophageal and musculoskeletal disorders are the most common non-cardiac causes of chest pain. Most of these conditions are benign with the exception of the rare and often forgotten diagnosis of oesophageal rupture (Boerhaave syndrome). No diagnosis can be made in approximately 10% of cases despite exhaustive investigation.

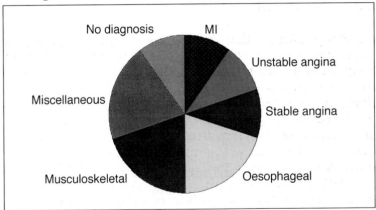

Figure 1.1 Diagnostic frequency of chest pain by aetiology.

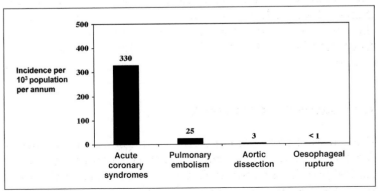

Figure 1.2 Life-threatening causes of acute chest pain-relative incidence.

Table 1.1 Causes of acute chest pain

	Common	Less common or rare
Cardiovascular	Acute coronary syndromes Pulmonary embolism	Aortic dissection Pericarditis Angina 2° to arrhythmia
Oesophageal	Gastro-oesophageal reflux Oesophageal spasm	Infective oesophagitis Oesophageal rupture
Respiratory	Pneumonia Pleurisy	Pneumothorax Pneumomediastinum
Musculoskeletal	Costochondritis Rib fractures Pain arising from intercostals or shoulder girdle muscles	Vertebral crush fractures
Others		Biliary tract disease Acute pancreatitis Perforated peptic ulcer Sickle cell crisis Herpes zoster

1.3 Diagnostic approach

The process begins in all patients with a rapid clinical assessment (including measurement of the vital signs and transcutaneous oxygen saturation) plus recording of a 12-lead ECG. Unless the ECG shows ST segment elevation diagnostic of acute myocardial infarction (see below) a chest radiograph is also needed as part of the initial evaluation. Selection of further investigations will then depend on the clinical picture.

In some cases the diagnosis may now be apparent from "pattern recognition", that is the presence of clinical, ECG, or radiographic features of high specificity for individual conditions. The most important examples of pattern recognition in patients presenting with acute chest pain are summarised in Box 1.1. Of course, many patients with these disorders will not exhibit such highly specific features, and then a systematic or hypothetico-deductive approach (thinking of possible diagnoses and testing for them) is required. In practice, it may still not be possible to make a definite early diagnosis in many cases of suspected acute coronary syndrome (by far the most common scenario). For this large and problematic subgroup, key management decisions (particularly with respect to admission/discharge) can be facilitated by the use of risk stratification algorithms to estimate the individual patient's short-term susceptibility to major/life-threatening cardiac events.

Box 1.1 Pattern recognition in acute chest pain

Acute myocardial infarction
- Pain, consistent with myocardial ischaemia, at rest for > 20 min; *and*
- ST segment elevation > 1 mm in 2 or more adjacent leads, not known to be old

Unstable angina
- Pain, consistent with myocardial ischaemia, on minimal exertion or at complete rest; *and*
- Relief with nitrates *or*
- ST depression > 1 mm *and/or* T wave inversion in 2 or more adjacent leads, not known to be old

Aortic dissection
- Abrupt severe anterior or posterior chest pain; *and*
- Major pulse asymmetry; *or*
- Aortic regurgitation; *and*
- No ST segment elevation

Oesophageal rupture
- Pain following vomiting; *and*
- Mediastinal gas on chest *x* ray (CXR); *and*
- No ST segment elevation

Pericarditis
- Pleuritic central chest pain; *and*
- Pericardial rub; or
- ST/T abnormalities consistent with pericarditis

Pneumothorax
- Abrupt pleuritic pain; *and*
- Visceral pleural line on CXR, with absent lung markings between this line and the chest wall

Musculoskeletal pain
- Localised chest wall pain; *and*
- Pain reproduced by pressure over the site of spontaneous pain; *and*
- Normal ECG and CXR

Based on these general principles, the diagnostic process can be approached in a series of steps:

Step 1: Confirming the obvious

Step 2: Identifying or excluding immediately life-threatening conditions

Step 3: Considering other specific diagnoses

Step 4: Deciding who can be discharged

1.3.1 Step 1: Confirming the obvious

The diagnosis will be obvious in a proportion of cases. This particularly applies to patients with acute chest pain suggestive of myocardial ischaemia (Box 1.2) in association with ST elevation (see Chapter 3) or those with typical pain and widespread ST depression (see Chapter 4). An extensive search through a long list of possible diagnoses is inappropriate: the emphasis here must be on speed. In patients with clear evidence of acute myocardial infarction and ST elevation, thrombolysis should be administered with a minimum of delay before a chest x ray is obtained and, if necessary, before the patient is transferred to the Coronary Care Unit (CCU).

1.3.2 Step 2: Identifying or excluding immediately life-threatening conditions

In patients in whom the diagnosis is unclear at presentation, the first priority is to exclude the four common conditions which present with acute chest pain and may result in sudden death (Figure 1.2) if not correctly identified and treated.

Acute coronary syndromes/myocardial ischaemia

The clinical features of acute myocardial ischaemia are well recognised (Box 1.2). However, the diversity of presentations of ischaemic chest pain gives rise to potential problems. Firstly, misdiagnosis may result if patients fail to use the classical descriptions such as "crushing pain", "heaviness", "chest tightness", etc., expected by doctors. Secondly, there is a tendency to classify patients as "cardiac" or "non-cardiac" early on in the history-taking process and then to search for corroborative evidence. It is important to keep an open mind as to the diagnosis, to give the patient ample opportunity to tell the story in his/her own words, and to be receptive to cues such as hand movements during descriptions of the pain. For example, three quarters of those who illustrate their pain by placing a flat hand or clenched fist on the sternum or by drawing both palms laterally across their chest are suffering from ischaemic chest pain (however, failure to provoke this sign does not exclude ischaemia).[1]

Box 1.2 Clinical features of myocardial ischaemia

- The pain is central and midsternal, and tends to radiate bilaterally: across or round the chest; into the sides of the neck and jaws; into the shoulders and down the inner or outer sides of the arms; occasionally through to the back between the shoulder blades. Radiation may be unilateral, and then more commonly to the left side than the right.
- Centrifugal radiation of the pain is the rule, but centripetal spread may occur, with pain starting in the wrists, upper arms, or jaw, and spreading to the chest.
- The pain is described in terms such as heavy, squeezing, constricting, aching, "a weight on the chest", "a band around the chest", or "like indigestion". It may be stinging, numbing, or burning. It is not sharp, shooting, or stabbing. The pain may be illustrated with a clenched fist held against the sternum.
- The severity of the pain is variable.
- The duration of pain in myocardial infarction is > 20 minutes and usually for several hours.
- Associated breathlessness is common. With myocardial infarction, there may also be weakness, sweating, nausea, and vomiting.
- Pain is not affected by deep inspiration or changes in posture (cf pericarditis).

The presence or absence of classical risk factors (smoking, hypertension, etc.) seems to be of surprisingly little value in making a diagnosis of acute myocardial ischaemia. In three large studies none of the classical risk factors emerged as independent predictors of the presence of an acute coronary syndrome.[2]

Diagnosing cardiac ischaemia may be more straightforward if there is any preceding history of angina pectoris. The cardinal feature is the relationship of the symptoms to exertion. The maxim that any discomfort experienced between the jaw and the umbilicus that starts with exertion and stops with rest should be considered ischaemic until proven otherwise, is worth remembering. Although myocardial ischaemia presenting as jaw and arm discomfort is well recognised, it is less commonly appreciated that these patients frequently admit to concomitant chest discomfort on direct questioning. The discriminatory value of associated features such as whether the pain radiates to the right or left arm, and the presence of nausea, etc., is poor and of little clinical value.[2]

In many cases, it is only possible to make a provisional diagnosis of suspected (rather than definite) acute coronary syndrome when the patient is initially assessed. It is in this group of patients that risk-stratification schemes may be of particular clinical utility (see below).

Aortic dissection and intramural haematoma

Problems with the diagnosis of aortic dissection and other acute aortic syndromes centre on unfamiliarity with a relatively rare condition (100 times less common than acute coronary syndromes) and the potential diversity of associated complications. Patients seldom present with a full constellation of signs; for example, classical features such as aortic regurgitation and demonstrable pulse deficits are each apparent in only 50% of cases of proximal dissection. Conversely, apparent mediastinal widening on the chest x ray (especially with an AP film) has poor specificity for aortic dissection in isolation, and too often is used to raise concerns about a clear cut diagnosis of acute myocardial infarction (see Chapter 3).

The possibility of aortic dissection must be considered in any patient with severe acute chest pain but no obvious ST segment shift; the disparity between the ECG and the severity of the symptoms should always trigger concern. The most important feature is the instantaneous onset of pain (in contrast to the pain of myocardial infarction which builds up over a period of several minutes). It is also not widely appreciated that the pain may radiate along the course of the aorta or its major branches. Proximal aortic dissection typically presents with retrosternal pain, whilst interscapular pain is more commonly associated with distal dissection. Other important clues *if present* include the finding of aortic regurgitation or associated neurological symptoms/signs (but absence of such features does not exclude dissection). One should be particularly vigilant in patients with conditions known to predispose to dissection such as hypertension, Marfan's syndrome, and pregnancy. Specific investigation of patients with suspected acute aortic syndromes is discussed in Chapter 7.

Pulmonary embolism

Minor pulmonary emboli typically present with pleuritic chest pain and the main differential diagnoses are pneumothorax, pneumonia, and chest wall pain. Patients with major pulmonary emboli (occlusion of ≥ 2 major lobar arteries) may develop retrosternal chest discomfort due to right ventricular ischaemia but this is almost always associated with dyspnoea and/or tachypnoea. The absence of dyspnoea/tachypnoea or pleuritic pain makes pulmonary embolism extremely unlikely (less than 3% of cases).

The relative rarity of pulmonary embolism presenting with ischaemic-type chest pain may result in it being overlooked as a possibility. Pulmonary embolism tends to be overdiagnosed in healthy patients and underdiagnosed in sick patients. The majority of patients with major emboli have a predisposing factor such as recent surgery, pregnancy, malignancy, prior thromboembolism, etc. A common pitfall is the failure to obtain arterial blood gases before the patient receives supplemental oxygen. Although correction for this is possible using the alveolar gas equation, firstly this tends to be neglected in the acute situation and secondly, the inspired oxygen concentration, at the time the sample was taken is usually not known. Once the diagnosis of pulmonary embolism is considered, the significance of relatively "minor" chest *x* ray abnormalities such as the presence of pleural effusions should not be underestimated. Further discussion of the investigation of patients with suspected pulmonary embolism is discussed in Chapter 8.[8]

Oesophageal rupture

The classical presentation is one of vomiting preceding severe chest pain (the opposite order to myocardial infarction), but this occurs in only a minority of cases. Although this is a rare condition, the diagnosis should be suspected in patients with unexplained chest pain and pleural effusions, pneumothoraces, particularly in patients who appear unexpectedly unwell or have unexplained leukocytosis.[3] It is more common in patients with chronic alcoholism or bulimia.

1.3.3 Step 3: Considering other specific diagnoses

Having excluded immediate life-threatening conditions, the next step is to consider alternative specific diagnoses. There are many potential conditions in this group (Table 1.1). Although the majority will declare themselves via the presence of associated features and do not usually present diagnostic difficulties, some deserve specific discussion.

Pericarditis

The central pleuritic chest pain that is worsened by lying down and relieved by sitting forward is well recognised as is the characteristic "concave upwards" ST segment elevation. Problems occur in differentiating the ECG changes from patients with acute infarction and from the changes of early repolarisation in young people.

Table 1.2 Comparison of the ECG features of acute myocardial infarction, early repolarisation, and pericarditis

ECG feature	Myocardial infarction	Early repolarisation	Pericarditis
ST morphology	Convex downwards	Concave upwards	Concave upwards
Distribution of ST elevation	Vascular distribution	Commonly septal, rarely limb leads	Non-vascular distribution
ST elevation V6	In inferolateral or anterolateral MI	Uncommon	Common
ST depression V1	In posterior MI	Rare	Common
ST/T evolution	Uniform in all involved leads	Does not occur	Various stages seem simultaneously
Pathological Q waves	Commonly develop	Never	Never

The cardinal feature is the fact that, in pericarditis, the ST elevation does not follow the characteristic vascular territories (anterior/inferior/posterior, etc.) seen in acute infarction. In addition there is usually a clear mismatch between the patient's clinical condition and the ECG in that there is ST elevation in numerous leads but the patient is not that unwell. If genuine doubt persists then echocardiography may be helpful as infarction on the scale suggested by the widespread ST elevation is always associated with a segmental contraction abnormality (Table 1.2).

Although idiopathic/viral pericarditis is the commonest aetiology it is important to consider other causes of pericarditis, and the possibility that a pericardial effusion in the context of acute chest pain could be secondary to aortic dissection, or complicating a late presentation of myocardial infarction. Patients should be carefully examined for signs of tamponade and echocardiography considered prior to discharge.

Oesophageal pain

In patients with undiagnosed acute chest pain following CCU admission, the incidence of oesophageal disorders (excluding rupture) is 70–90%.[4] Unfortunately, this is a difficult diagnosis to make with confidence on clinical criteria alone as both ischaemia and indigestion can occur after meals and, confusingly, both can be improved by belching. Oesophageal spasm may be provoked by exercise, whilst recumbancy may worsen both reflux and severe angina ("decubitus angina"). Occasionally, the pain of oesophageal spasm can be relieved by glyceryl trinitrate (GTN) (although less dramatically and over a longer time course than the pain of ischaemia). Oesophageal spasm has been associated with ECG changes and reflux can provoke angina ("linked angina"). Both conditions are common, and may co-exist in some patients. The presence of water brash (acid regurgitated into the mouth) is specific for reflux if it can be elicited. Disappointingly there is no straightforward answer to this dilemma and many of these patients will require admission in the first instance to rule out an acute coronary syndrome.

Musculoskeletal pain

Tenderness located in the region of the origin of the patient's spontaneous pain is the strongest evidence favouring this diagnosis, particularly when the quality of the pain evoked reproduces the spontaneous pain, and when present, this sign significantly reduces the likelihood of myocardial infarction.[2] A diagnosis of musculoskeletal chest pain should be avoided unless such local signs are present and the ECG and chest x ray are completely normal.

1.3.4 Step 4: Deciding whom to send home

As indicated previously, the most common problem is differentiating acute coronary syndromes from oesophageal or musculoskeletal causes. Ideally, only those patients with a definite diagnosis of a benign condition would be discharged directly from the emergency department. In reality, it is frequently not possible to establish the cause of acute chest pain with certainty on the basis of the initial assessment alone.

Making a specific diagnosis in patients with suspected acute coronary syndrome may be less important than the decision about whether hospitalisation is required or not. It is in this area that risk stratification schemes to estimate the individual's short-term risk of major adverse cardiac events (death, myocardial infarction, cardiac arrest, etc.) have become of increasingly important. A secondary issue then arises as to the appropriate level of care that the patient requires if admitted (i.e. CCU or general ward). In an attempt to rationalise this process, Goldman et al. have developed prediction rules which can provide a framework for decision making[5,6] (Figure 1.3). From their retrospective and prospective analysis of over 15 000 cases of acute chest pain the following key points emerge:

- Patients with ST elevation or pathological Q waves "not known to be old" are easily removed from the analysis as a high-risk group requiring admission and reperfusion (thrombolysis or primary PTCA)
- Patients with ST depression or T wave inversion in more than two leads form a group at "moderate risk" (8%) or "high risk" (16%) of major adverse cardiac events in the following 72 hours depending on the presence of additional risk factors (Box 1.3).

Box 1.3 "Additional" risk factors in patients with suspected ischaemic chest pain

- Systolic BP < 110 mmHg
- Crackles above both lung bases
- Worsening stable angina
- Post MI angina
- Angina following percutaneous transluminal coronary angioplasty (PTCA) or coronary artery bypass graft (CABG)
- Pain similar to prior myocardial infarction (MI)

- The event rate among patients with no ECG changes at presentation depends upon the number of risk factors present. With two or more additional risk factors, the event rate was still 8% ("moderate risk"), with one additional risk factor, the event rate was 4% ("low risk"), and with no additional risk factors, the chances of a major event over the next 72 hours falls to only 0.6% ("very low risk").

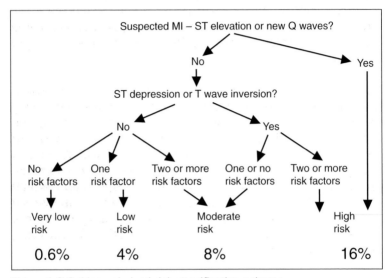

Figure 1.3 Goldman-derived risk stratification scheme.

In practice, approximately 50% of patients fall into the very low risk group, with 40% in the low and moderate risk groups and 10% in the high risk group.[6]

All patients with a risk in excess of 4% require admission, and those in the high risk group should be managed in a CCU. The placement of patients in the moderate risk category will depend on local facilities, but an admissions ward with ECG monitoring facility is usually appropriate.

Many patients within the low risk category and almost all patients in the very low risk category can be discharged from the emergency department and managed on an outpatient basis. Unless a confident diagnosis of non-cardiac chest pain has been made, these individuals should usually be started on appropriate medical therapy for a suspected acute coronary syndrome (e.g. aspirin, GTN, ß-blocker) and arrangements made for cardiology outpatient review and stress testing. They should also be advised about what to do if they experience further symptoms in the interim. The degree of urgency regarding clinical review depends on the individual case and local circumstances. Increasingly, these patients are being handled via dedicated chest pain clinics to ensure a rapid turnaround.

This approach may at first appear paradoxical when considered with the generally accepted fact that patients may present with a normal or non-diagnostic ECG but still go on to experience an infarct. However, one of the most important conclusions of the Goldman study is that, in the absence of the specified additional risk factors, these patients have an excellent prognosis: even if admitted to hospital they would not be candidates for active reperfusion therapy on current criteria,[7] and with such a low event rate, probably would not benefit from CCU admission, ECG monitoring, heparinisation, etc.

Whether or not one uses the prediction tool in practice, two clear messages emerge: patients with an abnormal ECG should *not* be sent home without very compelling reasons, and that proficiency in ECG interpretation is a prerequisite for rational decision-making. Studies of ECG interpretation skills do not give cause for optimism on the latter point and it may be that specific emphasis needs to be placed on developing such skills among junior doctors training in acute medicine.

1.4 Specific problems in the diagnosis of patients with chest pain

1.4.1 Chest pain and left bundle branch block

Patients presenting with an MI and left bundle branch block (LBBB) have a worse prognosis than patients with infarction and normal ventricular conduction (Box 1.4). This is true for patients both with acute LBBB (in whom there is usually a very proximal left anterior descending (LAD) coronary artery occlusion) and in patients with established LBBB in whom it is a marker of pre-existing ventricular disease.[8] This increased risk of death is reflected in a higher than average benefit from thrombolyis in this population. However, the diagnosis of infarction is difficult in the presence of abnormal ventricular activation. Analysis of the subset of patients with LBBB in GUSTO-1 revealed the following to be independent predictors of MI.[9]

Box 1.4 Predictors of MI in patients with LBBB

- > 1 mm ST elevation in leads with a positive QRS
- ST depression > 1 mm in V1, V2, or V3
- ST depression > 5 mm in leads with a negative QRS

The problem with these guidelines is that despite high specificity, their sensitivity for diagnosing MI is < 40%. The patients who benefited so dramatically from thrombolysis in clinical trials were not selected on the basis of these criteria and it would thus be incorrect to withhold thrombolysis from someone who did not meet the above criteria.

Another problem that arises is that although the presence of a conduction defect and chest pain increases a patient's risk of myocardial infarction by approximately three fold,[10] it does not guarantee it, emphasising the importance of a corroborating clinical history.

1.4.2 ECGs demonstrating "no acute changes"

The "no acute changes" comment is frequently seen on A&E notes and is potentially misleading. Even a "non acute" ECG may contain useful information as the presence of new Q waves increases the probability of an MI by up to 20-fold, but the presence of any Q wave still increases it four-fold. In addition, it is not possible to determine whether the changes are acute or not without a prior ECG, which is usually unavailable. Importantly, in the Goldman analysis the criterion is for "Q waves not known to be old" and thus those patients with Q waves of indeterminate age should strictly be in the high risk group. For these reasons a statement of what the ECG actually shows, new or old, is preferable.

1.4.3 Atypical symptoms but an abnormal ECG

The Goldman decision analysis provides a clear answer here, in that patients with chest pain and "ischaemic" ECGs have a high rate of adverse clinical events (8–16% over the ensuing 72 hours).[5] These patients should be admitted and failure to do so is a common source of litigation (in retrospect the atypical features of the history are soon forgotten but the accusingly abnormal ECG remains).

1.4.4 Role of troponins in deciding admission/discharge policy

There has been a protracted search for a single test that would reliably predict those patients with acute chest pain but no ST elevation who could be safely discharged home. Troponin T and I are subtle biochemical markers of myocardial necrosis (Table 1.3) and have been suggested as potential candidates for this role.[11,12] In the largest prospective study to date, only 0.3% of patients with negative troponin I levels died or experienced an MI over the following 30 days.[11] The attractiveness of troponin assays is in their inclusion of the subset of unstable angina patients who are most at risk of developing complications[13] (unlike CK assays which, by definition, are not elevated in unstable angina). However, to expect a single test to replace such a complex piece of clinical decision making is naïve. Firstly, two samples were required (the second 4 hours after the first) and analysis of patients with ST depression and negative troponin tests showed an upper confidence level of adverse events approaching an unacceptable 8%.[14] As troponin release may take 12 hours, sampling within 12 hours of the onset of chest pain may contribute to "false negative" results. Thus, whilst troponins can provide an additional safeguard in deciding which patients to send home they cannot replace the importance of the clinical history and a normal ECG.

Despite these limitations, many clinicians favour a protocol for patients with suspected acute coronary syndrome based on an abbreviated admission (8–12 hours) for observation, repeat

ECG analysis and measurement of troponin levels. All those without high risk features can be offered early discharge. Some A&E departments and acute medical units have introduced dedicated "short stay" areas specifically for this purpose, with access to predischarge exercise testing.

Table 1.3 Plasma markers of myocardial necrosis

Marker	Rise time	Peak	Return to baseline
Myoglobin	1–4 hours	6–7 hours	24 hours
Troponin I	3–12 hours	24 hours	5–10 days
Troponin T	3–12 hours	12–48 hours	3–4 days
CK	4–8 hours	12–24 hours	3–4 days
CK-MB	4–8 hours	18–36 hours	2–3 days
AST	8–12 hours	18–36 hours	3–4 days
LDH	8–12 hours	3–6 days	8–14 days

Note that the time to peak is shortened following successful reperfusion CK, creatine kinase; AST, aspartate transaminase; LDH, lactate dehydrogenase.

Plasma troponin level is of use for risk stratification of patients with suspected unstable angina in combination with clinical features and the ECG. This is discussed further in Chapter 4.

1.4.5 Atypical pain, normal ECG but raised enzymes/troponins

There are several other sources of "cardiac" markers that are frequently forgotten and produce diagnostic confusion. Plasma creatine kinase is present in skeletal muscle and is elevated by intramuscular injections, postoperatively and in marathon runners. Lactate dehydrogenase is present in erythrocytes and is therefore elevated by red cell breakdown such as pulmonary embolism and haemolytic anaemia. The clue tends to be an atypical progression over time and a disparity between a large enzyme rise and an apparently well patient. Note that for the diagnosis of myocardial infarction the enzyme level must be greater than twice the upper limit of normal. The MB fraction of creatine kinase (CK) is not entirely myocardial specific, particularly in the face of substantial elevations in total CK.

Although the troponins are more specific than traditional enzymes, positive results can also occur in pulmonary embolism, myocarditis, pulmonary embolism, and renal failure. In fairness, all of the above potentially require admission in their own right.

1.4.6 The patient who persistently returns

These patients soon become labelled as "malingerers" and their symptoms dismissed. However in retrospective analysis of inappropriate discharges, it is apparent that patients had frequently presented with a similar problem to another physician in the last week. There is a natural tendency to accept the prior diagnosis and to unconsciously contour the patient's symptoms to fit this. However, rather than accept the prior diagnosis, this should be taken as an opportunity to carefully re-evaluate the history. Often the passage of time and the patient's further exposure to the symptoms will have clarified the description of pain. The ECG should be repeated with particular emphasis on obtaining a recording during pain. Even in those without risk factors, coronary artery disease remains the commonest single cause of death in western society. Similar comments apply to the patient who is unwilling to go home following the diagnosis of non-cardiac chest pain in whom overnight admission is the preferred option.

1.4.7 Young patients with ST elevation and atypical symptoms

Patients of Caribbean origin may show persistent ST elevation in the anterior chest leads, which should be accepted as being a normal variant. Similarly young patients with high vagal tone may manifest "high take off" in the anterior leads. This normalises when vagal tone is reduced by exercise.

1.4.8 Patients with Marfan's syndrome

Patients with the Marfan phenotype who present with chest pain should be evaluated carefully to exclude the possibility of aortic dissection.

1.4.9 Atypical chest pains and mitral valve prolapse

Recent population studies have dismissed the belief that there is an association between mitral valve prolapse and atypical chest pain. Pain can occur at the point of chordal rupture but the accompanying severe mitral regurgitation will be clinically obvious.

1.4.10 Chest pain with ECGs evidence of left ventricular hypertrophy

Patients with left ventricular hypertrophy (LVH) (usually hypertensive) can present with ischaemic rest pain, frequently associated with atrial fibrillation. The ST segment depression associated with the electrical LVH can be confused with the dynamic ST depression of an acute coronary syndrome. Recognition that the finding of ST depression is not specific to acute coronary syndromes in the context of LVH is the key to correct diagnosis. These patients settle with control of the ventricular rate and attention should be directed towards identifying a stimulus for the tachycardia (i.e. heart failure, infection, etc.).

1.4.11 Role of non-invasive imaging in acute diagnosis

It is possible to further refine the diagnostic process by performing echocardiography (to look for segmental wall motion defects), myocardial contrast echocardiography (for segmental perfusion defects), or technitium[99] sestamibi scans[15] (again for segmental perfusion defects). However, recent studies have failed to demonstrate any additional benefit from the use of nuclear imaging compared to troponins.[16] In addition, the logistics of performing these tests in the A&E department and the fact that the costs are not dissimilar to those for overnight observation have prevented their adoption into routine clinical practice. Marginally more realistic in terms of UK practice is the use of the exercise ECG which has been demonstrated to be safe[17] and has been successfully used in the chest pain units in the USA.

Clinical cases

Case 1.1

A 33-year-old Afro-Caribbean man developed severe cramp-like chest and abdominal pain after taking "Ecstasy" and amphetamine. His ECG showed ST segment elevation (Figure 1.4). A diagnosis was made of acute myocardial infarction and thrombolysis was administered. There was no ECG evolution or enzyme release. Three months later he presented to another hospital following an episode of sharp left parasternal chest pain, associated with heaviness of the left arm, which lasted 40 minutes. Again, myocardial infarction was diagnosed and thrombolysis given. His ECG remained unchanged, and all other investigations, including echocardiography, were normal. The final diagnosis was non-specific chest pain and ST segment elevation due to early repolarisation.

ST elevation in the anterior leads is a normal variant in Afro-Caribbeans. This does not usually present problems in patients with atypical chest pain but, as this case demonstrates, can provide a major diagnostic dilemma in some patients. The absence of a contractile defect on echocardiography might have provided useful additional information here.

Case 1.2

A woman aged 50 developed severe pain in the left chest and shoulder after vomiting. Examination showed some tenderness of the thoracic spine, but no other abnormal signs. Her ECG was normal, and the chest radiograph, in the opinion of the doctor who saw her, was also normal. Musculoskeletal pain was diagnosed. She was given analgesia and discharged. She was found dead 12 hours later. A post-mortem examination revealed oesophageal rupture with food in the left mediastinum. Review of the chest radiograph showed mediastinal gas and small pleural effusions.

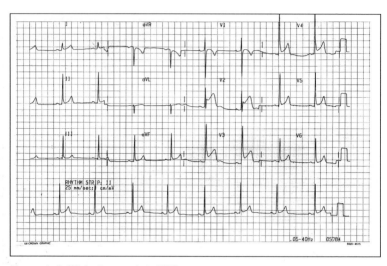

Figure 1.4 Clinical case 1.1: ECG.

> *A normal ECG does not guarantee the patient's safety. In retrospect the history of pain after vomiting should have aroused suspicion. Patients with chest pain and an abnormal chest x ray represent a potentially high risk group: small pleural effusions can occur in both oesophageal rupture, pulmonary embolism, aortic dissection, and aortic rupture.*

Case 1.3

A 73-year-old woman was woken by severe anterior chest pain which persisted. She was taking warfarin because of previous pulmonary embolism (INR on admission 2.6) and atrial fibrillation, and had been treated for hypertension for 15 years. Examination showed elevation of the jugular venous pressure, and normal peripheral pulses. Blood pressure was 140/70 mmHg, with 15 mmHg pulsus paradoxus. Her ECG showed minor ST/T wave abnormalities. Transthoracic echocardiography showed a small pericardial effusion, and normal left ventricular contraction, with concentric LV wall hypertrophy. No aortic intimal flap was seen. A diagnosis was made of pericarditis. She developed cardiac arrest with asystole 24 hours after admission. Post-mortem examination showed extensive aortic dissection, with haemopericardium due to rupture into the pericardial sac

Aortic dissection provides one of the greatest challenges in the diagnosis of chest pain as the penalties for failing to make the correct diagnosis are so high (see also Chapter 7). In retrospect, pericarditis of this severity, is usually accompanied by more dramatic ECG changes and a small effusion from viral pericarditis would not have produced detectable paradox (whereas even a small amount of blood introduced into the pericardial space at arterial pressure would). The failure of the pain to dramatically improve following a single dose of a non-steroidal anti-inflammatory drug might have raised suspicion that further investigation was necessary by CT or angiography.

Case 1.4

A 52-year-old woman with longstanding hypertension presented with a 24 hour history of intermittent chest discomfort. She was unsure of her current medications. Her ECG (figure 1.5a) was interpreted as demonstrating ST depression indicative of an acute coronary syndrome. Troponins were negative. Despite heparin and tirofiban, she continued to experience intermittent chest discomfort and was referred for urgent coronary angiography. This demonstrated left ventricular hypertrophy with normal coronary arteries. Her condition improved with appropriate control of her ventricular rate, achieved with β-blockade.

Poorly controlled atrial fibrillation may occasionally present with ill-defined chest discomfort, particularly in patients with left ventricular hypertrophy. ST depression (+/− T wave inversion) does not automatically indicate an acute coronary syndrome and requires cautious interpretation in the context of atrial fibrillation with digoxin (as in this patient) or in patients with left ventricular hypertrophy (as in figure 1.5b, whose chest discomfort was due to hypertrophic cardiomyopathy).

Summary: Common mistakes in the diagnosis of acute chest pain in accident and emergency departments

- Discharging patients with abnormal ECGs
- Attempting to make a diagnosis of musculoskeletal chest pain in the presence of "minor" ECG or chest x ray abnormalities
- Contouring patient's histories to fit preconceived ideas about the diagnosis
- Administering thrombolysis to patients without ST elevation or new LBBB
- Not considering acute aortic syndromes in patients with severe chest pain of abrupt onset and normal or non-diagnostic ECG
- Failing to consider pulmonary embolism as a diagnosis, despite the presence of risk factors
- Failing to account for the inspired O_2 concentration when analysing blood gases
- Reluctance to admit patients for overnight admission despite diagnostic uncertainty

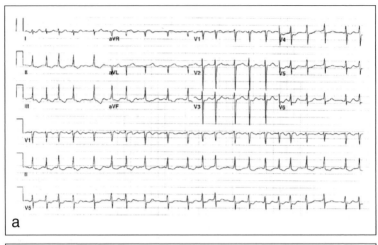

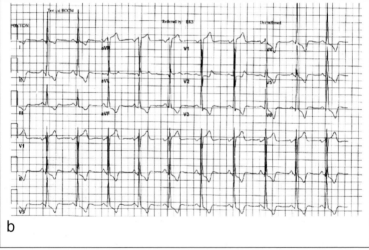

Figure 1.5 ECGs from Case 1.4: (a) on arrival and (b) the following day.

References

1 Edmondstone WM. Cardiac chest pain: does body language help the diagnosis? *BMJ* 1995;**311**:1660–1.
2 Panju M, Hemmelgarn BR, Guyatt GH, Simel DL. Is this patient having a myocardial infarction? *JAMA* 1998;**280**:1256–63.
3 Lemke T, Jagminas L. Spontaneous esophageal rupture: a frequently missed diagnosis. *Am Surg* 1999;**65**:449–52.
4 Panju M, Farkouh ME, Sackett DL, *et al*. Outcome of patients discharged from a coronary care unit with a diagnosis of "chest pain not yet diagnosed". *CMA J* 1996;**155**:552–3.

5 Goldman L, Cook EF, Johnson PA, *et al.* Prediction of the need for intensive care in patients who come to the emergency departments with acute chest pain. *N Engl J Med* 1996;**334**:1498–504.

6 Reilly B, Durairaj L, Husain S, *et al.* Performance and potential impact of a chest pain prediction rule in a large public hospital. *Am J Med* 1999;**106**:285–91.

7 FTT Collaborative Group. Indications for fibrinolytic therapy in suspected acute myocardial infarction: collaborative overview of early mortality and major morbidity results from all randomised trials of more than 1000 patients. Fibrinolytic Therapy Trialists' (FTT) Collaborative Group. *Lancet* 1994;**343**:311–22.

8 Wellens HJ. Acute myocardial infarction and left bundle-branch block – can we lift the veil? *N Engl J Med* 1996;**334**:528–9.

9 Sgarbossa EB, Pinski SL, Barbagelata A, *et al.* Electrocardiographic diagnosis or evolving acute myocardial infarction in the presence of left bundle-branch block. GUSTO-1 (Global Utilization of Streptokinase and Tissue Plasminogen Activator for Occluded Coronary Arteries) Investigators [published erratum appears in *N Engl J Med* 1996;**334**(14):931]. *N Engl J Med* 1996;**334**:481–7.

10 Wackers FJ. The diagnosis of myocardial infarction in the presence of left bundle branch block. *Cardiol Clin* 1987;**5**:393–401.

11 Hamm CW, Goldmann BU, Heeschen C, Kreymann G, Berger J, Meinertz T. Emergency room triage of patients with acute chest pain by means of rapid testing for cardiac troponin T or troponin I. *N Engl J Med* 1997;**337**:1648–53.

12 Hillis GS, Zhao N, Taggart P, Dalsey WC, Mangione A. Utility of cardiac troponin I, creatine-kinase MB mass, myosin light chain 1, and myoglobin in the early in-hospital triage of "high risk" patients with chest pain. *Heart* 1999;**82**:614–20.

13 Heeschen C, van den Brand MJ, Hamm CW, Simons ML. Angiographic findings in patients with refractory unstable angina according to troponin T status. *Circulation* 1999;**100**:1509–14.

14 Hlatky MA. Evaluation of chest pain in the emergency department. *N Engl J Med* 1997;**337**:1687–9.

15 Heller GV, Stowers SA, Hendel RC, *et al.* Clinical value of acute rest technetium-99m tetrofosmin tomographic myocardial perfusion imaging in patients with acute chest pain and nondiagnostic electrocardiograms. *J Am Coll Card* 1998;**31**:1011–17.

16 Kontos MC, Jesse RL, Anderson FP, Schmidt KL, Ornato JP, Tatum JL. Comparison of myocardial perfusion imaging and cardiac troponin I in patients admitted to the emergency department with chest pain. *Circulation* 1999;**99**:2073–8.

17 Kirk JD, Turnipseed S, Lewis WR, Amsterdam EA. Evaluation of chest pain in low-risk patients presenting to the emergency department: the role of immediate exercise testing. *Ann Emerg Med* 1998;**32**:1–7.

2: Acute coronary syndromes I: pathogenesis

CH DAVIES, Y BASHIR

2.1 Correlations between arterial pathology and clinical presentations

The acute coronary syndromes are a spectrum of conditions ranging from unstable angina to non-Q wave and Q wave infarction. Virtually all are initiated by the development of thrombosis on a plaque of coronary atheroma,[1] rare exceptions include coronary emboli from bacterial endocarditis and spontaneous coronary dissection.

The pathological sequelae of this thrombosis dictates the clinical presentation. The correlations between events in the arterial lumen and the ECG are imprecise but, perhaps surprisingly for a technique which is now over a century old, still form the basis of disease classification and management decisions.

2.2 Stable plaque formation and progression

Atheromatous plaques consist of an extracellular lipid-containing core surrounded by connective tissue in which numerous cholesterol laden macrophages are embedded.[2] Plaque formation is initiated by endothelial injury followed by lipid deposition; oxidation of this lipid then attracts monocytes which ingest lipid to become foam cells. Subsequent foam cell rupture releases large amounts of cellular debris and cholesterol, resulting in gradual plaque progression. The fibrous cap is the zone interposed between the lipid core and the vessel lumen (Figure 2.1).

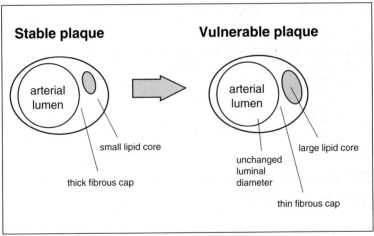

Figure 2.1 Transition from stable to vulnerable plaque. Adapted from Davies.[1]

Plaques are frequently found with increasing age in asymptomatic individuals. Flow limitation and stable angina do not occur until these occupy 50% of the luminal diameter. Matters are complicated by the fact that expansion of the adjacent vessel wall tends to accompany plaque development and thus luminal obstruction does not correlate with plaque volume. Continued extension of this process might be expected to eventually result in coronary occlusion and myocardial infarction. However, the gradual rate of progression provides ample time for the development of collaterals and infarction does not usually occur. At this stage, the resting ECG will be normal (although an exercise ECG may be abnormal).

2.3 Transition to vulnerable plaque

This relatively stable situation is disturbed by the transition from a stable to a vulnerable plaque[3] (Figure 2.1, Box 2.1).

Box 2.1 Factors favouring the transition from stable to vulnerable plaque

- Lipid core occupies > 50% of plaque volume
- Increase in macrophages
- Decrease in smooth muscle cells
- Thinning of the fibrous cap by macrophage derived metalloproteinases

---

Again, vulnerability does not necessarily equate with the degree of luminal obstruction and it is important to appreciate that even a vulnerable plaque may still not be apparent on coronary angiography.[4,5] Thus, in patients in whom angiography was performed prior to an ischaemic event it is frequently impossible to identify the plaque that subsequently results in vessel occlusion.

However at the same time as the severity of occlusive plaque disease increases so too does the presence of adjacent vulnerable plaques prone to disruption. Thus patients with severe triple vessel disease are more likely to harbour small rupture-prone plaques than a patient with single vessel disease.[6] This explains the apparent paradox whereby highly stenotic lesions are relatively safe, yet patients with these lesions are prone to acute coronary events.

2.4 Development of thrombosis

Thrombosis occurs by one of two clinically indistinguishable mechanisms; in the majority of cases, there is fissuring of an unstable plaque whilst in approximately one third there is endothelial erosion over a stable plaque.[7] The factors which trigger disruption of vulnerable plaques are less clearly understood than the mechanisms associated with the transition to vulnerability. The final link appears to be an increase in inflammatory activity within the plaque[8] and the trigger for this remains a matter of intense speculation. Fissuring of the plaque surface results in exposure of the intensely thrombogenic core to the circulation which misinterprets the situation as an external haemorrhage. A combination of fibrin, platelet aggregates, and red cells then forms within the fissured plaque, expanding its volume and, with larger tears, thrombus may then extend into the arterial lumen (Figure 2.2). In those cases where the initiating thrombosis was due to the endothelial erosion as opposed to plaque fissuring, platelets are deposited on the exposed sub-endothelial collagenous matrix and there is no contribution to luminal obstruction from haemorrhage within the plaque. At this stage there are several possible outcomes.

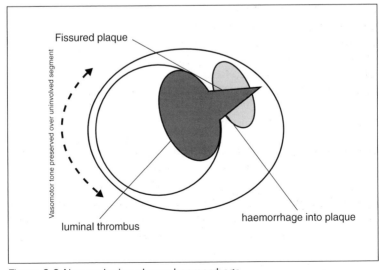

Figure 2.2 Non-occlusive plaque haemorrhage.

2.4.1 Non-occlusive thrombus: asymptomatic

Disruption of vulnerable plaques occurs relatively frequently,[9] but thrombus does not accumulate on the plaque surface and patients remain asymptomatic with a normal ECG, cardiac enzymes, and troponins. The relatively high frequency with which plaque fissuring occurs indicates the importance of the thrombotic response in determining subsequent clinical events.

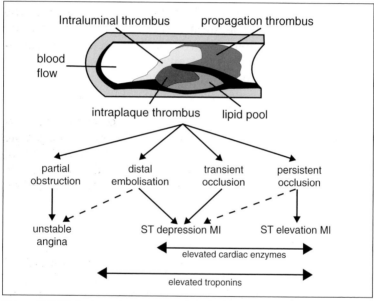

Figure 2.3 Clinical syndromes associated with the presence of intracoronary thrombus. Modified from Davies.[1]

2.4.2 Abrupt reduction in luminal diameter: unstable angina

The next possibility is that the thrombus produces a reduction in luminal diameter that falls short of complete occlusion. Under these circumstances the luminal clot tends to be platelet rich[10] (and as such, relatively resistant to thrombolysis[11]). The release of vasoactive substances from these platelets produces spasm of the smooth muscle in the adjacent arterial wall which further contributes to luminal narrowing. Luminal obstruction may be sufficient to produce an abrupt reduction in flow or even intermittent (10–20 minutes) occlusion, resulting in unstable angina (Figure 2.3). Several factors then determine the development of myocardial ischaemia.

The degree of luminal obstruction caused by the plaque/thombus complex

This will vary due to the dynamic interplay between the innate thrombotic and thrombolytic factors active on the plaque's surface. These tend to produce cyclical variations in the thrombus load.

Vascular tone of the adjacent arterial segment

Forty per cent of non-stenotic plaques are eccentric and thus there will be segments of arterial wall adjacent to the plaque where vascular tone remains an important determinant of vessel diameter. Platelet aggregation results in intense vasoconstriction of the vessel wall which is not held rigid by the disrupted plaque.

Myocardial oxygen demand

For a given degree of arterial narrowing the amount of myocardial ischaemia will depend on the myocardial oxygen demand, which will be determined by the product of rate and force of contraction.

The combination of these factors produces the characteristically intermittent and apparently unpredictable occurrence of the pain in unstable angina, with variations in arterial supply accounting for around 70% of ischaemic episodes and 30% attributable variations in metabolic demand.

Clinical history

Abrupt onset or deterioration in exertional angina or of angina occurring at rest.

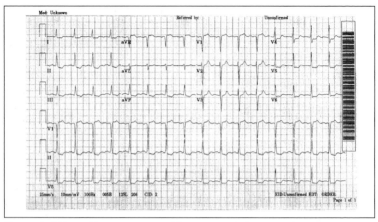

Figure 2.4 Unstable angina/non-ST elevation infarction. ST depression in leads I, II, III, aVF and V4–V6 with T wave inversion in II, III and aVF. Critical circumflex stenosis at angiography.

ECG

During periods of ischaemia this shows reversible ST depression (Figure 2.4) sometimes associated with T wave inversion which may persist after the resolution of the ischaemic episode. The ECG is frequently normal during pain-free periods (when there is insufficient luminal obstruction to cause ischaemia). The ECG can occasionally be normal during pain if ischaemia occurs in the electrically silent circumflex perfusion zone.

Cardiac enzymes

Normal.

Troponins

Normal or elevated (the latter defining a high risk group).

2.4.3 Intermittent occlusion or distal propagation of thrombus: non-Q wave infarction

A third possibility is that brief intermittent occlusion of the artery may occur due to luminal obstruction by thrombus for

< 1 hour followed by spontaneous thrombolysis, or there may be embolisation of thrombus from the plaque surface into the distal coronary bed.[12] Both of these processes result in non-Q wave infarction. The Q wave/non-Q wave differentiation does not necessarily equate with the pathological entities of transmural and non-transmural infarction[13] and these terms are no longer used. Non-Q wave infarction may also result from total coronary occlusion in the presence of collaterals supplying the myocardium which reduce the magnitude of infarction.

In a proportion of patients this embolisation of platelet-derived thrombi into the distal coronary circulation results in sudden death and this process appears to be the mechanism in 45% of cases of sudden death.[14]

Clinical history

Clinically indistinguishable from unstable angina.

ECG

Appearances are identical to those of unstable angina with reversible ST depression (although this tends to be deeper and more prolonged) with later T wave inversion.

Cardiac enzymes and troponins

Both elevated.

2.4.4 Stable occlusion: ST elevation infarction

Alternatively, the thrombus can completely occlude the artery, under these circumstances the thrombus tends to be rich in erythrocytes enmeshed in fibrin[10] (Figure 2.5). This results in complete obstruction to coronary flow for >1 hour and usually produces the clinical entity of ST elevation (Figure 2.6), although this is far from absolute and the presence of a collateral circulation may modify the extent of subsequent myocardial necrosis. Again, the process of occlusion is initially cyclical in many patients[15] resulting in a stuttering presentation of pain before occlusion becomes established. Total coronary occlusion also provides the second of the three mechanisms responsible for sudden cardiac death and is responsible for around 30% of cases.[14]

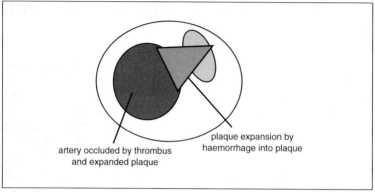

Figure 2.5 Occlusive plaque haemorrhage.

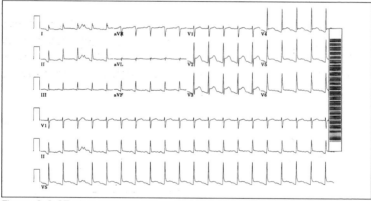

Figure 2.6 ST elevation infarction. ST elevation V2–V5. LAD occlusion at angiography.

Clinical history

Continuous pain lasting in excess of half an hour and usually much longer.

ECG

ST elevation, followed by eventual resolution with loss or R wave voltage and the formation of Q waves.

Cardiac enzymes and troponins

Elevated.

2.4.5 Acute reperfusion: ST segment resolution/non-resolution

Removal of the occlusive thrombus either by the thrombolysis (natural or pharmacological) or using angioplasty may produce restoration of arterial flow and ST segment resolution. However, the presence of platelet microthrombi and myocardial oedema in the capillary bed may prevent reperfusion occurring within the myocardium itself (the "no-reflow phenomenon"). Under these circumstances, the ST elevation persists (Figure 2.7). Conversely, if reperfusion occurs via collaterals despite persistent occlusion at the site of the fissured plaque, ST resolution occurs.

The fact that the ECG predicts occlusion at the level of the plaque but reperfusion at the level of the myocardium is initially confusing but provides further useful information as failure of ST resolution is associated with a less favourable prognosis.[16]

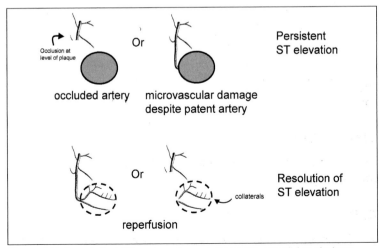

Figure 2.7 Correlating ST segment resolution with arterial pathology. Modified from Davies and Ormerod.[16]

2.5 Chronic resolution of thrombus and plaque remodelling

Chronic resolution of the plaque–thrombus complex occurs with a variable degree of incorporation of thrombus into the plaque substance (Figure 2.8). This can result in increases in plaque size (producing stable angina if luminal obstruction is >50%) or a return of the plaque to its previous dimensions and the patient to an asymptomatic state. This ability of plaques to progress rapidly, superimposed on the underlying development of gradual progression, produces the unpredictable variability in the development of atheroma. Following thrombolysis for acute myocardial infarction the average degree of luminal obstruction is >60%[17] and thus symptoms of ongoing ischaemia are not invariable. The clinical correlates of this are that many patients with acute coronary syndromes can be managed medically once the plaque has healed and do not invariably require mechanical intervention to reduce luminal obstruction by the residual plaque.

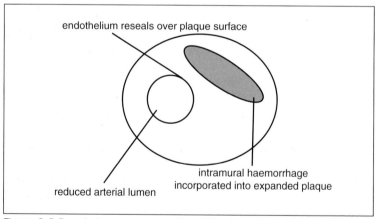

Figure 2.8 Resolution and remodelling following plaque haemorrhage.

2.6 Additional factors in the relationship between arterial pathology and clinical presentation

Although the above correlations between events on the plaque surface and subsequent clinical events provide a framework for understanding acute coronary syndromes, these mechanisms are an over-simplification and some additional processes need to be taken into account.

2.6.1 Relationship between initial ST shift and Q wave development

Classical ECG teaching states that ST elevation occurs when the myocardium nearest to the recording electrode is damaged ("epicardial ischaemia") whereas ST depression occurs where there is an intervening segment of normal myocardium ("subendocardial ischaemia"). It is tempting to simplify this situation into ST elevation resulting in Q wave infarction and ST depression producing non-Q wave infarction/unstable angina. Unfortunately, there is a crossover population with some patients who initially presented with ST elevation developing non-Q wave infarctions and a minority of those with ST depression subsequently developing Q waves. These inconsistencies in the relationship between arterial pathology and ECG findings tend not to produce problems in clinical practice as the response to the therapeutic strategies available has been defined on the basis of initial ST segment change (see Chapters 3 and 4).

2.6.2 Alternative mechanisms of non-Q wave infarction

A second inconsistency is that although the majority of patients with ST depression have either brief arterial occlusion or embolisation of platelet thrombi, in some proportion there is persistent occlusion of the epicardial artery combined with perfusion from collaterals. Importantly, in the setting of multivessel coronary disease, the collaterals themselves may be dependent on a critically stenosed vessel and intermittent ischaemia can then occur despite an occluded culprit vessel.

2.6.3 Unstable angina and no thrombus

Although the majority of studies of patients with unstable angina demonstrate intracoronary thrombus either angiographically, angioscopically, or at post mortem, this is not a universal finding.[18] Whilst some of these discrepancies are attributable to the timing of the investigation and the wide clinical spectrum of unstable angina, smooth muscle proliferation in the absence of plaque rupture may account for a proportion of cases[19] particularly in restenosis following angioplasty.

Summary

Q wave MI	Persistent occlusion >1 hour
Non-Q wave MI	Transient occlusion <1 hour Platelet emboli into distal coronary tree Persistent occlusion + collaterals
Unstable angina	Transient occlusion 10–20 minutes Platelet emboli into distal coronary tree Persistent occlusion + multivessel disease
Sudden ischaemic death	Persistent occlusion Platelet emboli into distal coronary tree No intramural thrombus – primary arrhythmia

References

1 Davies MJ. The pathophysiology of acute coronary syndromes. *Heart* 2000;**83**:361–6.
2 Stary HC, Chandler AB, Dinsmore RE, *et al.* A definition of advanced types of atherosclerotic lesions and a histological classification of atherosclerosis. A report from the Committee on Vascular Lesions of the Council on Arteriosclerosis, American Heart Association. *Circulation* 1995;**92**:1355–74.
3 Fuster V. Elucidation of the role of plaque instability and rupture in acute coronary events. *Am J Cardiol* 1995;**76**:24C–33C.
4 Mann JM, Davies MJ. Vulnerable plaque. Relation of characteristics to degree of stenosis in human coronary arteries. *Circulation* 1996;**94**:928–31.
5 Ambrose JA, Fuster V. The risk of coronary occlusion is not proportional to the prior severity of coronary stenoses. *Heart* 1998;**79**;3–4
6 Hangartner JR, Charleston AJ, Davies MJ, Thomas AC. Morphological characteristics of clinically significant coronary artery stenosis in stable angina. *Br Heart J* 1986;**56**:501–8.
7 Burke AP, Farb A, Malcolm GT, Liang YH, Smialek J, Virmani R. Coronary risk factors and plaque morphology in men with coronary disease who died suddenly. *N Engl J Med* 1997;**336**:1276–82.
8 Ross R. Atherosclerosis – an inflammatory disease. *N Engl J Med* 1999;**340**;115–26.

9 Kristensen SD, Ravn HB, Falk E. Insights into the pathophysiology of unstable coronary artery disease. *Am J Cardiol* 1997;**80**:5E–9E.

10 Mizuno K, Satomura K, Miyamoto A, *et al*. Angioscopic evaluation of coronary artery thrombi in acute coronary syndromes. *N Engl J Med* 1992;**326**:287–91.

11 Jang IK, Gold HK, Ziskind M, *et al*. Differential sensitivity of erythrocyte-rich and platelet-rich arterial thrombi to lysis with recombinant tissue-type plasminogen activator. A possible explanation for resistance to coronary thrombolysis. *Circulation* 1989;**79**:920–8.

12 Davies MJ, Thomas AC, Knapman PA, Hangartner IR. Intramyocardial platelet aggregation in patients with unstable angina suffering sudden ischemic cardiac death. *Circulation* 1986;**73**:418–27.

13 Phibbs B. "Transmural" versus "subendocardial" myocardial infarction: an electrocardiographic myth. *J Am Coll Cardiol* 1983;**1**:561–4.

14 Davies MJ, Bland JM, Hangartner JR, Angelini A, Thomas AC. Factors influencing the presence or absence of acute coronary artery thrombi in sudden ischaemic death. *Eur Heart J* 1989;**10**:203–8.

15 Hackett D, Davies G, Chierchia S, Maseri A. Intermittent coronary occlusion in acute myocardial infarction. Value of combined thrombolytic and vasodilator therapy. *N Engl J Med* 1987;**317**:1055–9.

16 Davies CH, Ormerod OIM. Diagnosis and management of failed thrombolysis. *Lancet* 1998;**351**:1191–6.

17 Hackett D, Davies G, Maseri A. Pre-existing coronary stenoses in patients with first myocardial infarction are not necessarily severe. *Eur Heart J* 1988;**9**:1317–23.

18 Waxman S, Mittleman MA, Zarich SW, *et al*. Angioscopic assessment of coronary lesions underlying thrombus. *Am J Cardiol* 1997;**79**:1106–9.

19 Flugelman MY, Virmani R, Correa R, *et al*. Smooth muscle cell abundance and fibroblast growth factors in coronary lesions of patients with nonfatal unstable angina. A clue to the mechanism of transformation from the stable to the unstable clinical state. *Circulation* 1993;**88**:2493–500.

3: Acute coronary syndromes II: myocardial infarction with ST elevation

CH DAVIES, Y BASHIR

3.1 Introduction

Realistically the approach to a patient presenting with chest pain and ST elevation is different from the situation of chest pain without ST elevation. In the presence of ST elevation the diagnosis is overwhelmingly likely to be myocardial infarction. Under these circumstances the emphasis should not be on considering an exhaustive list of differential diagnoses, but on rapid confirmation of the diagnosis swiftly followed by reperfusion therapy. The ECG will thus dictate the course of the subsequent clinical assessment and is considered first.

3.2 Correlations between site of infarction and ECG abnormalities

It is helpful to visualise the site of the arterial thrombus and the most probable location within the coronary circulation. For a given arterial occlusion the extent of infarction is determined by the proportion of myocardium supplied by the occluded vessel (which varies widely between individuals) and whether the occlusion is proximal or distal within the vessel. ST elevation is usually considered significant if it is >2 mm in the chest leads and >1 mm in the limb leads.

3.2.1 Anterior infarction

The anterior surface of the heart is supplied by the left anterior descending artery (LAD) and its occlusion results in anterior infarction with ST elevation in leads V2–V6 (Figure 3.1). The distal LAD may extend as far as the inferior surface of the heart resulting in simultaneous inferior infarction. With more proximal occlusion, the first diagonal branch is involved and lateral changes can also occur (Figure 3.2). The simultaneous occurrence of bundle branch block indicates even more proximal occlusion and is associated with a 2–3-fold increase in mortality (Figure 3.2). As the LAD is typically the largest of the three coronary arteries, anterior infarction results in a greater degree of myocardial damage than inferior infarction and is associated with increased mortality.

The occurrence of the various mechanical complications of infarction is also dependent upon the site of infarction.

Two-thirds of post-infarction ventricular septal defects follow anterior infarction (as a greater proportion of the intraventricular septum's supply is derived from the LAD) whereas three-quarters of cases of papillary muscle rupture occur in the setting of inferior infarction. Free wall rupture is equally common with either anterior or inferior rupture.

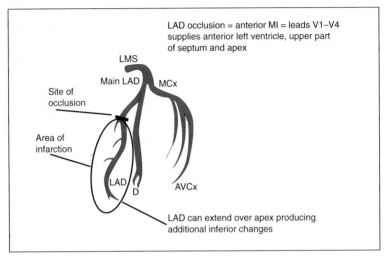

Figure 3.1 Mid-portion LAD occlusion=anterior infarction=leads V1–V4 The LAD supplies the anterior wall of the left ventricle and the upper portion of the septum in addition to the apex.

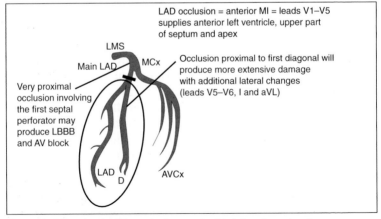

Figure 3.2 Proximal LAD occlusion=anterior infarction=leads V1–V5+/− lateral changes in V5, V6 and aVL. In addition, proximal occlusion may result in left bundle branch block, AV block.

3.2.2 Inferior infarction

Inferior infarction results in ST elevation in leads II, III, and atrioventricular fibrillation (VF). The diagnostic uncertainty in inferior infarction stems from the fact that the inferior surface of the heart is supplied by the right coronary artery (RCA) in two-thirds of patients, whilst in approximately one-third the inferior surface of the heart is supplied by the circumflex artery ("left dominance"). It is thus not possible to be certain whether a patient with an inferior infarction has occluded the circumflex or the right coronary artery (Figures 3.3 and 3.4). The site of occlusion can be associated with several additional features.

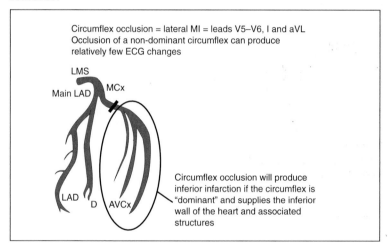

Figure 3.3 Circumflex occlusion=lateral infarction=leads V5, V6 and aVL. Occlusion of a dominant circumflex will produce inferior infarction= leads II, III and aVF. Occlusion of a non-dominant circumflex may be electrically silent.

3.2.3 Posterior infarction

True posterior infarction results from occlusion of the posterior descending artery (PDA) which is supplied by the right or circumflex artery, depending on which is dominant. The problem here is that posterior leads are not routinely recorded and the ST elevation is seen "upside down" as ST depression in the anterior leads. Any accompanying Q wave produces a dominant R wave in V1. The importance lies in appreciating that ECG changes of isolated PDA occlusion are indeed infarction and not merely "anterior ischaemia" and that combined inferior and posterior infarction (resulting from total occlusion of a very dominant RCA or circumflex) can represent a substantial infarction with significant potential for the development of complications.

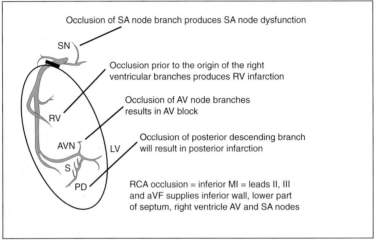

Figure 3.4 Right coronary occlusion=inferior infarction=leads II, III and aVF. The RCA supplies the inferior wall, the lower part of the septum, the right ventricle, the AV and SA nodes. Occlusion of a very dominant RCA will result in additional lateral changes (V5, V5 and aVL).

3.2.4 Right ventricular infarction

This results from RCA occlusion proximal to the origin of the right ventricular branches (Figure 3.4). The diagnosis of right ventricular infarction requires the use of right ventricular chest leads (placed on the right side of the chest in a mirror image to the usual configuration) – the presence of ST elevation in these leads signifies right ventricular involvement. These additional leads should be recorded at least once in all patients with inferior infarctions and repeated if cardiogenic shock develops.

3.2.5 Infarction with few ECG changes

This is frequently caused by circumflex occlusion. If the circumflex is dominant then the associated inferior wall changes are readily apparent. However the circumflex territory is relatively silent electrically as the commonly used chest positions do not extend laterally enough round the chest wall. For this reason isolated circumflex occlusion can result in only modest ECG changes despite significant myocardial necrosis. Recording additional chest leads V7, V8, etc. further laterally can occasionally be helpful in these circumstances.

3.2.6 Assessing infarct severity from the ECG

Despite the occasional lack of correlation for circumflex occlusion, the magnitude of the ST segment elevation generally correlates well with the extent of myocardial injury, both in terms of the number of leads involved and the degree of ST elevation. Patients with greater degrees of ST elevation are those who derive the most benefit from thrombolysis.[1] The presence of "reciprocal" depression (ST depression in leads remote from the ST elevation produced by the infarct related artery) is no longer perceived to be associated with an adverse prognosis in patients receiving thrombolysis.[2]

3.3 Clinical assessment

The differential diagnosis of chest pain has been discussed in Chapter 1. The assessment of most patients with chest pain and ECG evidence of ST elevation is straightforward and the current recommendation of a twenty minute "door to needle" time for thrombolysis should be achievable in the majority of patients.[3,4] There are four key questions to be answered.

3.3.1 Is there an alternative diagnosis?

It is important to ensure that this is indeed acute myocardial infarction, but in the presence of ST elevation this will be the diagnosis in the overwhelming majority of cases. Potential pitfalls include chronic ST elevation due to a left ventricular aneurysm (the ST elevation will be in leads with deep Q waves and little or no R waves), pericarditis and left bundle branch block (although the latter may still require consideration for thrombolysis). The most important differential diagnosis is that of aortic dissection, although pericarditis can occasionally cause confusion (Box 3.1).

Aortic dissection

Box 3.1 Differential diagnosis of ST elevation

- Myocardial infarction
- Acute pericarditis – atypical history and widespread ST changes in a healthy patient
- Left ventricular aneurysm – extensive Q waves in leads with ST elevation
- Afro-Caribbeans – atypical history, confined to V2, V3, lack of progression
- High vagal tone in young people – improves with exercise
- Acute myocarditis – rare, atypical history, does not conform to vascular territories

Aortic dissection can present with ST elevation and chest pain, but thrombolysis can be rapidly fatal due to haemorrhage into the aortic wall and pericardium.

In thoracic aortic dissection the pain is more commonly perceived to be intrascapular, is characteristically "tearing" in nature and its peak intensity occurs almost instantaneously after its onset. The characteristic clues on examination of discrepant blood pressures in each arm, absent peripheral pulses and the murmur of aortic regurgitation may all be absent. The assessment of mediastinal contour on portable chest x rays is frequently unhelpful, but the realisation that patients with a myocardial infarction and a normal ECG do not benefit from thrombolysis[5] has greatly simplified management. If ECG abnormalities are present in dissection they are usually those of ST depression secondary to hypertensive left ventricular hypertrophy and under these circumstances, even if the clinical history was misinterpreted as being due to myocardial infarction, thrombolysis would not be indicated. ST elevation can occasionally occur due to disruption of a coronary artery ostium. Although exceptions have occurred, anterior myocardial infarctions are rare in this context as acute disruption of the left main stem results in sudden death and the diagnostic uncertainty usually arises from inferior myocardial infarctions. If in doubt thrombolysis should be withheld and a CT scan of the thoracic aorta should be obtained (although it should be emphasised that a normal scan does not exclude aortic dissection, for further details see Chapter 7).

Pericarditis

Although the pleuritic pain of pericarditis is of a different character from that of myocardial infarction it can, on occasion, give rise to diagnostic difficulty. The "concave up" and "scooped" nature of the ST elevation are frequently not as distinct from the changes of myocardial infarction as might be imagined from the examples in ECG textbooks. More useful is the fact that the ST elevation is widespread, extending over the territories of several coronary arteries, in a patient who seems clinically well. Additional pointers are the lack of evolution over the hours following admission and in particular the lack of evolving Q waves.

This is one of the few instances where urgent cardiac enzymes are clinically useful as the failure of plasma creatine kinase (CK) to rise after 6 hours of chest pain in a patient with ST segment elevation makes myocardial infarction very unlikely. In the case of the localised pericarditis that can complicate a myocardial infarction, ECG changes occurring in addition to those of the infarct itself are uncommon, occurring in less than 4% of cases.[6]

3.3.2 What is the clinical severity of infarction?

It is important to identify high risk patients in whom more aggressive reperfusion strategies may be appropriate and who are also at higher risk of developing complications. Conversely, identification of low risk patients may prevent their exposure to the risks associated with inappropriate therapy. Independent predictors of mortality include: age, systolic BP < 120 mmHg, Kilip class (Table 3.1), heart rate and anterior infarction. The Kilip classification has recently been revalidated for use in patients receiving thrombolysis[7] (Table 3.1)

Table 3.1 Kilip classification

Class	Definition	30 day mortality
I	No S_3 and clear lungs	5%
II	S_3 or crackles < 50% of lungs	14%
III	Crackles > 50% of lungs	32%
IV	Shock	57%

Two important additional factors associated with increased mortality and not taken into account in the above analysis are the presence of widespread ST segment elevation[8] (as discussed above) and patients in whom thrombolysis is contraindicated.[9]

3.3.3 Is the time window appropriate for thrombolysis?

The FTT meta-analysis[5] and the results of the LATE[10] trial would suggest that thrombolysis is beneficial up to 12 hours from the onset of pain (30 lives saved per 1000 <6 hours and 20 per 1000 between 7 and 12 hours). The key question is the definition of onset as up to 50% of infarcts initially show intermittent coronary occlusion and it seems reasonable to time onset from the point at which pain no longer fluctuates rather than during any preceding period of unstable angina. Although not specifically assessed in a clinical trial a useful guideline is to consider thrombolysis in patients who are continuing to experience ischaemic pain.

3.3.4 Is there a contraindication to thrombolysis?

The contraindications to thrombolysis are well recognised (Box 3.2), although in general more patients have thrombolysis inappropriately denied than suffer harm because of failure to heed a contraindication. It is worth noting that contraindications have become less restrictive as clinical experience has accumulated over the past decade. It is also important to view these in the context of the clinical situation, i.e., a relative contraindication should not prevent thrombolytic administration in the context of widespread ST elevation and a short clinical history (where the potential for benefit from thrombolysis is large) whereas one might decide to withhold thrombolysis from a patient with a contraindication who was haemodynamically stable and pain free 11 hours after an inferior infarction. Similarly the local availability of primary angioplasty might well bias one against thrombolysis in the presence of a relative contraindication. Commonly cited but inappropriate reasons for withholding thrombolysis are listed below.

Box 3.2 Contraindications to thrombolysis

Absolute
- Prior haemorrhagic stroke
- Ischaemic stroke within one year
- Major trauma/surgery/head injury in preceding 3 weeks
- Gastrointestinal bleeding within the last month
- Known bleeding disorder
- Aortic dissection

Relative
- Warfarin with INR > 2.3
- Pregnancy
- Traumatic resuscitation
- Systolic BP > 180 mmHg despite treatment

Hypertension

Not a contraindication if it can be satisfactorily controlled (<180/100 mmHg), which is usually possible using a combination of opiates for pain relief and intravenous nitrates.

Hypotension

Not a contraindication, although it may mean that thrombolysis may be ineffectual and that mechanical revascularisation should be considered. This issue is discussed further in Chapter 6.

Menstruation

Not a contraindication.

Diabetic retinopathy

Concerns about retinopathy in diabetics are unfounded (of over 6000 diabetic patients in GUSTO-1 none experienced an intraoccular haemorrhage) and this does not represent a contraindication.[11]

Peptic ulceration

Active peptic ulceration is a contraindication, but previous symptoms of peptic ulceration that are now quiescent following treatment are not.

There are two contraindications specific to individual thrombolytic agents, alteplase is contraindicated in patients sensitive to gentamicin (which is used during manufacture) and streptokinase should not be used in patients who have received it previously. There has been some debate as to whether streptokinase could be repeated if the previous dose was administered less than 4 days or more than a year ago, but as the effects of antistreptokinase antibodies on thrombolytic performance remain uncertain it seem reasonable to use alteplase for all patients who have previously received streptokinase or one of its analogues such as anistreplase. Age is not a contraindication to thrombolysis for although the risks of haemorrhage are undeniably higher in the elderly the mortality associated with infarction also rises with age.

Myocardial infarction can occasionally present "silently" as heart failure, stroke or as an acute confusional state and under these circumstances thrombolysis is inappropriate.

Additional investigations

In addition to estimations of plasma electrolytes, glucose, cardiac enzymes, and a full blood count, it is important to measure plasma cholesterol in the first 24 hours after admission as it is subsequently artefactually depressed for up to 4 months.[12] Although plasma triglycerides cannot be accurately measured in a non-fasting sample, changes in plasma cholesterol are usually <10%. All patients should have a chest x ray to assess the presence of pulmonary oedema as clinical assessment can be unreliable.[13]

3.4 General management of myocardial infarction with ST elevation

Routine management based on current European[4] and American[3] guidelines is summarised in Box 3.3.

3.4.1 Use of aspirin

All patients should receive aspirin unless there is a specific contraindication such as unequivocal severe allergy or active peptic ulceration. Many patients who claim that they are "allergic" to aspirin give a very vague history of the allergy on closer questioning. As with thrombolysis it is commoner to see patients inappropriately denied treatment than to see patients in whom failure to heed a contraindication resulted in serious harm. The importance of aspirin is sometimes underplayed: the mortality reduction in ISIS-2 associated with aspirin was similar to that obtained with streptokinase (20 lives saved per 1000).[14] The dose of aspirin must be in excess of 150 mg (as an approximation to the 165 mg of ISIS-2) and there is some pharmacokinetic data to support the use of 300 mg as the initial dose to ensure early attenuation of platelet function. In any event, whatever the arguments about the most appropriate long term dose of aspirin, there is no data to support the use of a dose of 75 mg in acute infarction.

In patients who are genuinely intolerant of aspirin we would advocate the use of the ADP receptor antagonist clopidogrel 75 mg once daily. Although not formally tested in the setting of acute infarction, the results obtained in the CAPRIE trial of secondary prevention demonstrating a 19% reduction in myocardial infarction compared to aspirin are encouraging.

Box 3.3 Routine management of myocardial infarction

- IV access
- Aspirin 150 mg
- Analgesia: 2.5–5 mg diamorphine or 5–10 mg morphine iv
- Antiemetic: 10 mg metaclopramide iv (cyclizine 50 mg iv if required)
- Thrombolytic (or primary angioplasty)
- Adjunctive pharmacotherapy – ß-blockers, heparin (following alteplase)
- Oxygen?
- ACE inhibitors

Adequate analgesia is an essential part of management and it is important to add an antiemetic routinely. Additional antiemetic measures are sometimes required, particularly in the setting of inferior infarction, and cyclizine 50 mg iv 8 hourly is an alternative. Although prochlorperazine is occasionally used it is not licensed in the UK for intravenous use whilst intramuscular injections can distort plasma enzymes and result in substantial haematomas following thrombolysis. Oxygen is traditionally administered to patients following myocardial infarction although it is probably of no value in the absence of an oxygen saturation (assessed using pulse oximetry) of < 90%.

If pain is difficult to control with opiates then intravenous nitrates or β-blockers are often effective (for further details see below in section 3.5.4).

3.4.2 Specific issues related to thrombolysis

Choice of thrombolytic

The current choice lies between streptokinase (SK) and alteplase (tPA)[15] (see Box 3.4 for dosage schedules and Figure 3.5 for mechanisms of action) as there is no mortality advantage to be obtained from the use of anistreplase[16,17] or reteplase.[18] Streptokinase forms a complex with plasminogen to form "plasminogen activator" which promotes the conversion of plasminogen to plasmin. This in turn produces the breakdown of fibrin (Figure 3.5). Alteplase is a plasminogen activator in its own right, acting directly on plasminogen to form plasmin, it acts preferentially on plasminogen bound to fibrin with the theoretical advantage that its actions would be targeted to act at the site of clot formation minimising its systemic effects.[19] Unfortunately, this much publicised "fibrin specificity" is unable to distinguish between the fibrin in the occluded coronary artery and that preventing haemorrhage at the site of the pacing wire venepuncture. Alteplase produced a modest mortality benefit over streptokinase when administered with a relatively larger proportion of the dose given early during the course of the infusion ("front loaded") in the GUSTO-1 study[20] (7.3% to 6.3% – about one life saved per hundred treated). It may be that the benefits observed owe more to the differences in the infusion regimen rather than any differences in pharmacology[21] and this level of benefit seems insufficient to justify the routine use of alteplase given its increased cost and the increased rate of haemorrhagic stroke (an additional 3 per 1000 patients.[20] An alternative approach is to attempt to restrict the use of alteplase to higher risk patients such as those with higher Kilip class (except IV), anterior infarcts, hypotension (<120 mmHg), or tachycardia (>100/min).[22]

Table 3.2 Summary of key thrombolytic trials

Name	Therapy	Result
GISSI-1[28]	SK vs placebo	SK beneficial
ISIS-2[14]	SK vs placebo	SK beneficial
GISSI-2[17]	SK vs alteplase vs anistreplase	No difference
ISIS-3[16]	SK vs alteplase vs anistreplase	No difference
GUSTO-1[20]	Front loaded alteplase vs SK	Small benefit for alteplase
GUSTO-2B[29]	Alteplase vs PTCA	Small benefit for PTCA
GUSTO-3[18]	Alteplase vs reteplase	No difference

Box 3.4 Thrombolytic dosage schedules

Streptokinase	1.5 million units in 50 ml 5% dextrose infused over one hour
Alteplase	15 mg bolus 50 mg over 30 minutes (0.75 mg/kg) 35 mg over 60 minutes (0.5 mg/kg) followed by Heparin 5000 units bolus Heparin infusion for 48 hours (aiming for KCCT of 1.5–2×control)

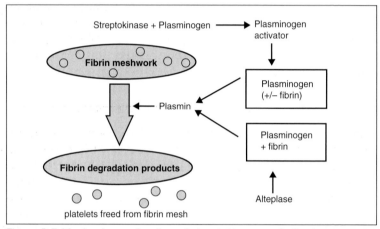

Figure 3.5 Mechanisms of action of streptokinase and alteplase.

Use of heparin

Although there is no benefit to heparin administration following streptokinase[16,17] there is convincing evidence that the higher patency rates achieved with tPA require heparin to prevent an increased rate of early reocclusion,[23] probably due to greater platelet activation following fibrin specific thrombolytics. There is no benefit from the routine use of heparin in patients ineligible for thrombolysis in the absence of a specific indication such as left ventricular thrombus, pulmonary embolism, etc.[24]

Complications of thrombolysis

Thrombolytic therapy results in an increase in the incidence of stroke (about 4 per 1000); of these two will be fatal (and are therefore already included in the mortality figures) and of the non-fatal strokes one will be disabling. The risk of stroke increases with age. Non-cerebral haemorrhage occurs in about 7 per 1000 patients and is particularly associated with vascular access. Arterial puncture should be avoided following thrombolysis and venous access obtained at sites which are readily compressed such as the jugular and femoral approaches. Severe haemorrhage will respond to the administration of fresh frozen plasma. Hypotension secondary to thrombolysis occurs in 3% of patients receiving streptokinase and 1% of those receiving alteplase; it usually responds to a reduction in the infusion rate. Allergic reactions are rare and respond to hydrocortisone 200 mg and chlorpheniramine 10 mg iv.

Thrombolysis for patients without ST elevation?

There is no evidence of benefit from thrombolysis in patients with normal ECGs[5] or unstable angina[25] and there is no prospective data to support its use in patients presenting with ST depression, despite the higher mortality of this group.[26] This reduces the usefulness of rapid screening of patients with chest pain and normal ECGs by creatine kinase estimations as, in the presence of a normal ECG, the result of the enzyme determination will not affect the decision on whether or not to administer thrombolysis.[27]

There is however good evidence to support the use of thrombolysis in patients with a typical history of myocardial infarction and left bundle branch block from the FTT meta-analysis where this group appeared to derive substantial benefit (30 lives saved per 1000).

The other patient group in whom thrombolysis should be considered is patients presenting with a true posterior infarction. The clues to the existence of a posterior MI as opposed to merely anterior ischaemia are the increased R wave height in V1, the fact that anterior ischaemia is usually more extensive than the limited changes in V1–V3 seen with posterior infarction and the frequent coexistence of an inferior infarction. The last potential problem is that anterior reciprocal ST depression can occasionally appear more prominent than the inferior ST elevation of the infarction itself. This can result in patients being initially misclassified as having unstable angina and not receiving thrombolysis.

3.4.3 The role of primary angioplasty

Primary angioplasty refers to the use of angioplasty (percutaneous transluminal coronary angioplasty, PTCA) instead of thrombolysis (see Table 3.3 for definitions of the terms used to describe PTCA at various time points during the course of infarction). Although there is evidence that primary PTCA may improve outcome in specialist centres,[30] attempts to reproduce these results in larger studies have been less encouraging.[29] Primary PTCA does however have an important role to play in patients with a contraindication to thrombolysis, a group with a mortality up to five times that of patients eligible for thrombolysis,[9] and if possible urgent transfer to a cardiothoracic centre should be arranged. The other group of patients in whom primary PTCA should be considered are those with cardiogenic shock.[31] For further discussion see Chapter 6.

There is no evidence of benefit from routine PTCA for all patients either immediately following thrombolysis or prior to discharge (Table 3.3).

Table 3.3 Benefits of routine PTCA

Name	Timing	Major trials	Evidence of benefit
Primary	*Instead* of thrombolysis	PAMI 1,[30] GUSTO 2b[29]	Possibly
Immediate	Immediately *following*	ESCG,[32] TAMI 5[33]	No
Rescue	Following *failed* thrombolysis	RESCUE[34]	Yes
Early	<24 hours – all patients	TIMI 2,[35] SWIFT[36]	No
Late	>24 hours – all patients	TOPS[37]	No

3.4.4 Use of β-blockers

The benefits of β-blockers are less significant than those of thrombolysis (6 lives saved per 1000). Although the TIMI-2B trial demonstrated a benefit from the early use of metroprolol following tPA and there is recent support for the use of carvedilol,[38] most of the convincing evidence for the use of ß-blockers predates the thrombolytic era.[39] However, there are no grounds to believe that the benefits of β-blockade are negated by the use of thrombolytics; in fact the reverse is likely to be true. The chief benefit of early iv β-blockade is a reduction in cardiac rupture,[39] a condition which is more common in patients receiving thrombolysis. There is a perception that early β-blockade is currently underused and, as with thrombolysis, more patients are inappropriately denied β-blockade than are harmed due to administration in the presence of a minor contraindication.

There is most experience with atenolol[39] and metoprolol[40] (Box 3.5). The short plasma half life of metoprolol (3–7 hours) has the advantage that, should haemodynamic deterioration occur, the effects are relatively short lived. β-blockers are contraindicated in heart failure, shock, obstructive airways disease, heart block, and in patients already receiving calcium antagonists. They are not contraindicated in diabetes and can be used cautiously in patients with non-critical peripheral vascular disease.

Box 3.5 Use of β-blockers in myocardial infarction

Metoprolol	5 mg iv every 2 minutes if heart rate >60/min to a maximum of 15 mg. If well tolerated give 50 mg orally 15 minutes later. Followed by 50 mg bd for 48 hours and 100 mg bd thereafter.
Atenolol	5 mg iv followed by a further 5 mg 10 minutes later if heart rate >60/min. If well tolerated give 50 mg orally 15 minutes later. Followed by 50 mg od for 48 hours and 100 mg od thereafter.

3.4.5 Use of ACE inhibitors

There is clear evidence of benefit from the use of ACE inhibitors in patients with evidence of left ventricular impairment or overt heart failure following MI,[41–43] there is also evidence for a much smaller benefit when ACE inhibitors are administered early on to the infarct population as a whole.[44,45] The unresolved question is whether to adopt the late/selective strategy (quantification of LV function before deciding if ACE inhibition is appropriate) or the early/nonselective approach (ACE inhibitors for all after the first 24 hours).[46] The advantage of the late/selective approach is that therapy is targeted at the group most likely to benefit; the disadvantage is that the facilities to provide quantification of LV function are frequently unavailable and that some of the benefits of ACE inhibitor therapy occur in the first few days following infarction before a decision is likely to have been made. The proponents of the early/non-selective approach point to its simplicity and the fact that LV rupture in particular is reduced by early ACE inhibition.

Although either policy is acceptable, current opinion favours starting all patients on an ACE inhibitor and assessing LV function 4–6 weeks after discharge when this can be stopped if the ejection fraction is in excess of 40%. Recent direct comparisons of early and delayed ACE inhibition in smaller studies supports this approach.[47] Starting doses of ACE inhibitors are captopril 6.25 mg, ramipril 2.5 mg, trandolapril 0.5 mg, and lisinopril 5 mg. In patients with heart failure and hypotension the (unlicensed) paediatric dose of captopril 2 mg is useful for initiating treatment. Although the evidence for the use of ACE inhibitors post MI relates to those described above there is no reason to believe that this is not a class effect. Renal function should be monitored but a plasma creatinine of < 20 micromol/l is not a contraindication.[48]

3.5 Management of specific problems

3.5.1 Management of failed thrombolysis and indications for cardiac catheterisation

Patients in whom pain continues following thrombolysis and in whom previously elevated ST segments do not resolve by > 50%, particularly in the presence of extensive ST elevation, form a group at increased risk of subsequent complication.[8] In angiographic terms, even with "front loaded" alteplase, thrombolysis achieves an open artery with adequate flow in less than 60% of patients.[49] This may reflect either resistance to the production of a lytic state or extensive plaque haemorrhage with the result that the occlusion is not predominantly due to intraluminal thrombus (Figure 3.6).

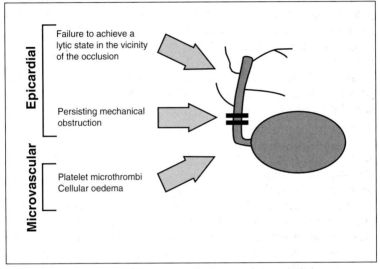

Figure 3.6 Mechanisms responsible for failure of thrombolytics to produce myocardial reperfusion. From Davies and Ormerod.[8]

Despite an extensive literature, and promising results using myoglobin, biochemical markers currently have no clinical role in the diagnosis of reperfusion[8] and the diagnosis should be made on the failure of the ST segment to resolve on a 12 lead ECG 90 minutes after starting thrombolysis. This can be measured as either the ST elevation in the worst single lead or as the total sum of ST elevation.

Attempts have been made to improve arterial patency with both repeat thrombolysis using tPA[50,51] or PTCA.[34] Although both strategies have been successful in these small trials, there remains uncertainty as to the role of either therapy in the general clinical setting. In particular the use of combination

(SK+tPA) thrombolysis was not associated with clinical benefit in GUSTO-1 (administered non-selectively to all patients and not specifically targeted at those who failed to reperfuse) but was associated with a doubling of the intracranial haemorrhage rate.[20] This provides clear evidence of the potential risks of increasing the intensity of thrombolysis for all infarcts, but as we do not know the benefits in a large population it is impossible to assess the risk/benefit ratio of this approach. Similarly the favourable outlook following successful rescue PTCA should be set against the high mortality associated with failed rescue PTCA. Further studies are needed to decide on the correct approach. What is clear is that this selective approach of targeting more aggressive treatment to those at higher risk is likely to yield greater benefits than attempts to increase the intensity of reperfusion therapy for the infarct population as a whole.

Despite these uncertainties, attempts at achieving reperfusion following unsuccessful thrombolysis should certainly be considered if there is evidence of ongoing ischaemia (i.e. ischaemic pain) or haemodynamic compromise (increasing tachycardia or falling BP) and failure of ST segment resolution. The choice between repeat tPA and rescue PTCA will largely be dictated by local availability. Cardiac catheterisation is also indicated if ischaemic pain recurs after initially settling despite appropriate medical measures (see below).

3.5.2 Management of bradycardia and sinus tachycardia

Bradycardia

This is discussed in Chapter 12.

Sinus tachycardia

This is frequently a manifestation of an extensive infarct[7,52] and it is a mistake under these circumstances to β-block the patient without first performing a chest x ray to exclude occult pulmonary oedema. Other causes of tachycardia to consider are volume depletion (in particular gastrointestinal haemorrhage following thrombolysis), pulmonary embolism, and fever. In the absence of an underlying cause patients should be β-blocked in an attempt to reduce myocardial oxygen demand and limit infarct size.

3.5.3 Diabetes

Patients with diabetes have an almost two-fold increase in early mortality and reinfarction compared to non-diabetics.[53] In the DIGAMI[54] study, patients with a blood glucose > 11.0 mmol/l on admission or with known diabetes received glucose and insulin. Compared to patients receiving standard therapy, one year mortality in the treated group was reduced by 52%.

After achieving blood glucose within the target range for 24 hours, patients should be transferred to a tds subcutaneous regimen and in the DIGAMI study this was continued for a minimum of three months.

Despite these impressive results, the DIGAMI regimen is cumbersome and unfamiliar to most units. The amount of glucose infused is relatively modest and it is likely that the observed benefits are due largely to improved glycaemic control as opposed to the effects of a pharmacological effect from increased glucose flux into the myocardium. Many units have adopted a pragmatic approach and substituted their standard IV sliding scale insulin regimen. See Appendix for further details.

3.5.4 Recurrent chest pain

The differential diagnosis of recurrent chest pain following a myocardial infarction is shown in Table 3.4.

Table 3.4 Differential diagnosis of recurrent chest pain following myocardial infarction

Pain	Characteristics
Residual pain from infarction	24–36 hours post MI, dull ache, "bruised", pain continuous with infarct pain, ECG shows continued evolution from initial MI
Recurrent ischaemia	Clear worsening of pain after initial improvement, ECG sometimes shows evidence of recurrent ST elevation of ST depression
Rupture of ventricular septal defect (VSD)	Sudden recurrence of ischaemic like pain associated with haemodynamic deterioration $+/-$ murmur
Pericarditis	Pleuritic, positional, $+/-$ pericardial rub, ECG changes rare
Pulmonary embolism	Pleuritic, associated hypoxia, $+/-$ pleural rub, uncommon since thrombolysis
Sub-acute cardiac rupture	Pleuritic, transient hypotension, new T wave changes, CRP > 20 mg/dl
Rib fractures	Following traumatic resuscitation

Pain due to recurrent ischaemia

There are two pathological mechanisms for continuing ischaemia, one is that the original infarct-related artery has partially reperfused, leaving a severe enough stenosis to produce renewed ischaemia in the original infarct territory. This implies that there is at least some viable myocardium in the area of the initial infarct and will of course be more common following a non-Q wave infarction. The second possibility is that the patient has multi-vessel coronary disease and that occlusion of one coronary has unmasked ischaemia in other territories. The significance of recurrent ischaemia under either of these circumstances is firstly that the patient has further myocardium at risk in a situation where they have already suffered myocardial damage and secondly that ischaemia provoked under these resting conditions is likely to cause substantial limitation when the patient is mobilised. Due to the confounding effects of the changes still evolving from the original infarction, ECG evidence of ischaemia is frequently absent under these circumstances, although if present this is associated with a worse prognosis.

Recurrent pain + recurrent ST elevation

This occurs in up to 10% of patients who receive thrombolysis but only 3–4% of patients receiving aspirin and thrombolysis, underscoring the importance of not withholding aspirin because of a minor contraindication. Pain associated with recurrent ST elevation should be managed with repeat thrombolysis or PTCA as described above (management of failed thrombolysis).

Recurrent pain + ST depression or unchanged ECG

Unfortunately patients with recurrent ischaemia were specifically excluded from the various trials examining the role of PTCA in the peri-infarct period (Table 3.3) and there is a paucity of data on which to base recommendations. In the first instance, patients presenting with recurrent ischaemia associated with ST depression or insignificant ECG changes can frequently be settled with an intensification of medical management.

- Ensure that aspirin has been given and that if not the reasons for withholding it were genuine.
- Attempt to introduce a β-blocker and if this has already been done, ensure that the pulse rate is < 60/minute.
- Add intravenous nitrates as glyceryl trinitrate (GTN) 0–10 mg/hour titrated against BP response (aim for BP ↓ < 30% of systolic).
- Start heparin-5000 unit bolus and then KCCT adjusted to 1.5–2 × control.

If the patient continues to experience recurrent ischaemia despite the above regimen then cardiac catheterisation is appropriate. If they settle then heparin should be withdrawn after 48 hours and oral nitrates substituted for the iv GTN. If they remain asymptomatic then a pre-discharge exercise test should be performed to ensure that inducible ischaemia is not present at low workload (in which case cardiac catheterisation would still be appropriate).

Pain due to rupture of ventricular septal defect

Patients not infrequently experience pain at the moment of VSD rupture, associated with evidence of haemodynamic compromise and some ST segment re-elevation. This can mimic coronary re-occlusion leading to repeat thrombolysis with potentially disastrous consequences if urgent repair of the VSD is required. The presence of a new murmur should suggest the diagnosis and the need for urgent echocardiography.

Pain due to post-infarct pericarditis

Pericarditis typically occurs 48–72 hours following the initial infarction, and is associated with more substantial Q wave infarctions. A pericardial effusion is present in approximately 40% of patients, although given the high frequency of pericardial effusion following infarction this is of limited diagnostic use. The dramatic response to a non-steroidal anti-inflammatory is diagnostically useful.

Pain due to subacute rupture

The incidence of early cardiac rupture has been *increased* by the use of thrombolytics, and usually presents as unheralded electromechanical dissociation. Subacute cardiac rupture occasionally presents with pleuritic chest pain associated with transient hypotension, transient T wave changes[55] and often CRP level >20 mg/dl,[56] prior to the catastrophic event of rupture. Under these circumstances echocardiography should be performed to determine whether there is evidence of subacute rupture with a view to surgery.

3.5.5 New murmur

A soft murmur of mitral regurgitation in an otherwise well patient, due to papillary muscle dysfunction, is very common. This is easily differentiated from the severely ill patient with a ventricular septal defect or severe mitral regurgitation secondary to chordal rupture and a loud murmur. Diagnostic difficulties arise in patients with cardiogenic shock in whom the intensity of the murmur does not correlate with the severity of the haemodynamic disturbance. All patients with either a loud murmur or haemodynamic compromise should undergo echocardiography on the coronary care unit. Well patients with soft murmurs can safely have echocardiography deferred. The central clue to a mechanical complication of infarction on echocardiography is the presence of relatively well preserved left ventricular function in a patient with evidence of haemodynamic compromise. The presence of a flail or severely prolapsing mitral valve leaflet will be readily apparent, but ventricular septal defects, particularly those in the distal septum, may be harder to visualise. For further details please see Chapter 6 on the management of cardiogenic shock.

> **Box 3.7 Causes of a new murmur following myocardial infarction**
>
> - Pericarditis
> - Papillary muscle dysfunction
> - Papillary muscle rupture
> - Ventricular septal defect

Ventricular septal defect

Occurs in 1–2% of infarctions and without surgery carries a high mortality. Diagnosis is by echocardiography, confirmed if necessary by a saturation step up in the right ventricle at right heart catheterisation. Coronary angiography should be performed prior to surgery if possible as almost half of the patients will have multivessel disease. Emergency repair is required in the presence of haemodynamic compromise, although the operative mortality remains high at 30–50%.[57]

Severe mitral regurgitation due to infarction of a papillary muscle

This occurs in 2–4% of patients and is usually associated with significant stenoses of the right and circumflex coronaries with involvement of the posteromedial papillary muscle. Although the diagnosis of severe mitral regurgitation can be made using transthoracic echocardiography, transoesophageal echo is often required to confirm the exact mechanism of regurgitation as this will dictate whether valve replacement or repair is required at the time of surgery.

3.5.6 Atrial fibrillation

This complicates 15–20% of infarctions, is frequently a marker of more extensive myocardial damage and is associated with significant increases in both mortality and stroke.[58] The standard advice is that all arrhythmias associated with haemodynamic compromise should receive immediate DC cardioversion. Atrial fibrillation is rarely associated with severe enough compromise to justify this approach and even if one were to adopt this strategy the rate of failure to sustain sinus rhythm would be high as it is frequently paroxysmal.

The first step is to attempt to identify any predisposing cause such as left ventricular dysfunction and to ensure that this is adequately treated, a chest x ray or echocardiography may be worthwhile at this stage. The serum K^+ should be rechecked and maintained > 4.5 mmol/l, if necessary with insertion of a central line to infuse a concentrated K solution. The patient should be anticoagulated unless there are specific contraindications (heparin 5000 U IV followed by an infusion aiming for a KCCT 1.5−2×control). There are three options for controlling the ventricular rate, none of which is ideal:

Amiodarone
IV loading: 300 mg over 1 hour in 50 ml 5% dextrose, followed by 900 mg over the following 24 hours.
Oral: 400 mg tds for 7 days simultaneously with the IV regimen.

The advantage of amiodarone is that it has the greatest potential to produce reversion to sinus rhythm. Its disadvantages are a slow onset of action, the potential for acute toxicity and the need to administer it via a central line. Although usually well tolerated by patients with impaired

left ventricular function the diluent used in the intravenous formulation can occasionally worsen severe heart failure (a diluent free preparation will shortly be available). Blood should be taken for thyroid function tests prior to administering amiodarone.

Metoprolol

IV 5–15 mg followed by 50 mg orally as described above. Although their well recognised role in mortality reduction makes these an attractive option, many of the patients in atrial fibrillation will have significantly impaired LV function and acute β-blockade may not be practicable.

Digoxin

Oral loading: 0.5 mg tds for 24 hours and then 0.25 mg daily thereafter.

IV loading: 0.5 mg over 30 minutes instead of first oral dose and then continued as above.

The advantages of digoxin are its convenience and familiarity and the fact that it is not a negative inotrope. Against this are its relatively slow onset of action and suggestions of an increased mortality when digoxin is used in the post-infarction setting.[59] Further management is discussed in Chapter 9.

3.5.7 Heart failure and cardiogenic shock

These are discussed in Chapters 5 and 6.

3.5.8 Drugs to use with caution in acute infarction

Calcium antagonists

There is very little convincing evidence of benefit from the routine use of calcium antagonists in myocardial infarction and suspicion of harm in some patients.[3] Verapamil has a minor role in place of β-antagonists in patients without evidence of LV dysfunction.[60]

Lidocaine (lignocaine)

The use of prophylactic lidocaine in an attempt to reduce the frequency of VF is no longer recommended, due to an increase in overall mortality,[61] and there is little enthusiasm for the treatment of ventricular ectopics. It continues to have a role in the initial management of sustained ventricular tachycardia (VT) with a BP > 90 mmHg.

Magnesium

Although the results of further studies are awaited (particularly in patients ineligible for thrombolysis) there is no current evidence to support the use of magnesium except in the treatment of resistant ventricular tachycardia or proven magnesium deficiency.[44]

Case 3.1

A 70-year-old woman presented to her local hospital with an acute anterior infarction. The ECG showed ST elevation in V2–V5 and she received streptokinase and aspirin. There was little resolution of her ST segments following thrombolysis but her pain settled with supplemental opiates and she remained haemodynamically stable. Five days after admission she developed further chest pain associated with recurrent ST elevation in V2–V5 associated with hypotension (BP 95/70) and tachycardia.

A diagnosis of recurrent infarction was made and she received alteplase with heparin. There was no resolution of her ST segments, her hypotension did not improve and she was transferred with a view to immediate coronary angiography. On arrival she was additionally noted to have a pansystolic murmur at the left sternal edge. Echocardiography demonstrated an extensive anterior infarction with an abrupt hinge point at the junction of the infarcted and non-infarcted tissue, with colour flow confirming the presence of a ventricular septal defect with a left to right shunt. Coronary angiography demonstrated severe 3 vessel disease with persistent occlusion of the LAD. She died following attempted VSD repair and coronary bypass surgery.

The formation of a post infarct VSD may be associated with recurrent pain and ST segment elevation leading to a mistaken diagnosis of recurrent coronary occlusion and the administration of repeat doses of thrombolytics. In addition to complicating surgical haemostasis there is a suspicion that thrombolytic administration may further soften the infarcted myocardium and hamper operative repair. In the thrombolytic era the outlook for patients with post infarction VSDs appears to be worse than would be predicted from past surgical series.

Case 3.2

A 67-year-old man was admitted with an acute anterior infarction for which he received streptokinase, aspirin and subsequently lisinopril without ECG evidence of reperfusion. Seventy-two hours following admission he developed atrial fibrillation at a rate of 140/min. He was otherwise well, but his blood pressure fell to 106/70 mm. Heparin was initiated and two oral potassium supplements were administered. On the basis that he was haemodynamically compromised by the atrial fibrillation he was anaesthetised, and cardioverted back to sinus rhythm with a 200J shock. Following this his systolic blood pressure improved to 115 mmHg, but he reverted back to atrial fibrillation one hour later. Chest x ray at this point revealed interstitial oedema. His condition improved with intravenous diuretics and digoxin and he spontaneously reverted back to sinus rhythm 36 hours later.

Although the dictum that "haemodynamically compromising arrhythmia = DC shock" is broadly correct, matters are frequently less straightforward in acute atrial fibrillation complicating infarction. In particular, the role cardioversion is less clear than in patients who present with acute onset AF as their sole problem (see Chapter 9). Unless the environment that created the AF (atrial pressure overload, sepsis, hypoxia etc) is corrected then fibrillation tends to recur. In the majority of patients, the haemodynamic compromise genuinely attributable to the AF is modest compared to the effects of the ventricular dysfunction that predisposed to its occurence. Recognition and treatment of an initiating/aggravating mechanism (in this case unrecognized heart failure) with slowing of the ventricular response with the positively inotropic digoxin might have been a better option. The use of β-blockers was precluded by the relative hypotension. One should be particularly reluctant to consider cardioversion in patients who have paroxsysmal AF due to the overwhelming likelihood of swift recurrence. If restoration and maintenance of sinus rhythm is considered essential then aggressive correction of predisposing factors combined with appropriate intravenous K^+ replacement and possibly intravenous amiodarone should be considered.

Case 3.3

A 50-year-old woman with a past history of hypertension was making an uneventful recovery following an inferior infarction previously for which she had received streptokinase. She developed transient recurrent chest pain on the morning of the sixth hospital day. The nursing observations revealed a pulse of 45/min and a BP of 90/70 at this point, but on review 30 minutes later on the morning ward round both of these had resolved and an ECG showed merely the expected changes consistent with resolving infarction. The possibility of pulmonary embolism was raised, but arterial blood gases were normal and she was reassured accordingly.

Six hours later her team were called to her cardiac arrest – there was pulseless electrical activity (PEA). Echocardiography during the arrest demonstrated ventricular rupture and subsequent tamponade. Resusciation was unsuccessful.

A syndrome of pre-rupture prior to the fatal event of free wall rupture is occasionally encountered. In theory early recognition of this might permit surgical repair although in practice this is very difficult to achieve – the best protection we have against rupture is the early use of β-blockers and possibly ACE inihbitors. Paradoxically, thrombolytic use is associated with an increase in the incidence of rupture, particularly within the first 24 hours of admission.

Case 3.4

A 75-year-old woman presented with a 12 hour history of intermittent chest pain associated with ECG evidence of 2 mm ST depression in V2–V5. Because of the severity of the chest pain and the fact that infarction (as opposed to angina) was felt to be occurring, she received streptokinase. Her pain and ECG changes both resolved, although her troponins rose to > 50 micrograms/l and her CK peaked at 400 IU/l. Eighteen hours after administration of streptokinase, her pain and ECG changes returned. Cardiac catheterisation revealed a severe, thrombus containing, ulcerated proximal plaque in her LAD (but with preserved flow as opposed to complete occlusion) which was successfully stented.

Thrombolysis is not beneficial in the absence of ST elevation (or new left bundle branch block) and is indeed actually harmful in non-ST elevation infarction and unstable angina due to increased platelet activation. The platelet predominance of the non-occlusive thrombi found in non-ST elevation syndromes require treatment with tirofiban or eptifibatide plus heparin. Interestingly, current evidence suggests that, despite the excellent performance of abciximab during angioplasty and stenting, it does not have a role in the management of patients outside the cath lab.

Summary

Chest pain + ST elevation = myocardial infarction until proven otherwise (the diagnosis is rarely in doubt)

Risk stratification can be accomplished using simple clinical and ECG variables

All patients should receive aspirin and a β-blocker in the absence of specific contraindications

ST elevation → thrombolysis, ST depression or normal ECG → no thrombolysis

Alteplase should be reserved for high risk patients or patients who have previously received streptokinase

Primary angioplasty should be strongly considered in patients with a contraindication to thrombolysis or those in cardiogenic shock

Unless LV function can be assessed early, all patients should receive an ACE inhibitor pending echocardiography

Patients with diabetes should receive intensive control of blood glucose

Transcutaneous pacing has reduced the need for transvenous pacing, the only indication now being symptomatic bradycardia unresponsive to atropine

Only patients with evidence of continuing ischaemia or a mechanical complication of infarction require early cardiac catheterisation

References

1 Mauri F, Maggioni AP, Franzosi MG, *et al.* A simple electrocardiographic predictor of the outcome of patients with acute myocardial infarction treated with a thrombolytic agent. A Gruppo Italiano per lo Studio della Sopravvivenza nell'Infarto Miocardico (GISSI-2)-Derived Analysis [published erratum appears in *J Am Coll Cardiol* 1995;**25**(3):805]. *J Am Coll Cardiol* 1994;**24**:600–7.

2 Stevenson RN, Ranjadayalan K, Umachandran V, Timmis AD. Significance of reciprocal ST depression in acute myocardial infarction: a study of 258 patients treated by thrombolysis. *Br Heart J* 1993;**69**:211–14.

3 Ryan TJ, Anderson JL, Antman EM, *et al.* ACC/AHA guidelines for the management of patients with acute myocardial infarction: executive summary. A report of the American College of Cardiology/American Heart Association Task Force on Practice Guidelines (Committee on Management of Acute Myocardial Infarction). *Circulation* 1996; **94**:2341–50. *This should be read with the 1999 update:* Ryan TJ, Antman EM, Brooks NH, *et al.* 99 update: ACC/AHA Guidelines for the Management of Patients With Acute Myocardial Infarction: Executive Summary and Recommendations: A report of the American College of Cardiology/American Heart Association Task Force on Practice Guidelines. *Circulation* 1999;**100**:1016–30.

4 Acute myocardial infarction: pre-hospital and in-hospital management. The Task Force on the Management of Acute Myocardial Infarction of the European Society of Cardiology. *Eur Heart J* 1996;**17**:43–63.

5 Indications for fibrinolytic therapy in suspected acute myocardial infarction: collaborative overview of early mortality and major morbidity results from all randomised trials of more than 1000 patients. Fibrinolytic Therapy Trialists' (FTT) Collaborative Group [published erratum appears in *Lancet* 1994;**343**(8899):742]. *Lancet* 1994;**343**:311–22.

6 Krainin FM, Flessas AP, Spodick DH. Infarction-associated pericarditis. Rarity of diagnostic electrocardiogram. *N Engl J Med* 1984;**311**:1211–14.

7 Lee KL, Woodlief LH, Topol EJ. Predictors of 30-day mortality in the era of reperfusion for acute myocardial infarction. Results from an

international trial of 41.021 patients. GUSTO-I Investigators. *Circulation* 1995;**91**:1659–68.

8 Davies CH, Ormerod OJM. Diagnosis and management of failed thrombolysis. *Lancet* 1998;**351**:1191–96.

9 Cragg DR, Friedman HZ, Bonema JD, *et al.* Outcome of patients with acute myocardial infarction who are ineligible for thrombolytic therapy. *Ann Intern Med* 1991;**115**:173–77.

10 Late Assessment of Thrombolytic Efficacy (LATE) study with alteplase 6–24 hours after onset of acute myocardial infarction [see comments]. *Lancet* 1993;**342**:759–66.

11 Mahaffey KW, Granger CB, Toth CAA, *et al.* Diabetic retinopathy should not be a contraindication to thrombolytic therapy for myocardial infarction: review of occular haemorrhage incidence and location in GUSTO-1. *J Am Coll Cardiol* 1997;**30**:1606–10.

12 Durrington PN. Biological variation in serum lipid concentrations. *Scand J Clin Lab Invest Suppl* 1990;**198**:86–91.

13 Timmis AD. Routine chest radiographs in admissions to coronary care. *Lancet* 1995;**345**:652–3.

14 Randomised trial of intravenous streptokinase, oral aspirin, both, or neither among 17 187 cases of suspected acute myocardial infarction: ISIS-2. ISIS2 (Second International Study of Infarct Survival) Collaborative Group. *Lancet* 1988;**2**:349–60.

15 Boersma E, Simons ML. Reperfusion strategies in acute myocardial infarction. *Eur Heart J* 1997;**18**:1703–11.

16 ISIS-3: a randomised comparison of streptokinase vs tissue plasminogen activator vs anistreplase and of aspirin plus heparin vs aspirin alone among 41 299 cases of suspected acute myocardial infarction. ISIS-3 (Third International Study of Infarct Survival) Collaborative Group [see comments]. *Lancet* 1992;**339**:753–70.

17 Six-month survival in 20 891 patients with acute myocardial infarction randomized between alteplase and streptokinase with or without heparin GISSI-2 and International Study Group. Gruppo Italiano per lo Studio della Sopravvivenza nell'Infarto. *Eur Heart J* 1992;**13**:1692–7.

18 Califf RM. The GUSTO trial and the open artery theory *Eur Heart J* 1997; **18** supplement F:2–10.

19 Gersh BJ, Opie LH. Antithrombotic agents: platelet inhibitors, anticoagulants and fibrinolytics, in Opie LH, ed. *Drugs for the heart.* Saunders: Philadelphia, 1997:248–87.

20 An international randomized trial comparing four thrombolytic strategies for acute myocardial infarction. The GUSTO investigators. *N Engl J Med* 1993;**329**:67–82.

21 Friedman HF. Streptokinase vs alteplase in acute myocardial infarction. *J Roy Soc Med* 1996;**89**:427–30.

22 Califf RM, Woodlief LH, Harrell FE Jr, *et al.* Selection of thrombolytic therapy for individual patients: development of a clinical model. GUSTO-I Investigators. *Am Heart J* 1997;**133**:630–9.

23 Hsia J, Hamilton WP, Kleiman N, Roberts R, Chaitman BR, Ross AM. A comparison between heparin and low-dose aspirin as adjunctive therapy with tissue plasminogen activator for acute myocardial infarction. Heparin-Aspirin Reperfusion Trial (HART) Investigators [see comments]. *N Engl J Med* 1990;**323**:1433–7.

24 Collins R, MacMahon S, Flather M, *et al.* Clinical effects of anticoagulant therapy in suspected acute myocardial infarction: systematic overview of randomised trials. *BMJ* 1996;**313**:652–9.

25 Effects of tissue plasminogen activator and a comparison of early invasive and conservative strategies in unstable angina and non-Q-wave

myocardial infarction. Results of the TIMI IIIB Trial Thrombolysis in Myocardial Ischemia [see comments]. *Circulation* 1994;**89**:1545–56.

26 Langer A, Goodman SG, Topol EJ, *et al*. Late assessment of thrombolytic efficacy (LATE) study: prognosis in patients with non-Q wave myocardial infarction. *J Am Coll Cardiol* 1996;**27**:1327–32.

27 Timmis AD. Will serum enzymes and other proteins find a clinical application in the early diagnosis of myocardial infarction? [see comments]. *Br Heart J* 1994;**71**:309–10.

28 Long-term effects of intravenous thrombolysis in acute myocardial infarction: final report of the GISSI study. Gruppo Italiano per lo Studio della Streptochi-nasi nell'Infarto Miocardico (GISSI). *Lancet* 1987;**2**:871–4.

29 A clinical trial comparing primary coronary angioplasty with tissue plasminogen activator for acute myocardial infarction. The Global Use of Strategies to Open Occluded Coronary Arteries in Acute Coronary Syndromes (GUSTO IIb) Angioplasty Substudy Investigators. *N Engl J Med* 1997;**336**:1621–8.

30 Grines CL, Browne KF, Marco JM. PAMI: A comparison of immediate angioplasty with thrombolytic therapy for acute myocardial infarction. *N Engl J Med* 1993,**328**:673–9.

31 Berger PB, Holmes DR, Jr., Stebbins AL, Bates ER, Califf RM, Topol EJ. Impact of an aggressive invasive catheterization and revascularization strategy on mortality in patients with cardiogenic shock in the Global Utilization of Streptokinase and Tissue Plasminogen Activator for Occluded Coronary Arteries (GUSTO-I) trial. An observational study. *Circulation* 1997;**96**:122–7.

32 Simons ML, Arnold AE, Betriu A, *et al*. Thrombolysis with tissue plasminogen activator in acute myocardial infarction: no additional benefit from immediate percutaneous coronary angioplasty. *Lancet* 1988;**1**:197–203.

33 Califf RM, Topol EJ, Stack RS, *et al*. Evaluation of combination thrombolytic therapy and timing of cardiac catheterization in acute myocardial infarction. Results of thrombolysis and angioplasty in myocardial infarction – phase 5 randomized trial. TAMI Study Group. *Circulation* 1991;**83**:1543–56.

34 Ellis SG, da Silva ER, Heyndrickx G, *et al*. Randomized comparison of rescue angioplasty with conservative management of patients with early failure of thrombolysis for acute anterior myocardial infarction. *Circulation* 1994;**90**:2280–4.

35 Rogers WJ, Baim DS, Gore JM, *et al*. Comparison of immediate invasive, delayed invasive, and conservative strategies after tissue-type plasminogen activator. Results of the Thrombolysis in Myocardial Infarction (TIMI) Phase II-A trial [see comments]. *Circulation* 1990;**81**:1457–76.

36 SWIFT trial of delayed elective intervention v conservative treatment after thrombolysis with anistreplase in acute myocardial infarction. SWIFT (Should We Intervene Following Thrombolysis?) Trial Study Group. *BMJ* 1991;**302**:555–60.

37 Ellis SG, Mooney MR, George BS, *et al*. Randomized trial of late elective angioplasty versus conservative management for patients with residual stenoses after thrombolytic treatment of myocardial infarction. Treatment of Post-Thrombolytic Stenoses (TOPS) Study Group. *Circulation* 1992,**86**:1400–6.

38 Basu S, Senior R, Raval U, van der Does R1 Bruckner T, Lahiri A. Beneficial effects of intravenous and oral carvedilol treatment in acute myocardial infarction. A placebo-controlled, randomized trial. *Circulation* 1997;**96**:183–91.

39 Randomised trial of intravenous atenolol among 16 027 cases of suspected acute myocardial infarction: ISIS-1. First International Study of Infarct Survival Collaborative Group. *Lancet* 1986;**ii**:57–66.

40 Hjalmarson A, Elmfeldt D, Herlitz J, *et al.* Effect on mortality of metoprololin acute myocardial infarction. A double-blind randomised trial. *Lancet* 1981;**ii**:823–27.

41 Hall AS, Murray GD, Ball SG. Follow-up study of patients randomly allocated ramipril or placebo for heart failure after acute myocardial infarction: AIRE Extension (AIREX) Study. Acute Infarction Ramipril Efficacy. *Lancet* 1997;**349**:1493–7.

42 Kober L, Torp Pedersen C, Carlsen JE, *et al.* A clinical trial of the angiotensin converting-enzyme inhibitor trandolapril in patients with left ventricular dysfunction after myocardial infarction. Trandolapril Cardiac Evaluation (TRACE) Study Group [see comments]. *N Engl J Med* 1995;**333**:1670–6.

43 Pfeffer MA, Braunwald E, Moye LA, *et al.* Effect of captopril on mortality and morbidity in patients with left ventricular dysfunction after myocardial infarction. Results of the survival and ventricular enlargement trial. The SAVE investigators. *N Engl J Med* 1993;**327**:669–77.

44 ISIS-4: a randomised factorial trial assessing early oral captopril, oral mononitrate, and intravenous magnesium sulphate in 58 050 patients with suspected acute myocardial infarction. ISIS-4 (Fourth International Study of Infarct Survival) Collaborative Group. *Lancet* 1995;**345**:669–85.

45 Six-month effects of early treatment with lisinopril and transdermal glyceryl trinitrate singly and together withdrawn six weeks after acute myocardial infarction: the GISSI-3 trial. Gruppo Italiano per lo Studio della Sopravvivenza nell'Infarto Miocardico. *J Am Coll Cardiol* 1996;**27**:337–44.

46 Lindsay HS, Zamari AG, Cowan JC. ACE inhibitors after myocardial infarction: patient selection or treatment for all? [published erratum appears in *Br Heart J* 1995;**74**(2):206]. *Br Heart J* 1995;**73**:397–400.

47 Pfeffer MA, Greaves SC, Arnold JM, *et al.* Early versus delayed angiotensin-converting enzyme inhibition therapy in acute myocardial infarction. The healing and early after load reducing therapy trial. *Circulation* 1997;**95**:2643–51.

48 Cohn JN. The management of chronic heart failure. *N Engl J Med* 1996; **335**:490–8.

49 Simes RJ, Topol EJ, Holmes DR, Jr., *et al.* Link between the angiographic sub study and mortality outcomes in a large randomized trial of myocardial reperfusion. Importance of early and complete infarct artery reperfusion. GUSTO-I Investigators. *Circulation* 1995;**91**:1923–8.

50 Mounsey JP, Skinner JS, Hawkins T, *et al.* Rescue thrombolysis: alteplase as adjuvant treatment after streptokinase in acute myocardial infarction. *Br Heart J* 1995;**74**:348–353.

51 De Belder. Failed thrombolysis. *Heart* 2001;**85**:104–12.

52 Crimm A, Severance HW, Jr., Coffey K, McKinnis R, Wagner GS, Califf RM. Prognostic significance of isolated sinus tachycardia during first three days of acute myocardial infarction. *Am J Med* 1984;**76**:983–8.

53 Kjekshus J. Treating the diabetic patient with coronary disease. *Eur Heart J* 1996;**17**:1298–301.

54 Malmberg K. Prospective randomised study of intensive insulin treatment on long term survival after acute myocardial infarction in patients with diabetes mellitus. DIGAMI (Diabetes Mellitus, Insulin Glucose Infusion in Acute Myocardial Infarction) Study Group. *BMJ* 1997;**314**:1512–15.

55 Oliva PB, Hammill SC, Edwards WD. Cardiac rupture, a clinically

predictable complication of acute myocardial infarction: report of 70 cases with clinicopathologic correlations. *J Am Coll Cardiol* 1993;**22**:720–6.

56 Anzai T, Yoshikawa T, Shiraki H, *et al.* C-reactive protein as a predictor of infarct expansion and cardiac rupture after a first Q-wave acute myocardial infarction. *Circulation* 1997;**96**:778–84.

57 Pellerin M, Bourassa MG. Postinfarction ventricular septal rupture [editorial; comment]. *Eur Heart J* 1996;**17**:1778–9.

58 Crenshaw BS, Ward SR, Granger CB, Stebbins AL, Topol EJ, Califf RM. Atrial fibrillation in the setting of acute myocardial infarction: the GUSTO-I experience. Global Utilization of Streptokinase and TPA for Occluded Coronary Arteries. *J Am Coll Cardiol* 1997;**30**:406–13.

59 Simons M, Leclerc G, Safion RD, Inser JM, Weir L, Baim D. Relation between activated smooth-muscle in coronary lesions and restenosis after angioplasty. *N Engl J Med* 1993,**328**:608–13.

60 Effect of verapamil on mortality and major events after acute myocardial infarction (the Danish Verapamil Infarction Trial II – DAVIT ll) [see comments]. *Am J Cardiol* 1990;**66**:779-85.

61 MacMahon S, Collins R, Peto R, Koster RW, Yusuf S. Effects of prophylactic lidocaine in suspected acute myocardial infarction. An overview of results from the randomized, controlled trials. *JAMA* 1988; **260**:1910–16.

4: Acute coronary syndromes III: chest pain with ST depression or a normal ECG

CH DAVIES, BK SHIVELY

4.1 Introduction

Acute coronary syndromes associated with ST depression or non-specific ECG changes encompass a continuum of clinical presentations ranging from unstable angina to non-Q wave myocardial infarction. These entities cannot be differentiated on initial presentation.[1,2] As discussed in Chapter 2, the most common cause is partial luminal obstruction due to platelet rich ("white") thrombus (Figure 4.1). Ischaemia in these patients is due to the combined effects of increasing luminal obstruction from progressive thrombus accumulation, micro fragmentation with distal embolisation, and intermittent vasoconstriction. Importantly, the presence of partial luminal occlusion produces a set of problems distinct from those of ST elevation associated infarction. Firstly, acute problems due to the loss of functioning myocardium such as shock and heart failure are less common in the absence of ST elevation – the fact that the artery is not completely occluded minimises myocardial loss. Unfortunately, this is counter balanced by the potential for the artery to close completely at a later date producing further damage. Thus early mortality is higher in ST elevation infarction and later re-infarction is more common in non-ST elevation syndromes, and overall mortality is similar between the two groups by one year. Secondly, the presence of a predominantly platelet based thrombus significantly shifts the anti-thrombotic regimens required away from the use of thrombolytics. Another important difference between ST depression and ST elevation infarction is the fact that ST depression can occur in the context of a wider spectrum of pathologies (Figure 4.1). This heightens the importance of considering a broader range of possibilities in the differential diagnosis such as the exacerbating factors fever, anaemia, etc.

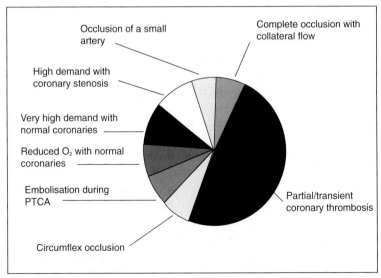

Figure 4.1 Aetiology of acute coronary syndromes presenting as ST depression.

4.2 Clinical presentations

Unstable angina is an unsatisfactory amalgam of conditions spanning angina of recent onset, increasing frequency of stable angina, and angina at rest (Box 4.1).

Box 4.1 Spectrum of unstable angina presentations
- Angina at rest
- New onset angina
- Deteriorating stable angina
- Post MI angina

4.2.1 Risk stratification

There are two distinct clinical problems at presentation, firstly whether this is an acute coronary syndrome and secondly an assessment of the risk posed by the condition. Patients present in one of three groups.

Group 1: ST elevation

Confusingly, approximately one-third of patients who are subsequently shown to have suffered a non-Q wave infarction initially present with ECG evidence of ST elevation. This crossover group represents patients with occluded epicardial arteries at presentation who subsequently achieve satisfactory myocardial reperfusion (either spontaneously or with thrombolysis) and should be managed as outlined in Chapter 3.

Group 2: ST depression and T wave inversion

These patients do not present any serious diagnostic dilemma, the goal here is to achieve risk stratification. ST depression confers a significantly worse outlook than T wave inversion even if this occurs in the anterior chest leads.

Group 3: No acute ECG changes

This group comprises patients with unstable coronary disease and non-diagnostic ECGs but also patients with non-cardiac chest pain. The problem here is to stabilise patients who do have unstable coronary disease whilst achieving a definite diagnosis as to whether coronary disease is present or absent in those that do not. A balance must be achieved between failing to treat patients with life threatening disease adequately and exposing patients with more benign conditions to the risks of treatment from which they cannot derive benefit. Whilst a normal ECG in pain does not exclude unstable angina (for example in the circumflex territory) it identifies a particularly low risk subgroup.

Almost all of the data about management is derived from Group 2 patients as most clinical trials have required ECG changes or enzyme rises as inclusion criteria. This results in the formation of a high risk population enabling benefits to be demonstrated or refuted using the minimum number of patients. Unfortunately the results of these cannot necessarily be extrapolated to the much larger group of patients in Group 3 in whom the risk/benefit ratio remains unknown.

Diagnostic difficulty can arise in patients presenting for the first time. For example, patients with pre-existing exertional angina will readily identify that the pain at rest is similar to their "usual" angina, whereas when patients have only a single episode of pain their descriptions tend to be less classical. The most diagnostic features are the duration of pain (daily episodes of pain, each lasting for many hours for the past 10 days are not due to angina) and whether there is any exercise limitation between episodes of pain. Prompt recording of ECGs when patients experience pain and documentation on the ECG of the level of pain are important factors in achieving an early diagnosis. Patients in Groups 2 and 3 require secondary clinical risk stratification on the basis of the clinical presentation, the ECG and troponin levels indicated below.

Low risk (< 5% risk of MI)

New onset angina. Deteriorating exercise tolerance in stable angina.

Intermediate risk (9% risk of MI)

Angina at rest.

High risk (> 17% risk of MI)

Prolonged angina at rest with ECG changes. The risk is increased further by:

- Increasing severity of ST depression (depth of depression and number of leads) and in particular the presence of fluctuating ST changes.[3]
- Evidence of infarction (enzyme rise or troponin T > 0.06 µg/l).[4]
- Recent infarction.
- Recurrence of angina after initially settling.
- Presence of heart failure.
- Hypotension (systolic BP < 105 mmHg).

The gradation of risk produced by the relationship between the severity of the ECG changes and the degree of troponin T elevation can be appreciated from Figure 4.2 (although less than 20% of UK hospitals currently have access to troponin assays). The ability of the ECG to stratify risk should come as no surprise and follows logically from the Goldman risk stratification in the diagnosis of chest pain discussed in Chapter 1. Additional diagnostic tests should include:

- Chest x ray (to look for heart failure).
- FBC (to ensure that any deterioration has not been precipitated by anaemia).
- Cholesterol (for secondary risk modification if the patient is eventually discovered to have coronary disease).

4.3 Management

4.3.1 Home or hospital?

The first decision is whether the patient can be managed as an outpatient or whether admission to hospital is required. Although this will depend on local circumstances (both social

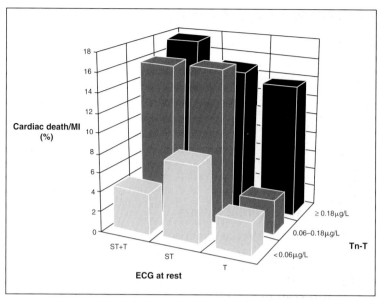

Figure 4.2 The relationship between the risk of cardiac death/MI to the presence of ECG abnormalities and troponin T levels. Note that even when both are negative the risk is not insignificant from Lindahl et al.[30]

and organisational), patients with recent onset exertional angina and those with a deteriorating exercise tolerance can be managed as outpatients. In these patients, medication can be optimised and early outpatient review arranged. With patients whose medical management is already optimal, outpatient coronary angiography may be appropriate, whilst in patients presenting for the first time an outpatient exercise ECG will be required either to confirm the diagnosis or for further risk stratification. In those admitted to hospital, patients in the high risk group merit admission to a coronary care unit, whereas those in the intermediate and low risk groups can safely be managed on a general admissions ward.

4.3.2 Medical management

Patients in acute pain should receive appropriate analgesia as previously described in Chapter 2. Also ensure the following, described below, are covered:

- Correction of precipitants.
- Reducing myocardial O_2 demand.
- Antiplatelet therapy.
- Antithrombin therapy.
- Load reduction/vasodilatation.

Control of precipitating factors

The possibility that ischaemia may be provoked or aggravated by anaemia, pain, fever, or hypoxia should always be considered. Failure to spot these conditions may have catastrophic results (i.e. using heparin in someone whose primary problem is gastrointestinal haemorrhage).

Reducing myocardial oxygen demand

Myocardial oxygen demand can be clinically assessed by the "double product" (systolic blood pressure×heart rate). A value of < 12 000 is an essential first step in management and a value of less than 7000 is desirable, equating to a systolic BP in the region of 120 mmHg with a heart rate of 50–60 mmHg. This combination of hypotension and relative bradycardia is achieved with β-blockade, which achieves a reduction in the progression to MI of the order of 13%.[5] Treatment should be initiated with IV metoprolol (administered in 5 mg increments every 5 minutes to a total of 15 mg). The decision as to whether IV therapy is required before oral treatment (metroprolol 25–50 mg tds) will clearly depend on the patient's evaluated risk. However, in general, blockers are under utilised in the management of unstable angina. The exact choice of agent can be left to personal preference and familiarity. Although the question of β subtype selectivity seems to matter little, drugs with intrinsic sympathetic activity should be avoided and there are advantages to using drugs with shorter half lives. If hypertension requires control in its own right (which is unusual) then IV glyceryl trinitrate (GTN) combined with β-blockade is the first choice in the acute situation (see below).

Antiplatelet therapy – first line

First line management is aspirin and, as with the treatment of ST elevation infarction, it is important that the first dose is at least 150 mg (300 mg is recommended in the National Service Framework). As with ST elevation MI, the results of aspirin treatment are impressive with a two to threefold reduction in MI and death.[6,7] In those who are genuinely aspirin intolerant, the ADP antagonist clopidogrel 75 mg once daily is an alternative.

Antiplatelet therapy – second line (Table 4.1)

Both inhibitors of cyclo-oxygenase and the ADP antagonists used as first line treatment are limited by the fact that they antagonise platelet aggregation triggered from single stimuli (thromboxane and ADP respectively) leaving the platelets still responsive to other factors such as epinephrine (adrenaline), collagen adhesion, etc. The more recently developed antagonists of the glycoprotein IIb/IIIa receptor (the final common pathway of attachment) circumvent this (Figure 4.3). The gpIIb/IIIa antagonists can be divided into the monoclonal antibody abciximab and the synthetic antagonists triofiban and eptifibatide.

Table 4.1 Second-line antiplatelet therapy

	Structure	Binding	Major trial
Abciximab	antibody	irreversible	CAPTURE[8] GUSTO-4 TACTICS TIMI
Tirofiban	peptide	reversible	PRISM[9] PRISM-plus[10]
Eptifibatide	peptide	reversible	PURSUIT[11]

Abciximab is a potent, expensive and irreversible antagonist of the gp IIb/IIIa receptor which in addition may mitigate against neutrophil mediated reperfusion damage. Given its antibody based structure, there is continuing uncertainty as to whether repeat administration is feasible. Abciximab's primary role is during angioplasty, where it is highly effective and there is evidence from the EPISTENT trial to support its use during

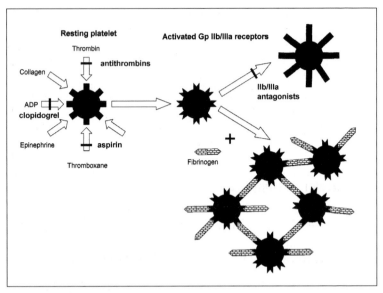

Figure 4.3 Sites of action of anti-platelet drugs. With multiple potential stimuli for aggregation, use of drugs acting at this point only produces partial inhibition of platelet function. By contrast, drugs acting on the glycoprotein IIb/IIIa receptor protect from multiple potential stimuli. Modified from Madan et al.[29]

coronary intervention in all patients with unstable symptoms. However there is also evidence from the CAPTURE[8] trial that in unstable patients in whom the coronary anatomy is known but in whom PTCA is not being performed for 24 hours, that treatment with abciximab significantly improves outcomes (particularly in troponin positive patients[12]). This situation occurs when a patient has undergone diagnostic catheterisation in a facility that does not perform percutaneous transluminal coronary angioplasty (PTCA), to which they are then transferred the following day with abciximab used to stabilise them in the interim (a policy inelegantly known as "drip and ship"). This would be unusual in the UK as most catheter labs that do not perform PTCA will not study unstable patients. The prospect of administering abciximab to a patient without knowing whether the coronary anatomy is even suitable for PTCA is not attractive, particularly as this might jeopardise its use during a subsequent PTCA. Thus in practice, current use of abciximab is restricted to its role during PTCA, a policy recently confirmed by the GUSTO-4 ACS trial. By contrast there is a role for the synthetic antagonists eptifibatide[11] and tirofiban[9,10] which have both been demonstrated to reduce recurrent ischaemia by small but significant margins in high risk patients (predominantly troponin positive). As neither of these binds the gp IIb/IIIa receptor irreversibly their effect is less prolonged than abciximab and as both are synthetic they will not jeopardise future use of abciximab. Currently the use of both agents is limited to patients with refractory symptoms associated with dynamic ST segment depression[13] but they are increasingly used in all patients with ST shift or positive troponins. Investigations into the potential for oral IIb/IIIa antagonists have been disappointing and they have no current clinical role.

Indirect antithrombin therapy – unfractionated heparin

Unfractionated heparins are glycosaminoglycans ranging in molecular weight from 3 to 30 KDa. They act by binding to antithrombin III and potentiating its inhibition of thrombin (IIa) and factor Xa (Figure 4.4) in addition to inhibiting platelet aggregation. Unfortunately, heparin binds extensively to other plasma proteins, is a relatively weak inhibitor of clot bound thrombin, and is inhibited by platelet factor 4. Very occasionally heparin induced thrombocytopenia develops. Despite widespread use, the evidence of benefit from unfractionated heparin is surprisingly poor with many contradictory studies. A recent meta-analysis suggested a 33% reduction in MI or death for heparin and aspirin compared to aspirin alone which supports its inclusion in almost all practice guidelines.[14] The problems of achieving an adequate therapeutic response to heparin are well recognised and to have any chance of achieving therapeutic consistency a nurse led dose adjustment protocol is essential.

Unfractionated heparin dosage

- 80 units/kg bolus
- 18 units/kg/hour
- Aim for KCCT 1.5 to 2.5 × control

As almost all of the data supporting the use of heparins is derived from patients with either ST depression or elevated cardiac enzymes, its use is not recommended in patients with chest pain who do not fall into these categories.

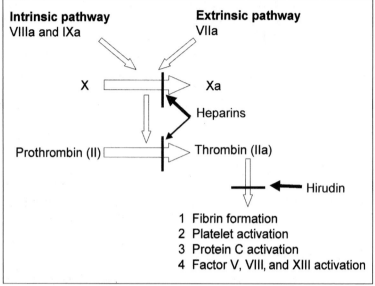

Figure 4.4 Sites of action of drugs on the coagulation cascade. Low molecular weight heparins with increased activity against factor Xa appear to be superior to those with lower anti Xa:IIa ratios.

Indirect antithrombins – low molecular weight heparins

These short chain fragments inhibit factors Xa and IIa in varying degrees, have more predictable effects and longer plasma half lives. They tend to have less anti-platelet activity than unfractionated heparin although in an era where additional additional antiplatelet inhibition is standard this is unlikely to be important. Interestingly the relative inhibition of factors Xa and IIa differs between the available compounds, and those with greater degrees of anti Xa activity appear superior, whilst those with lower Xa/IIa ratios behave in a similar fashion to unfractionated heparin.[15]

Xa:IIa ratios of low molecular weight heparins	
Tinzaparin	1.9
Dalteparin	2.7
Nadroparin	3.6
Enoxaparin	3.8

The attraction of superior efficacy combined with the ease of subcutaneous administration and the lack of requirement for monitoring has resulted in the widespread abandonment of unfractionated heparins. Unfractionated heparins still have a role in the management of patients pre and post PTCA or coronary artery bypass graft (CABG) where their short half life permits rapid discontinuation of anticoagulation. It is important to note that the doses required for unstable angina treatment are higher than those used in deep vein thrombosis (DVT) treatment and that twice daily dosage is required.

Direct antithrombins – hirudin

The potential attraction of compounds which directly inhibit thrombin as opposed to heparin is their ability to inhibit fibrin bound thrombin. However, this has to be set against the fact that although thrombin itself is inhibited, thrombin formation continues (see Figure 4.3). Initial studies of direct antithrombins were associated with unacceptable rates of haemorrhage However, in the recent OASIS-2[16] trial, recombinant hirudin (lepirudin) was superior to unfractionated heparin. The significance of this result is difficult to interpret as a similar improvement could potentially have been obtained by the use of low molecular weight heparins in this trial. In addition, the fact that hirulog infusions lack the convenience of subcutaneous administration has meant that their current role is limited to patients with heparin induced thrombocytopenia.

Load reduction/vasodilatation

This is principally achieved with IV nitrate preparations, which act via multiple mechanisms including a reduction in ventricular preload secondary to venodilatation, some reduction in afterload due to vasodilatation, a reduction of coronary spasm, and potentially an inhibition of platelet aggregation. Given their widespread use there is a surprising paucity of evidence of benefit, however, this primarily reflects a lack of studies as opposed to negative trials. Intravenous GTN (1–10 mg/hour) is particularly useful in the acute control of ischaemic episodes and can be titrated against pain until limited by hypotension (drop in systolic BP of > 30 mmHg, or a 30% fall or 105 mmHg, whichever is the least). There is no justification for using proprietary preparations of longer acting preparations such as isosorbide dinitrate as these offer no benefit when used as an infusion and indeed the prolonged duration of action may prove troublesome if there is a sudden change in the patient's haemodyanmic state. Similarly, patients find buccal preparations difficult to tolerate and these are not recommended. Tolerance rapidly develops after 24 hours due to increased vascular superoxide and endothelin production, and although this process can be attenuated by co-administration of vitamin C, this is rarely required in acute coronary syndromes. Firstly, the GTN dose can easily be increased (tolerance to the hypotensive effects develops simultaneously and it is this that is usually the dose limiting factor) whilst secondly, patients who continue to demonstrate pain and ST shifts after 24–48 hours clearly require urgent revascularisation (see below).

4.3.3 Mechanical revascularisation

There are several issues surrounding the role of mechanical revascularisation (CABG or PTCA) for patients with non-ST elevation acute coronary syndromes and this has been a contentious topic for much of the last decade. Revascularisation can be attempted either early, in patients who have failed to settle with medical management or later in those who have settled but in whom non-invasive testing identifies them to be at high risk of subsequent ischaemic events.

Early revascularisation	Continuing ischaemia
Late revascularisation	Those with positive stress tests Severe pre-existing angina For all patients?

Although the use of revascularisation in patients who fail to settle has never been formally tested in a clinical trial, there is almost universal agreement that it is appropriate. It is vital to appreciate that the entire debate about the appropriateness of revascularisation in non-ST elevation coronary syndrome has specifically *excluded* these patients. However, the undoubted benefits of timely revascularisation in patients with persistent ischaemia has to be set against the fact that the risks of angiography, PTCA and CABG are all substantially higher earlier on in the course of the illness. This is due to magnitude of the thrombus load at the site of the fissured plaque and the intensity of platelet activation at this time. Thus the problem with early revascularisation is in selecting the 20% of patients who are not going to settle without exposing the majority of patients to the risks of unnecessary intervention. These high risk patients can be identified using the same criteria that are applied to the initial risk stratification, although recurrent ischaemia despite prior intensive treatment should also be included[17] (Box 4.2).

Box 4.2 Indications for early angiography

- Recurrent chest pain with dynamic ST segment shifts despite optimal medical management
- Recurrent chest pain when unfractionated heparin is withdrawn at 48 hours
- Ischaemia+haemodynamic instability (either pulmonary oedema or hypotension)

The important point here is that medical therapy should genuinely be optimal before angiography is considered (Figure 4.5); patients are not infrequently referred for angiography after anti-platelet or β-blocker therapy has been withheld due to a minor contraindication. Not only does this potentially expose the patient to the risks of unnecessary revascularisation, but the hazards of angiography itself tend to be higher in inadequately stabilised patients. Angiography is also required in patients who continue to experience pain without dynamic ST segment shift; although these patients have a better overall prognosis than those with ST shifts (many of them in fact have non-cardiac pain), some have circumflex obstruction producing ischaemia in the electrically silent lateral LV wall (Figure 4.1) and these divergent entities can be difficult to differentiate clinically. Lastly, there should be a lower threshold for proceeding to angiography in patients who have experienced an enzyme rise and who continue to experience ongoing ischaemia. These patients usually have critical ischaemia in the context of impaired left ventricular function and have a high risk for subsequent events and the potential to derive significant prognostic benefit from revascularisation.

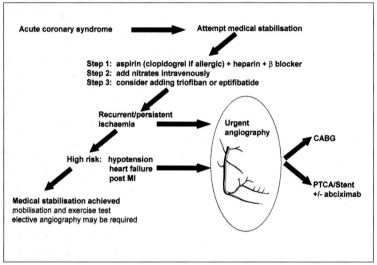

Figure 4.5 Treatment strategies in the initial management of non-ST elevation acute coronary syndromes. In general, the use of heparin and second line antiplatelet agents should be restricted to those with ST segment shift or elevated cardiac enzymes/troponin. It is important to appreciate that optimal medical stabilisation should be attempted in all patients prior to angiography.

A detailed discussion of whether all of the 80% patients who settle with medical management require angiography and subsequent revascularisation prior to hospital discharge is beyond the scope of this book. However, the data from the three trials which have attempted to answer this question is often cited in support of a more general policy of non-invasive management of acute coronary syndromes and the available evidence merits review. Neither the TIMI 3B[18] or VANQWISH[19] trials demonstrated significant benefit from a policy of early revascularisation compared to a policy of revascularisation restricted to patients with evidence of inducible ischaemia at low workload (<6 minutes) during exercise ECG or nuclear perfusion scanning. However both of these trials have significant limitations; in TIMI 3B the number of patients in the *conservative* strategy group undergoing angiography was substantial (63%), whilst in VANQWISH[19] although the differences in the proportions catheterised in each group were slightly more appropriate (44% vs 33%), less than half of those in the invasive group were actually revascularised and any benefit from this was negated by a high CABG mortality (8%). More recently the FRISC II[20] trial achieved an adequate separation between the two strategies (96% vs 10%) and demonstrated a significant benefit from an invasive strategy in terms of a reduced incidence of myocardial infarction[20]. The results of the recent TIMI-18 TACTICS trial also strongly support this policy. On the basis of these latter trials it seems likely that in future a higher proportion of patients will undergo coronary angiography following initial medical stabilisation. It is important to appreciate however that patients in FRISC II underwent a minimum of 48 hours of intensive medical stabilisation prior to angiography (with the exception of those with refractory ischaemia) and that this trial does not produce a mandate for abandoning the established principle of initial medical stabilisation.

The question of how revascularisation should be achieved is largely dependent upon the coronary anatomy. Traditionally, three vessel and left main disease has been treated surgically whilst "non-prognostic" single and double vessel disease has been treated with PTCA The advent of coronary stenting combined with the use of abciximab and concerns about the high CABG mortality in VANQWISH have tended to increase the proportion of patients treated with PTCA/stenting and even left main stem stenosis is no longer an absolute contraindication to PTCA.[21] This policy is particularly attractive in patients with more substantial non-Q wave infarction in whom PTCA to the culprit lesion may permit CABG at a later date remote from the occurrence of infarction.

4.4 Problems in non-ST elevation acute coronary syndromes

4.4.1 Failure to respond to medical management

This group comprises patients who have refractory ischaemia, those who have received suboptimal medical management and those with non-cardiac pain. After first confirming that the history is indeed compatible with myocardial ischaemia, it is worth checking that the medical therapy is optimal. Common problems include a failure to ensure a therapeutic KCCT/APPT when using unfractionated heparin, absent or inadequate β-blockade and occluded drips resulting in subcutaneous nitrate administration. Many patients with minor contraindications to β-blockade such as peripheral vascular disease, conducting system disease or chronic airflow limitation can safely receive metoprolol (25–50 mg tds) during an acute ischaemic episode. As noted above, diltiazem (90 mg MR bd) provides a useful bradycardia in patients with genuine contraindications such as asthma.

If pain persists despite these measures, urgent angiography is indicated. However, in the UK there may be a delay of 7–14 days before this can be performed and the question then arises as to which patients can wait over this period and which patients need angiography within the next 12 hours. As a general rule patients with haemodynamic instability merit urgent attention, followed by those with dynamic ST segment shifts, while those with chest pain and normal ECGs can usually wait without excessive risk.

4.4.2 Use of intra-aortic balloon pumping

The potential use of intra-aortic balloon pumping in the management of patients with refractory ischaemia who are not hypotensive is often neglected. By reducing left ventricular work and potentially increasing coronary perfusion, balloon pumps can stabilise high risk patients during angiography and can be particularly useful while preparations for emergency surgery are undertaken. Coronary surgery is technically demanding and whilst it can be performed in the middle of the night it is often preferable to stabilise the patient with a balloon pump and place the patient first on the morning operating list.

4.4.3 Ensuring adequate antiplatelet therapy

As with the management of ST elevation infarction it is essential that patients receive aspirin and that this is not withheld because of ill defined fears of "allergies" or prior dyspepsia. With respect to "allergy" only a history of urticarial rash should be accepted as a definite contraindication – patients may need some convincing on this point but this is time well spent. As indicated above, clopidogrel is an alternative for those who are genuinely aspirin intolerant. Two further points require clarification, firstly that the prior use of a non-steroidal anti-inflammatory drug does not obviate the need for aspirin (these are all reversible inhibitors whose efficacy as anti-platelet agents in this situation is unknown). Secondly, that in all of the major trials of second line anti-platelet agents, aspirin administration continued in addition to the agent under investigation. This is necessary because aspirin's additional role of reducing vascular reactivity by thromboxane inhibition is not covered by drugs acting on platelet aggregation in isolation. Finally, a cautionary note in patients managed without platelet antagonists comes from the landmark trial of Theroux *et al.* in which patients managed with heparin but without aspirin tended to settle but then demonstrated a dramatic recurrence of ischaemia after heparin was discontinued[22] It would be unusual to encounter a patient managed without platelet antagonists in current practice but, were this to occur, one should be particularly vigilant for this effect following heparin withdrawal.

4.4.4 Use of thrombolysis in the absence of ST elevation/LBBB

Although it at first appears counterintuitive, thrombolysis is of no value in patients without ST elevation (or new left bundle branch block)[23]. The fact that the balance of pathophysiology of non-ST elevation syndromes is platelet- as opposed to thrombus-mediated means that the platelet activating properties of alteplase are not outweighed by its thrombolytic efficacy. The TIMI 3B trial showed clear increases in death, MI, and bleeding in alteplase treated patients with unstable angina or non-Q wave infarction[18] and in the light of this the only indication to administer thrombolysis would be the development of new ST elevation or LBBB.

4.4.5 Unstable angina complicated by haemorrhage

In reality this is much more of a problem than in the thrombolytic treatment of patients with ST elevation who tend to have a single very intense period of haemorrhagic risk early on in the course of their illness. In non-ST elevation syndromes the period of anticoagulation is much more protracted producing an extended opportunity for problems to develop. Minor bleeding occurs in 4% of heparin treated patients and is rarely a problem. By contrast, major haemorrhage which occurs in 1% of patients, usually manifesting as gastrointestinal haemorrhage, is a significant source of morbidity and mortality. The combination of haemorrhage and ischaemia is very difficult to stabilise as both pathologies require opposing management strategies. Based on experience the gastrointestinal haemorrhage is usually the more life-threatening of the two. Anticoagulation should be discontinued and meticulous care should be taken to ensure replacement of circulating volume and red cell mass. Early endoscopy to define the bleeding point and to explore the possibility of local sclerotherapy should be undertaken.

4.4.6 The role of calcium antagonists

The potential for calcium antagonists is much smaller than is commonly imagined. There is clear evidence from both the HINT[24] study and a subsequent meta-analysis that nifedipine in isolation actually *increases both infarction and mortality rates.*[25] This is believed to occur due to a combination of unopposed reflex tachycardia and a significant negative inotropic effect. Given this unfavourable profile, the use of nifedipine is not recommended even in combination with β-blockade and patients admitted on nifedipine should have this discontinued.

The evidence for calcium antagonists that slow the heart rate is more complex and there is evidence of benefit from the use of diltiazem[26] in unstable angina and from verapamil in non-Q wave infarction. However, these benefits are substantially less well established than those of β-blockade and are only indicated in patients with genuine contraindications to the use of β-blockers. They do not have a role as additional therapy in those patients who have not stabilised despite maximal tolerated medical therapy: these patients require angiography. In particular it should be emphasised that calcium antagonists should be avoided in patients with impaired left ventricular function as are all significantly negative inotropes.

4.4.7 Role of potassium channel activators

Although there is some data to support the use of potassium channel activators such as nicorandil, the role of these drugs remains uncertain. In particular, there is no evidence that the addition of nicorandil to patients already receiving maximal medical therapy improves outcome; as discussed above these patients require angiography. Nicorandil contains a nitrate moiety and it is illogical to use it simultaneously with nitrates.

4.4.8 Duration of heparin therapy

We recommend that, once started, heparin should be continued for a minimum of 48 hours as, on a mechanistic basis, it seems improbable that brief pulses of anticoagulation will be beneficial. However, beyond this point use of heparin is associated with adverse outcomes, probably due to delays in performing angiography.[27] In other words, if patients have not settled at this time despite optimal medical therapy then angiography should not be delayed whilst a further period of heparin administration is attempted. Whilst angiography is being arranged heparin therapy should be continued in an attempt to reduce PTCA complications and this is an appropriate point to add a second line anti-platelet agent if this has not already been done. Long term use of low molecular weight heparins (>1 month) in an attempt to produce "plaque passivation" is not currently recommended after the disappointing results of the FRISC II study.[28]

4.4.9 Management of coronary spasm

Spasm is frequently invoked as a cause of unstable symptoms often accompanied by the assumption that this is a benign condition. In reality, the most common cause of spasm is thrombus overlying a fissured coronary plaque (the majority of Prinzmetal's original patients had severe coronary disease). Spasm in normal coronary arteries is recognised angiographically but its relationship to symptoms is unclear. Overall the diagnosis is best avoided in the absence of angiographic proof; it should certainly not be regarded as a mandate for failing to treat an acute coronary syndrome aggressively or for the administration of calcium antagonists (particularly nifedipine in the absence of a β-blocker).

4.4.10 Differences in the management of non-Q wave infarction and unstable angina

It makes little difference to the initial management whether patients have a non-Q wave MI or unstable angina. Although more prolonged pain and intense ECG changes tend to be associated with infarction there is no certainty in the majority of cases until the enzyme results return; patients are therefore managed identically for the first 12–24 hours. Occasionally the enzyme release can be unexpectedly large for the ECG changes, particularly for posterior and lateral infarctions. Under these circumstances the focus of attention needs to shift to the severity of left ventricular damage along the lines previously described in Chapter 3. This point is underscored by the fact that 20% of patients with post MI cardiogenic shock initially presented with a ST depression associated infarction.

Clinical cases

Case 4.1

A 75-year-old retired headmaster presented with episodes of ischaemic sounding chest discomfort and a long history of dyspeptic symptoms. His ECG during pain showed bifasicular block with inferior Q waves. His pain settled with aspirin, heparin, and cautious β-blockade. He developed melena 36 hours later and became hypotensive with a Hb of 7.2 g/dl. Endoscopy demonstrated a large oesophageal ulcer with evidence of recent haemorrhage.

At this point the conflicting requirements of his two life-threatening pathologies provide a major dilemma. Experience suggests that the GI bleeding usually poses the greatest immediate threat. Heparin was discontinued and he underwent coronary angiography 72 hours later. This demonstrated critical three vessel disease. He remained in hospital for a further 4 weeks until endoscopic healing of the oesophageal ulcer had occurred before undergoing CABG. He remains well 5 years later.

Case 4.2

A 56-year-old man presented with recurrent episodes of chest pain. During an episode of pain the ECG was reported as showing no evidence of ischaemia (Figure 4.6). Despite a convincing history, he was felt to have non-cardiac pain. His pain failed to settle and he underwent coronary angiography. This revealed an isolated critical stenosis in the proximal circumflex that was successfully treated with PTCA and a stent.

Despite the absence of ST segment shift, the ECG demonstrates tall, peaked and symmetrical T waves in the anterior chest leads, which may occur in circumflex ischaemia. These are deep posterior T waves seen "upside down" anteriorly (holding the ECG backwards and upside down against a bright light may make it more obvious). The concept of a dominant R wave in V1 representing a posterior Q wave is well recognised but the "tall T wave sign" is less commonly appreciated. It should be noted that tall anterior T waves are occasionally seen in young people as a normal variant due to high vagal tone.

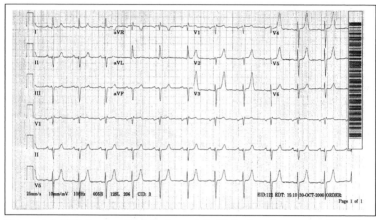

Figure 4.6 ECG from patient in Case 4.2. Note the absence of ST segment changes but the commonly ignored presence of peaked and symmetrical T waves in V2 and V3.

Further reading

Braunwald E, Antman EM, Beasley JW, *et al*. ACC/AHA Guidelines for the management of patients with unstable angina and non-ST segment elevation myocardial infarction. *J Am Coll Cardiol* 2000;**36**:970–1062.

Summary

- Risk stratification can be achieved by a combination of clinical features, ECG, and troponin T levels
- All patients should receive a trial of intensive medical management with aspirin, β-blocker and heparin and 80% will subsequently settle under medical management
- Current evidence favours the use of low molecular weight heparins with high Xa:IIa ratios
- Thrombolysis is harmful in the absence of ST elevation or new LBBB
- The use of second line anti-platelet agents is restricted to patients with dynamic ST shifts or elevated troponins (triofiban and eptifibatide) or during angioplasty/stenting (abciximab)
- Hirudin is only indicated for patients with heparin induced thrombocytopenia
- Patients with recurrent ischaemia or haemodynamic compromise should undergo urgent coronary angiography
- All medically managed patients should undergo non-invasive stress testing prior to hospital discharge

References

1 Yeghiazarians Y, Braunstein JB, Askari, A, Stone PH. Unstable angina pectoris. *N Engl J Med* 2000;**342**:101–14.

2 Fox KAA. Acute aortic syndromes – clinical spectrum and management. *Heart* 2000;**84**:93–100.

3 Schechtman KB, Capone RJ, Kleiger RE, *et al*. Risk stratification of patients with non-Q wave myocardial infarction. The critical role of ST segment depression. The Diltiazem Reinfarction Study Research Group. *Circulation* 1989;**80**:1148–58.

4 Hamm CW, Goldmann BU, Heeschen C, Kreymann G, Berger J, Meinertz T. Emergency room triage of patients with acute chest pain by means of rapid testing for cardiac troponin T or troponin I. *N Engl J Med* 1997;**337**:1648–53.

5 Yusuf S, Wittes J, Friedman L. Overview of results of randomized clinical trials in heart disease. I. Treatments following myocardial infarction. *JAMA* 1988;**260**:2089–93.

6 Theroux P, Ouimet H, McCans J, *et al*. Aspirin, heparin, or both to treat acute unstable angina. *N Engl J Med* 1988;**319**:1105–11.

7 Anonymous. Risk of myocardial infarction and death during treatment with low dose aspirin and intravenous heparin in men with unstable coronary artery disease. The RISC Group. *Lancet* 1990;**336**:827–30.

8 Anonymous. Randomised placebo-controlled trial of abciximab before and during coronary intervention in refractory unstable angina: the CAPTURE Study. *Lancet* 1997;**349**:1429–35.

9 Anonymous. A comparison of aspirin plus tirofiban with aspirin plus heparin for unstable angina. Platelet Receptor Inhibition in Ischemic Syndrome Management (PRISM) Study Investigators. *N Engl J Med* 1998;**338**:1498–505.

10 Inhibition of the platelet glycoprotein IIb/IIIa receptor with tirofiban in unstable angina and non-Q-wave myocardial infarction. Platelet Receptor Inhibition in Ischemic Syndrome Management in Patients Limited by Unstable Signs and Symptoms (PRISM-PLUS) Study Investigators. [Published erratum appears in *N Engl J Med* 1998;**339**(6):415]. *N Engl J Med* 1998;**338**:1488–97.

11 Inhibition of platelet glycoprotein IIb/IIIa with eptifibatide in patients with acute coronary syndromes. The PURSUIT Trial Investigators. Platelet Glycoprotein IIb/IIIa in Unstable Angina: Receptor Suppression Using Integrilin Therapy. *N Engl J Med* 1998;**339**:436–43.

12 Hamm CW, Heeschen C, Goldmann B, *et al*. Benefit of abciximab in patients with refractory unstable angina in relation to serum troponin T levels. c7E3 Fab Antiplatelet Therapy in Unstable Refractory Angina (CAPTURE) Study Investigators [published erratum appears in *N Engl J Med* 1999;**341**(7):548]. *N Engl J Med* 1999;**340**:1623–9.

13 Ryan TJ, Antman EM, Brooks NH, *et al*. 1999 update: ACCIAHA Guidelines for the Management of Patients With Acute Myocardial Infarction: Executive Summary and Recommendations: a report of the American College of Cardiology/American Heart Association Task Force on Practice Guidelines (Committee on Management of Acute Myocardial Infarction). *Circulation* 1999;**100**:1016–30.

14 Oler A, Whooley MA, Oler J, Grady D. Adding heparin to aspirin reduces the incidence of myocardial infarction and death in patients with unstable angina. A meta-analysis. *JAMA* 1996;**276**:811–15.

15 Antman EM, Cohen M, Radley D, *et al*. Assessment of the treatment effect of enoxaparin for unstable angina/non-Q-wave myocardial infarction. TIMI IIB-ESSENCE meta-analysis. *Circulation* 1999;**100**:1602–8.

16 Effects of recombinant hirudin (lepirudin) compared with heparin on death, myocardial infarction, refractory angina, and revascularisation procedures in patients with acute myocardial ischaemia without ST elevation: a randomised trial. Organisation to Assess Strategies for Ischemic Syndromes (OASIS-2) Investigators. *Lancet* 1999;**353**:429–38.

17 Stone PH, Thompson B, Zaret BL, *et al.* Factors associated with failure of medical therapy in patients with unstable angina and non-Q wave myocardial infarction. A TIMI-IIIB database study. *Eur Heart J* 1999;**20**:1084–93.

18 Anonymous. Effects of tissue plasminogen activator and a comparison of early invasive and conservative strategies in unstable angina and non-Q wave myocardial infarction. Results of the TIMI IIIB Trial. Thrombolysis in Myocardial Ischemia. *Circulation* 1994;**89**:1545–56.

19 Boden WE, O'Rourke RA, Dai H, Crawford MH, Blaustein AS, Deedwania PC. Outcomes in patients with acute non-Q wave myocardial infarction randomily assigned to an invasive as compared with a conservative management strategy. *N Engl J Med* 1998;**388**:1785–92 (Abstract).

20 Invasive compared with non-invasive treatment in unstable coronary artery disease: FRISC ll prospective randomised multicentre study. FRagmin and Fast Revascularisation during InStability in Coronary artery disease Investigators. *Lancet* 1999;**354**:708–15.

21 Davies CH, Banning AP, Channon KM, Ormerod OJM. Coronary stenting of unprotected left main stem stenoses in elderly; patients unsuitable for coronary surgery. *Int J Cardiol* 1997;**62**:13–18.

22 Theroux P, Waters D, Lam J, Juneau M, McCans J. Reactivation of unstable angina after the discontinuation of heparin. *N Engl J Med* 1992;**327**:141–45.

23 FTT Collaborative Group. Indications for fibrinolytic therapy in suspected acute myocardial infarction: collaborative overview of early mortality and major morbidity results from all randomised trials of more than 1000 patients Fibrinolytic Therapy Trialists' (FTT) Collaborative Group. *Lancet* 1994;**343**:311–22

24 Early treatment of unstable angina in the coronary care unit: a randomised, double blind, placebo controlled comparison of recurrent ischaemia in patients treated with nifedipine or metoprolol or both. Report of The Holland Interuniversity Nifedipine/Metoprolol Trial (HINT) Research Group. *Br Heart J* 1986;**56**:400–13.

25 Yusuf S, Wittes J, Friedman L. Overview of results of randomized clinical trials in heart disease. II. Unstable angina, heart failure, primary prevention with aspirin and risk factor modification. *JAMA* 1988;**260**:2259–63.

26 Gobel EJ, Hautvast RW, van Gilst WH, *et al.* Randomised, double-blind trial of intravenous diltiazem versus glyceryl trinitrate for unstable angina pectoris. *Am J Cardiol* 1995;**346**:1653–7.

27 Klein LW, Wahid F, VandenBerg BJ, Parrillo JE, Calvin JE. Comparison of heparin therapy for < or = 48 hours to > 48 hours in unstable angina pectoris. *Am J Cardiol* 1997;**79**:259–63.

28 Long-term low-molecular-mass heparin in unstable coronary-artery disease: FRISC II prospective randomised multicentre study. FRagmin and Fast Revascularisation during InStability in Coronary artery disease. Investigators [published erratum appears in *Lancet* 1999;**354**(9188):1478]. *Lancet* 1999;**354**:701–9.

29 Madan M, Berkowitz SD, Tcheng JE. Glycoprotein IIb/IIIa integrin blockade. *Circulation* 1998;**98**:2629–35.

30 Lindahl B, Venge P, Wallentin L. Relation between troponin T and the risk of subsequent cardiac events in unstable coronary artery disease. The FRISC study group. *Circulation* 1996;**93**:1651–7.

5: Acute pulmonary oedema

CH DAVIES

5.1 Introduction

Pulmonary oedema is so commonly encountered that it rarely merits much thought. Breathless patients with basal crackles swiftly receive furosemide (frusemide) (often combined with amoxicillin, just in case); most seem to improve and the matter receives little further thought. This intellectually lax strategy is, by now, too ingrained to eradicate from the clinical repertoire. However in a proportion of patients this approach leads to serious problems of both inadequate and inappropriate treatment. If these errors are to be avoided, a more systematic approach to the acutely breathless patient with interstitial shadowing on their chest x ray is required.

5.2 Clinical presentation

The distribution of lung water is maintained by an equilibrium between osmotic and hydrostatic forces across the endothelial and alveolar membranes[1] (Figure 5.1). Accumulation of excess lung water may occur due to increases in the resistance to lymphatic or venous drainage, damage to the endothelium (originating either systemically or from the alveolus), or rarely, due to negative pressure applied to the alveolus. Due to excess capacity within the lymph drainage system, lung water initially rises only slowly with increasing pulmonary venous pressure. At first, water accumulates in the peribronchial tissues, followed by progressive accumulation around the margins of the alveolus, producing alveolar thickening. When this alveolar thickening reaches a critical threshold there is an abrupt change in endothelial-alveolar permeability and the alveolus floods. The approximate correlations between these events, the chest x ray appearances and, in the case of a haemodynamic mechanism, the left atrial pressure[1,2] are listed in Table 5.1.

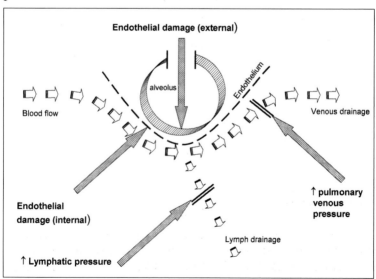

Figure 5.1 Potential processes in the development of pulmonary oedema.

Table 5.1 Chest *x* ray appearances and left atrial pressures in pulmonary oedema

Stage	Chest *x* ray	Approximate left atrial pressure
Pre oedema		
↑ flow in vessels	Upper lobe diversion	12–15
Distended lymphatics	Kerley lines	
Interstitial oedema		
Fluid in	Fluid in fissures	
peri-alveolar spaces	Peribronchial cuffing	15–20
	Micronoduli	
	Hilar blurring	19–24
Alveolar oedema		
Alveolar flooding	Fluffy hilar shadowing	
	"Bat's wing"/"Butterfly" shadowing	>25
	Pleural effusions	
	Loss of lung volume	

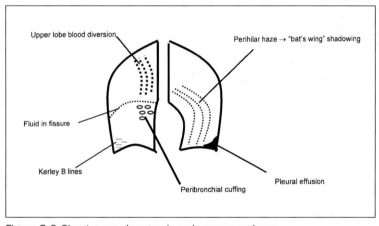

Figure 5.2 Chest *x* ray changes in pulmonary oedema.

5.3 Diagnosis

During the pre-oedema phase, the most noticeable signs are those of sympathetic activation. Most prominent is a persistent sinus tachycardia and, in the context of impaired left ventricular function, this should always arouse suspicion of impending pulmonary oedema. Interstitial oedema results in breathlessness, wheezing, and cough. The association between pulmonary oedema and an unproductive cough is insufficiently appreciated – ACE inhibitors are often mistakenly discontinued when what is actually required is an intensification of treatment. With the onset of alveolar oedema the fine pulmonary crackles caused by the abrupt opening of small airways is replaced by the coarse bubbling of free fluid, whilst the dry cough gives way to frothy and then blood stained sputum. If untreated, cardiogenic shock and death follow. The diagnostic process can be approached in five stages (Figure 5.3)

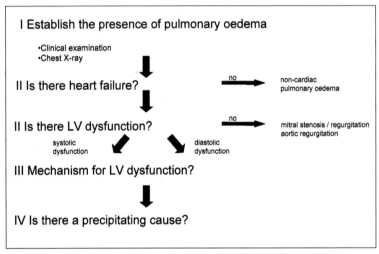

Figure 5.3 Diagnostic strategy in acute pulmonary oedema.

5.3.1 Establishing the presence of pulmonary oedema

Problems arise due to the poor correlation between the existence of lung crackles and the presence of pulmonary oedema combined with the difficulty in assessing the presence of added heart sounds and the level of the jugular venous pressure (JVP) in many acutely ill patients. In the face of these obstacles, the chest x ray assumes a central role in diagnosis

(Figure 5.2) although, on occasion, this too may be misleading. Problems arise due to an occasional lead phase (<12 hours) that occurs before an elevated left atrial pressure is translated into oedema accumulation and conversely, and a more prominent lag phase (hours to days) during resolution during which fluid is resorbed. Both cardiomegaly and upper lobe blood diversion are less prominent with the more acute onset of pulmonary oedema. The presence of chronic obstructive airways disease may result in patchy changes as fluid accumulates only in the residual islands of lung parenchyma. Similarly, positive pressure ventilation may attenuate the appearance of oedema, followed by rebound accumulation on extubation. Unilateral pulmonary oedema may result from prolonged lateral decubitus positioning, or from unilateral thromboembolism.

5.3.2 Is there heart failure?

Having established the presence of pulmonary oedema, the next step is to establish whether there is heart failure. The fact that pulmonary oedema is so commonly due to heart failure leads to the tacit assumption that this is a universal causation. It is important to briefly consider the possibility of non-cardiogenic pulmonary oedema[3] (NCPO, effectively the adult respiratory distress syndromes) as failure to do so is potentially disastrous. Unfortunately the causes are legion and most are exceedingly rare (see Box 5.1).

As a differential diagnosis, this list appears overwhelming (and it is far from complete). However, in practice these diagnoses do not present as "pulmonary oedema of unknown origin" requiring a diagnosis to be made from this list, they present as a complication of a pre-existing fulminant illness. All that is required is an appreciation that NCPO can complicate almost any fulminant illness.

Box 5.1 Causes of non-cardiogenic pulmonary oedema

Endothelial damage (external)
Smoke inhalation
Aspiration – gastric contents, fresh or salt water

Endothelial damage (internal)
Septicaemia (especially gram negative)
Malaria
Pancreatitis
Burns
Post transfusion
Head injury
Hepatic/renal failure
Pulmonary embolus: thrombus, fat, amniotic fluid
Drugs: opioids, paraquat, bleomycin, ritodrine, cocaine
Post bypass, post cardioversion
High altitude

Obstructed lymphatic drainage
Lymphangitis carcinomatosa
Post lung transplantation (reimplantation response)

Reduced airways pressure
Obstructive sleep apnoea
Acute airways obstruction
Rapid relief of pneumothorax/pleural effusion

Table 5.2 Clinical clues to the presence of non-cardiogenic pulmonary oedema

	Cardiogenic	Non-cardiogenic
History	Cardiac event Orthopnoea	Severe non-cardiac illness
Examination	Cool peripheries S_3, JVP ↑ "Moist" crackles	Usually warm peripheries JVP ↓, no S_3 "Dry" and more extensive crackles
ECG	Usually abnormal	Usually normal
CXR	Perihilar distribution	Peripheral distribution
PCWP	> 20 mmHg	< 20 mmHg
Echo	Almost always abnormal	Usually normal

There are some clinical clues that may alert one to the presence of NCPO[3] (Table 5.2). In NCPO there is no upper lobe blood diversion or peribronchial cuffing, alveolar shadowing tends to be more peripheral (often with basal sparing), septal lines absent, and heart size normal. Unfortunately, these changes are rarely distinctive enough to be of genuine diagnostic value. Lastly, the absence of a third heart sound in NCPO, although useful in theory, is very difficult to judge in an acutely distressed patient.

5.3.3 Is there evidence of left ventricular dysfunction?

The causes of cardiogenic pulmonary oedema not associated with left ventricular dysfunction are also rare. However, as with NCPO, their importance lies in the requirement for radically different medium and long term management (Box 5.2). They emphasise the need to make a specific diagnosis of the mechanism of heart failure in all patients in the convalescent phase.

> **Box 5.2 Cardiogenic pulmonary oedema not associated with left ventricular dysfunction**
>
> - Mitral regurgitation
> - Mitral stenosis:
>   rheumatic/congenital
>   thrombosed prosthetic valve
> - Left atrial myxoma (rare)
> - Pulmonary venous obstruction (very rare)

As a rule aortic valve disease only presents with pulmonary oedema once left ventricular failure has supervened. Acute valve failure should always raise the possibility of infective endocarditis, whilst in patients with a prosthetic mechanical valve, valve thrombosis should be considered.

5.3.4 Defining a mechanism for left ventricular dysfunction

Although an exhaustive list of potential causes of left ventricular dysfunction appears overwhelming, the acute choice lies between systolic dysfunction due to coronary disease (accounting for > 50%), isolated diastolic dysfunction (accounting for up to 30%) and valvular disease (Figure 5.4). These categories are not mutually exclusive (systolic dysfunction frequently co-exists with diastolic dysfunction).

Differentiating coronary from myopathic disease

In the acute situation, this differentiation matters little: acute revascularisation is never required for acute left ventrlcular dysfunction in the absence of shock or continuing chest pain. It is important to remember that the combination of unstable angina and heart failure carries a poor prognosis and is an indication for urgent angiography as discussed in Chapter 4. A dramatic example of this is ischaemic mitral regurgitation where transient circumflex ischaemia produces intermittent torrential mitral regurgitation. The clue is the association of ischaemia and severe heart failure in the presence of well preserved left ventricular function between acute episodes.

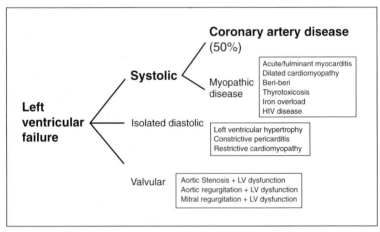

Figure 5.4 Mechanisms of left ventricular dysfunction.

The ECG may offer useful clues: ischaemic left ventricular dysfunction severe enough to produce pulmonary oedema will almost invariably be associated with either ST segment shifts or extensive Q waves. Unlike troponins, minor (<2×upper limit) elevations of cardiac enzymes are frequent and do not indicate an ischaemic aetiology.

Unfortunately, almost none of the myriad causes of dilated cardiomyopathy and acute myocarditis have specific treatments. There is currently no evidence to support the use of immunosuppression in the management of acute myocarditis.[4,5] Biopsy only makes a specific diagnosis in 15% of patients,[6] rarely alters management, and it is not recommended. The only exceptions to this are beri-beri which requires iv thiamine and the prompt initiation of treatment in thyroid heart disease.

Differentiating systolic from isolated diastolic failure

In contrast to systolic heart failure where there is a failure of adequate contraction, in diastolic heart failure the primary problem is a failure of adequate relaxation: effective pumping requires both processes. Impaired diastolic function frequently accompanies systolic failure but there remains uncertainty as to how commonly it occurs in isolation. The most common aetiology is hypertensive left ventricular hypertrophy, however it also occurs in restrictive cardiomyopathy (such as amyloid) and in constrictive pericarditis. The distinction is diagnostically important as measures of systolic function (basically how well the ventricle squeezes) form the basis of standard echocardiographic assessment of ventricular function. The combination of heart failure with a normal ejection fraction on echo provokes considerable confusion. Estimates of the proportion of patients in this category approach one-third.[7]

Although the differentiation can only be made with specialised echo techniques,[8] certain clinical clues may help (Table 5.3) and in particular, the presence of left ventricular hypertrophy on echo should raise suspicion.

The systolic/diastolic differentiation carries surprisingly few implications for acute management. Patients with diastolic heart failure require high filling pressures to maintain cardiac output and as such are particularly sensitive to the effects of excess diuresis. In addition, they are also sensitive to inappropriate tachycardia (poorly controlled atrial fibrillation in particular), although digoxin is not the first choice in this situation as it worsens diastolic function.

109

Table 5.3 Clinical clues to help in differentiating systolic from isolated diastolic failure

	Systolic failure	Diastolic failure
History	Coronary disease	Hypertension
Examination	S_3	S_4 ↑ ↑ BP
CXR	Cardiomegaly	
ECG	Q waves Low R wave voltages ST elevation	Electrical LVH

Differentiating valvular from non-valvular disease

Patients with mitral valve disease and aortic regurgitation in combination with left ventricular dysfunction usually respond to initial medical management at which point the physical signs become manifest. In patients with mitral stenosis, control of heart rate and avoidance of vasodilators is important, whilst intra-aortic balloon pumping is contraindicated in patients with significant aortic regurgitation. The most feared valvular lesion in heart failure is aortic stenosis; a very narrow valve orifice combined with left ventricular failure produces an inaudible murmur and an inappropriately low Doppler gradient. The circulation is critically balanced and initiating diuretics tend to produce hypotension and renal failure: the only way out of this vicious spiral is aortic valve surgery (confirmation of the adage that "mechanical problems need mechanical solutions"). This reinforces the importance of performing echocardiography as soon as possible after admission in all patients with unexplained heart failure and immediately in those who deteriorate despite medical management.

5.3.5 Identifying a predisposing cause

The majority of patients admitted with pulmonary oedema will already have been documented to have impaired left ventricular function and, in these, it is important to identify the factors which precipitated admission[9] (Figure 5.5).

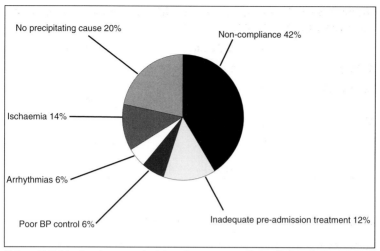

No precipitating cause 20%

Non-compliance 42%

Ischaemia 14%

Arrhythmias 6%

Poor BP control 6%

Inadequate pre-admission treatment 12%

Figure 5.5 Mechanisms underlying decompensation of chronic heart failure.

5.4 Management

Cardiac output is determined by the relationship between preload, afterload and contractility. The normal heart is essentially preload dependent (Starling relationship – Figure 5.6) and afterload independent (Figure 5.7). Raising the venous pressure increases the cardiac output, altering blood pressure has little effect. Heart failure produces pulmonary oedema secondary to an elevated LV filling pressure and/or impaired perfusion secondary to reduced cardiac output (Figure 5.6). In heart failure the ventricle becomes less preload dependent (it is no longer able to respond to increased venous pressure by elevating output – Figure 5.6) but more afterload sensitive (increases in blood pressure depress cardiac output – Figure 5.7). Manipulation of the pre- and afterloads can be achieved either by reducing the total circulating volume (diuresis, venesection) or by increasing the system's capacity (veno- and vasodilators) whilst contractility may be augmented by vasodilators. In practice, management can be considered in three steps ("hopeful", "struggling", and "desperate").

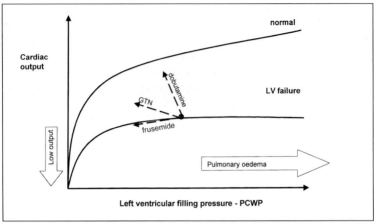

Figure 5.6 Relationship between preload and cardiac output in normal and failing hearts.

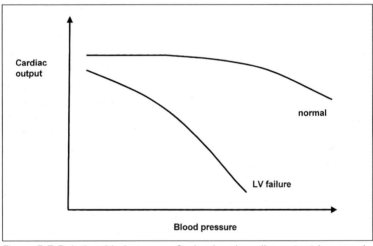

Figure 5.7 Relationship between afterload and cardiac output in normal and failing hearts.

5.4.1 Step 1

Posture and oxygen

The need for patients with acute pulmonary oedema to sit upright should not need re-iterating. In reality unless they are so severely unwell as to be neurologically obtunded, they will not adopt any other posture. Similarly the administration of a high percentage of inspired oxygen as the next step is commonsense. An excessive fear of co-existing CO_2 retention is still pervasive resulting in administration of low dose oxygen to patients with little chance of CO_2 retention and in whom this fear would rapidly be resolved by blood gas analysis (repeated if necessary 30–45 minutes later).

Loop diuretics

Intravenous administration of a loop diuretic will be required for all patients with acute pulmonary oedema. There is no compelling reason to use any other agent than furosemide (frusemide). The initial dose should be determined on the basis of whether the patient is currently receiving furosemide (generally the initial iv dose should be double the usual daily oral dose) and the level of renal dysfunction. If the patient normally takes bumetanide then the ratio of oral furosemide is 1 mg bumetanide to 40 mg furosemide. Furosemide should be administered at a rate of less than 4 mg/min and the use of an infusion pump is needed for any dose >50 mg. There are many reports of the adverse effects of diuretics emphasising the risk of excessive diuresis and hypovolaemia. However, in general it is more common to see patients under diuresed with inadequately treated pulmonary oedema. Problems with over diuresis are more likely in patients with acute heart failure who will not have received furosemide previously and who have little genuine expansion of their plasma volume; in these caution against overdiuresis is warranted. By contrast, patients with an acute decompensation of chronic heart failure will have significant fluid overload, will already be receiving diuretics, and in these diuretic dose is frequently inadequate.

Nitrates

In anything other than mild heart failure, venodilatation and vasodilatation should be initiated with intravenous nitrates. This is most conveniently achieved with IV GTN 1–10 mg/hr titrated to achieve a drop in systolic BP of >30 mmHg, or a 30% fall or 105 mmHg whichever is the least. Nitrates are particularly useful in patients with acute (as opposed to decompensated chronic) heart failure as in these patients there is no generalised fluid overload. In general, acute nitrate administration is underutilised in acute heart failure and it may have advantages over the use of furosemide in isolation, with preservation or even increases in cardiac output.[10] In particular, the vasodilatory actions of furosemide have probably been overstated. Acute use of sublingual GTN may be worthwhile whilst the infusion in prepared, but buccal nitrates are uncomfortable and should be avoided. For this relatively acute situation, nitrate tolerance is not a problem as the infusion will be discontinued within 12–18 hours of initiation. Rebound haemodynamic deterioration following discontinuation, however, does occur and it is important to ensure that patients are adequately observed whilst the dose is weaned at a rate of 1–2 mg/hr. Nitroprusside is now rarely needed in this situation.

Opioids

By contrast, there is significant overuse of opioids. The traditional rationale for opioid use is as an anxiolytic and venodilator combined with a blunting of medullary CO_2 sensitivity that reduces the sensation of breathlessness. Although a small dose of diamorphine 2.5 mg or morphine 5 mg (in combination with metoclopramide 10 mg) is helpful in distressed patients, opioids should be seen only as an adjunct and not as a primary treatment of acute pulmonary oedema. If acute venodilatation is required, then this should be achieved with intravenous nitrates.

5.4.2 Step 2

The beneficial effects of the first line measures start to appear after 30 minutes and the diuresis should be maximal after 60–90 minutes. The patient should be reassessed at this point and the majority of patients will have undergone a gratifyingly dramatic improvement in their condition. The tachycardia will be subsiding and peripheral perfusion will have improved. One of the benefits of not having used excessive opioids is that the patient will not be excessively obtunded at this point and a clearer history of the events precipitating admission will emerge. However, a proportion of patients will not have improved and this is an ominous prognostic sign.

Escalating diuretic dosage

If no diuresis has occurred then a urinary catheter should be inserted to exclude mechanical obstruction and provide accurate information about subsequent urine output. The initial diuretic dose should be doubled, by now the electrolytes will have returned and it may become clear that there is significant renal impairment. The dose escalation required to overcome the substantial diuretic resistance of renal impairment is frequently underestimated: doses of 250 and 500 mg are not uncommon. It should be noted that the bumetanide:frusemide dose ratio of 1:40 does not hold in renal failure and that furosemide (frusemide) is the clear drug of choice under these circumstances.

Low dose dopamine

Despite a lack of trial data, clinical experience strongly favours the use of low dose (< 2.5 micrograms/kg/min) dopamine in patients refractory to diuretics. At this dose the mechanism of action is via renal artery vasodilatation with antagonism of the Na^+ symporter in the proximal tubule and problems associated with subsequent weaning are unusual. The major disadvantage is the need to obtain central venous access, although this is probably not an unreasonable step at this point in the management of such a critically ill patient and will allow confirmation of the raised central venous pressure.

Dobutamine

Increasing myocardial contractility will reduce pulmonary oedema even in the absence of hypotension but entails all the disadvantages of inotopes discussed in Chapter 6. A dose of 5–10 micrograms/kg/min is usually required. Paradoxical hypotension due to β_2-mediated vasodilation can occur, whilst sinus tachycardia and atrial fibrillation are both common. One advantage of dobutamine is that, as it lacks α-adrenergic activity it can be administered peripherally; as such it can provide useful palliation in patients in whom obtaining central access is not appropriate.

Continuous positive airway pressure (CPAP)

CPAP is significantly underused, probably because it is cumbersome, noisy, difficult to organise, and poorly tolerated by patients. However, the addition of CPAP (5–10 cm of water) may produce dramatic improvements and reduce the need for full mechanical ventilation by one-third.[11] Alternatively, full face mask biphasic intermittent positive airway pressure ventilation (BiPAP) may be better tolerated, although there is less experience with this.

Sequential nephron blockade

With furosemide (frusemide) doses >80 mg, there is a compensatory increase in ion transport by the remaining tubular symporters (Figure 5.8) and, as a result, the response to furosemide tends to decline with subsequent doses. To minimise this effect, bendroflumethiazide (bendrofluazide) 2.5 mg should be added orally, cautiously followed by amiloride 10 mg or spironolactone 25 mg in patients who remain refractory. It should be emphasised that these measures are aimed at maintaining as opposed to initiating a diuresis.

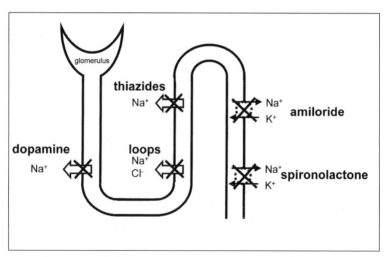

Figure 5.8 Sequential nephron blockade.

5.4.3 Step 3

Patients who continue to deteriorate despite the above, require reassessment before proceeding further as the measures outlined below will be appropriate in only a minority of cases. The crucial issues are whether a reversible or mechanical cause for pulmonary oedema is likely to exist and an assessment of the patient's preceding quality of life. It is in those patients in whom aggressive intervention is felt to be *inappropriate* that the use of larger doses of opioids, traditionally administered in Step 1, should now be considered in order to palliate distress.

Venesection

Although frequently dismissed as outmoded, venesection still has a place. Removal of 200–300 ml may produce a dramatic improvement. This is particularly worth considering in situations where absolute (as opposed to relative) volume overloading has occurred, such as following overtransfusion. As this occurs at lower degrees of venous tone, the amount of fluid removal required to produce resolution of pulmonary oedema is significantly larger than in acute pulmonary oedema due to left ventricular dysfunction. It follows that nitrates will not be particularly helpful under these circumstances and that removal of sufficient fluid with diuretics may be difficult. Venesection should also be considered in patients who develop pulmonary oedema due to the contrast load associated with coronary angiography; the arterial sheath provides ready access to the circulation.

Intra-aortic balloon pumping (IABP)

The use of an IABP tends to be neglected in patients who are not hypotensive, but may produce dramatic improvements in patients with acute left ventricular failure. The use of IABP needs careful consideration, as unless a clearly reversible mechanism for heart failure can be identified, patients will inevitably deteriorate once support is removed. An IABP can be particularly useful to stabilise patients during coronary angiography or angioplasty. Further use of IABPs is discussed in Chapter 6.

Mechanical ventilation (IPPV)

Although mechanical ventilation may dramatically improve a patient's condition by improving oxygenation and reducing the work of breathing, it is only usually appropriate as part of a co-ordinated management plan when a reversible cause for heart failure has been identified or whilst investigation is undertaken. Similarly, ultrafiltration, though undeniably effective, is rarely appropriate or tolerated.

5.5 Specific problems

5.5.1 Pulmonary oedema presenting as bronchospasm

Airway narrowing in pulmonary oedema occurs due to a combination of increased reactivity of bronchial smooth muscle with a late contribution from physical narrowing of airways by fluid accumulation. On examination, pulmonary crackles are masked by wheeze and the intense sympathetic activation is equally compatible with either severe asthma or heart failure. A chest x ray will resolve the issue, even if eosinophilic shadowing is present in asthma it is rarely as prominent as the alveolar oedema required to produce bronchospasm. The bronchospasm will resolve with standard heart failure management, if there is genuine doubt then nebulised salbultamol will treat both pathologies. Although effective, the high risk of arrhythmias precludes the use of aminophylline.

5.5.2 Heart failure, atrial fibrillation and digoxin

In patients with atrial fibrillation, any tachycardia will be disproportionately fast. Elevated ventricular rates over many months may produce heart failure in the absence of structural heart disease, but this is unusual. Far more common is a situation of progressive structural heart disease (ischaemic or valvular) associated with insidious atrial dilatation in which the development of atrial fibrillation is simply the last straw. This is a particular problem in patients in whom diastolic dysfunction is present as, during tachycardia, the proportion of the cardiac cycle devoted to cardiac filling is disproportionately shortened relative to systole, mitral stenosis is the classic example of this. Acute cardioversion in these patients is not an option: quite apart from the thromboembolic risks, the heart will never hold sinus rhythm until the left atrial pressure is reduced. Digoxin is the ideal drug under these circumstances combining atrioventricular blocking activity with a mild positive inotropic effect. As discussed in Chapter 9 the problem is the slow onset of action, which is why it is important to consider it during step 1 if atrial fibrillation is present. Although the protracted onset of action makes digoxin of little use in the immediate management of heart failure, one of the few clear answers to emerge from the trials of digoxin in sinus rhythm is that discontinuation is associated with clinical deterioration.

5.5.3 Administering diuretics to patients with hypotension/renal impairment

There is occasional reluctance to administer diuretics to patients with even mild hypotension for fear that furosemide's (frusemide's) vasodilatory properties will exacerbate this. There are two reasons to discard these worries. The steep first portion of the Starling relationship (Figure 5.6) ensures that cardiac output will not fall dramatically whilst filling pressures remain > 10 mmHg. Secondly it is unclear where this strategy leads to: without a diuresis the patient will only deteriorate and thus withholding diuretics is not a realistic option. For patients with significant hypotension (systolic < 100 mmHg), additional measures will be required as discussed in Chapter 6,[9] but diuretics will still be required in the presence of pulmonary oedema.

Similarly, the presence of mild to moderate renal failure should not prevent diuretic administration because of a fear of precipitating a further decline in renal function. Short of dialysis the only method to improve the patient's symptoms is by achieving a diuresis, even if this is at the expense of deterioration in renal function. Interestingly, the assumption that a reduction in circulating fluid volume inevitably equates to a decline in renal function is incorrect; more commonly renal dysfunction transiently regresses after starting treatment due to improvements in intrarenal haemodynamics

5.5.4 Management of patients on β-blockers

An increasing proportion of patients admitted with pulmonary oedema due to decompensation of chronic left ventricular dysfunction will be receiving β-blockers. Although these clearly reduce both mortality and the likelihood of hospital admission significantly,[12] if an acute deterioration does occur it can be difficult to manage. The problem centres on whether to attempt to continue the β-blocker whilst treating the acute decompensation. The advantage of doing this is that the effort undertaken during the many weeks of careful dose titration will not be lost; the obvious disadvantage being the possibility that re-establishing haemodynamic control will be more difficult or even impossible. For minor episodes of decompensation, β-blockers can generally be continued, although the dose should be reduced by one titration increment. If there is any doubt or the patient fails to respond rapidly to iv diuretics then they should be discontinued and, if appropriate, recommenced as an outpatient.

This is distinct from the approach to patients receiving Ca^{2+} antagonists. These are significantly more negatively inotropic than commonly perceived, devoid of any mortality benefits in heart failure and should be discontinued.

5.5.5 Initiation of ACE inhibitors

The traditional approach to heart failure management is to stabilise patients with diuretics and then to initiate ACE inhibitors in the convalescent phase. The disadvantage of doing this is that the circulating plasma volume will by then be depleted and the risks of hypotension and renal dysfunction accentuated. For this reason, as long as hypotension is not a problem, the first dose of ACE inhibitor should be administered 8–12 hours following admission. A useful additional effect is that these will also help to stem the potassium losses associated with intensive diuresis. Similar comments apply to the use of the newer angiotensin II receptor antagonists. The benefits of renin-angiotensin inhibition in this group of patients are such that every possible effort should be made to initiate treatment. If borderline hypotension is a problem then the unlicensed paediatric formulation of captopril (2 mg tds) provides an ultra low starting dose from which up titration can be achieved over the following weeks. In particularly difficult cases the addition of oral digoxin as a positive inotrope can occasionally be a useful adjunct to starting ACE inhibitor treatment.

5.5.6 Managing potassium and magnesium losses

A similar rationale applies to the management of potassium and magnesium levels. There is a tendency to worry about potassium depletion 24–36 hours after the onset of diuresis when the plasma K^+ falls when unpalatable and inefficient potassium supplements are administered. An alternative strategy is to attempt to minimise urinary K^+ losses during the initial diuresis by co-administering amiloride 10 mg od or spironolactone 25 mg simultaneously with the iv loop diuretic. The use of spironolactone is particularly attractive as there is now convincing evidence that patients will require this following discharge. Careful monitoring of plasma K^+ is essential whichever strategy is adopted.

5.5.7 Pulmonary oedema and a "normal" echocardiogram

The first possibility is that the patient has non-cardiogenic pulmonary oedema and under these circumstances measurement of the pulmonary capillary filling pressure is appropriate. Although pulmonary oedema in the context of a normal echo should raise the suspicion of non-cardiogenic pulmonary oedema, the converse that systolic dysfunction equals the presence of cardiogenic pulmonary oedema does not invariably hold true (see below). The next most likely possibility is that although left ventricular function is normal, there is a mechanical problem that has been missed such as mitral regurgitation: if the echo doesn't seem to fit the rest of the clinical picture it is always worth repeating or re-reporting it. Lastly there is the possibility that although systolic function is normal, there is abnormal diastolic function – as indicated above, standard echocardiography does not assess diastolic function.

5.5.8 Indications for Swan-Ganz catheterisation

Swan-Ganz insertion is only rarely required in patients with a combination of radiographic pulmonary oedema and an appropriate mechanism for heart failure identified by echocardiography. Although frequently recommended[13] in patients who are deteriorating despite maximal medical treatment they rarely alter management under these circumstances and there are continuing concerns about the potential for harm.[14] However, measurement of pulmonary capillary wedge pressure (PCWP) has a pivotal role in identifying patients with non-cardiogenic pulmonary oedema in whom a low PCWP ($< 0.57 \times$ plasma albumin) in the presence of widespread pulmonary shadowing is virtually diagnostic. There are several caveats here, firstly that the results of PCWP interpretation are likely to be conclusive prior to the use of diuretics as these can lower PCWP values below this critical threshold. Secondly, since venous pressure is a product of volume $\times$ vascular tone it is important to investigate the effect of volume loading on borderline values; in an underfilled system PCWP or central venous pressure (CVP) will remain static or even fall following 250 ml 0.9% saline infused over 15 minutes. Lastly, although the normal PCWP is < 8 mmHg, the optimal level in left ventricular MI is 17 mmHg and only in excess of 25 mmHg is pulmonary oedema considered inevitable; in patients with pre-existing left ventricular impairment this latter threshold may rise as high as 30 mmHg due to endothelial thickening and improved lymphatic drainage.

5.5.9 Deciding on the appropriateness of treatment

Despite a relatively good acute prognosis (5–10% mortality), the poor medium and long term prognosis of heart failure is now well recognised. The quality of life for patients between acute episodes is very variable, with some achieving excellent palliation whilst others experience substantial suffering. During an episode of acute decompensation, it may be difficult to decide on the appropriateness of intensive management in those who do not respond to the Step 1 measures outlined above. Discussions with relatives and, if possible, the patient may help to clarify the appropriate level of intervention. Recent research highlights the problems associated with these discussions: almost a quarter of patients changed their minds about whether they wished to undergo resuscitation during a subsequent acute deterioration.[15]

Clinical cases

Case 5.1

A 64-year-old man with a prior history of aortic valve surgery was referred with a diagnosis of an occluded aortic prosthesis producing left ventricular failure and pulmonary oedema.

Clinical examination revealed no evidence of elevated central venous pressure and a soft ejection systolic murmur at the base. An absence of prosthetic valve clicks had been noted at his referring hospital and this was confirmed. Auscultation of his lungs revealed widespread inspiratory crackles.

Oxygen saturation on room air was 89%. A chest x ray revealed widespread alveolar shadowing occupying both lung fields, but no caridiomegaly. Echocardiography revealed normal left ventricular systolic function, left ventricular hypertrophy and a normal gradient across a bioprosthetic aortic valve (the presence of the bioprosthesis explaining the absence of a prosthetic click). A diagnosis of diastolic heart failure was made and treatment started with diuretics.

The patient continued to deteriorate despite diuretics and a Swan-Ganz catheter was inserted. This demonstrated a PCWP of 5 mmHg. Subsequent lung biopsy demonstrated the presence of aggressive pulmonary fibrosis.

Not all patients with alveolar shadowing have cardiogenic pulmonary oedema and our techniques for quantifying diastolic dysfunction (misleadingly suggested here by the presence of left ventricular hypertrophy) are too crude to be useful clinically. The possibility of non-cardiogenic pulmonary oedema, though rare, should always be considered in patients not responding to diuretics.

Case 5.2

A 70-year-old woman presented with acute breathlessness. On examination there was evidence of severe pulmonary oedema with no evidence of valvular heart disease. Chest x ray confirmed the presence of alveolar pulmonary oedema whilst her ECG showed sinus tachycardia with electrical left ventricular hypertrophy.

Her condition improved slightly with intravenous diuretics but this was accompanied by a slight fall in blood pressure and abruptly deteriorating renal function.

Echocardiography demonstrated critical aortic stenosis with a peak gradient of 35 mmHg, severely impaired left ventricular function and valve area of 0.5 cm^2 (normal > 3.0 cm^2). She underwent successful aortic valve replacement.

In severe, end stage aortic stenosis, there is so little flow across the valve that the characteristic murmur becomes inaudible and will certainly be missed in a critically ill patient. At the same time the slow rising carotid pulse is indistinguishable from the low volume pulse of severe left ventricular failure. It is for this reason that all patients with heart failure require echocardiography.

Patients with critical aortic stenosis are intolerant of volume depletion (even if they are in pulmonary oedema) and tend to become hypotensive and develop renal failure when treated with diuretics.

The low flow across the aortic valve results in a low Doppler gradient even in the presence of a severely narrowed valve. Thus low gradients in the presence of impaired ventricular function may represent severe stenosis: a less flow dependent measure such as valve area is required under these circumstances.

Case 5.3

A 60-year-old man was referred with unilateral pulmonary oedema. He was known to have poor left ventricular function secondary to severe three vessel coronary artery disease. He was initially referred to hospital with episodes of recurrent syncope: these episodes corresponded to periods of ventricular tachycardia (VT). Whilst an inpatient he had suffered a further syncopal episode of VT which had been successfully terminated with a 200 J shock.

The following day he developed breathlessness associated with right sided interstitial shadowing on his chest x ray. Echocardiography demonstrated very poor left ventricular systolic function with an estimated ejection fraction of 20%. Neither the patient's clinical condition nor the chest x ray appearances improved with IV diuretics. Various exotic causes of unilateral pulmonary oedema were considered.

Re-examination of the circumstances of the episode of VT revealed that it had occurred immediately following the patient's evening meal and that aspiration was the most likely diagnosis. The patient improved with appropriate antibiotics and subsequently underwent successful revascularisation with implantation of an internal cardioverter/defibrillator.

Again, not all lung shadowing in patients with severely impaired left ventricular function is due to left ventricular failure. Echocardiography in isolation cannot make the diagnosis of heart failure. A variation on this theme occurs in patients with poor LV function who develop pulmonary fibrosis secondary to amiodarone toxicity.

Summary

Pulmonary oedema is not always due to heart failure.

Heart failure is not always due to left ventricular failure.

Left ventricular failure is not always due to ischaemic heart disease.

Patients who deteriorate or fail to respond require urgent echocardiography to define a mechanism for heart failure. All patients require definition of a mechanism prior to discharge.

Normal systolic function on echo does not exclude heart failure and neither does impaired systolic function diagnose it.

Treatment of acute left ventricular failure should primarily be by manipulation of the circulation, not by indiscriminate use of opioids.

Intravenous nitrates are underused in the management of acute left ventricular failure.

Sequential nephron blockade with potassium sparing diuretics is preferable to the use of potassium supplements.

Low dose dopamine frequently overcomes acute diuretic resistance.

References

1 Morgan PW, Goodman LR. Pulmonary edema and adult respiratory distress syndrome [published erratum appears in *Radiol Clin North Am* 1991;**29**(6):ix]. *Radiol Clin North Am* 1991;**29**:943–63.
2 Baumstark A, Swensson RG, Hessel SJ, *et al.* Evaluating the radiographic assessment of pulmonary venous hypertension in chronic heart disease. AJR 1984;**142**:877–84.
3 Sibbald WJ, Cunningham DR, Chin DN. Non-cardiac or cardiac pulmonary edema? A practical approach to clinical differentiation in

critically ill patients. *Chest* 1983;**84**:452–61.

4 Karliner JS. Fulminant myocarditis. *N Engl J Med* 2000;**342**:734–5.

5 Latham RD, Mulrow JP, Virmani R, Robinowitz M, Moody JM. Recently diagnosed idiopathic dilated cardiomyopathy: incidence of myocarditis and efficacy of prednisone therapy. *Am Heart J* 1989;**117**:876–82.

6 Felker GM, Hu W, Hare JM, Hruban RH, Baughman KL, Kasper EK. The spectrum of dilated cardiomyopathy. The Johns Hopkins experience with 1278 patients. *Medicine* 1999;**78**:270–83.

7 Vasan RS, Levy D. Defining diastolic heart failure: a call for standardized diagnostic criteria. *Circulation* 2000;**101**:2118–21.

8 Anonymous. How to diagnose diastolic heart failure. European Study Group on Diastolic Heart Failure. *Eur Heart J* 1998;**19**:99–103.

9 Michalsen A, Konig G, Thimme W. Preventable causative factors leading to hospital admission with decompensated heart failure. *Heart* 1998;**80**:437–41.

10 Northridge D. Frusemide or nitrates for acute heart failure? *Lancet* 1996;**347**:667–8.

11 Pang D, Keenan SP, Cook DJ, Sibbald WJ. The effect of positive pressure airway support on mortality and the need for intubation in cardiogenic pulmonary edema: a systematic review. *Chest* 1998;**114**:1185–92.

12 Davies CH, Bashir Y. Beta-blockers for heart failure – time to think the unthinkable? *Quart J Med* 1999;**92**:673–8.

13 Anonymous. Guidelines for the evaluation and management of heart failure. Report of the American College of Cardiology/American Heart Association Task Force on Practice Guidelines (Committee on Evaluation and Management of Heart Failure). *Circulation* 1995;**92**:2764–84.

14 Connors AFJ, Speroff T, Dawson NV, *et al.* The effectiveness of right heart catheterization in the initial care of critically ill patients. SUPPORT Investigators. *JAMA* 1996;**276**:889–97.

15 Stevenson LW. Rites and responsibility for resuscitation in heart failure: tread gently on the thin places. *Circulation* 1998;**98**:619–22.

6: Cardiogenic shock

CH DAVIES

Shock complicates 7–10% of myocardial infarctions. The mortality of cardiogenic shock remains between 70 and 90% and has only declined slightly[1] at a time when the mortality for infarction as a whole has significantly improved and much uncertainty remains as to the optimal treatment strategy.

6.1 Diagnosis

The diagnosis is frequently straightforward in that a patient who has suffered an extensive myocardial infarction presents with hypotension (defined as a systolic BP < 90 mmHg for > 30 minutes). The majority of patients who develop shock do so within 48 hours of admission, with less than 10% shocked on arrival.[2] Shock is more common in patients with a history of previous infarction, diabetes, and those patients who experience recurrent infarction during admission.[3,4]

The first step in the diagnostic process is confirmation of hypotension with a manual blood pressure cuff as automatic

BP equipment is frequently unreliable in shocked patients. Next, assess whether hypotension is associated with tissue hypoperfusion (signifying a worse outlook[5]) or warm peripheries (suggesting vasodilatation due to drugs or sepsis). If there is any doubt, insert a urinary catheter and monitor urine output: a flow <30 ml/hr indicates impaired renal perfusion.

Shock may occur because of inadequate contractility or due to inadequate circulating volume, either absolute as in haemorrhage or relative due to vasodilatation. The differentiation between these two states relies on an assessment of central venous pressure (CVP). The well recognised problem in post infarct patients is that because myocardial damage may have disproportionately affected one or other of the ventricles, central venous pressure will not necessarily reflect the left ventricular filling pressures. As a result, assessment of the CVP/JVP (jugular venous pressure) cannot be relied upon to resolve the hypovolaemia/pump failure dilemma accurately. The presence of clinical evidence of pulmonary oedema and left ventricular third sound should, in theory, resolve this issue but in practice both signs are too insensitive. The traditional solution to resolve potential disparity between left and ventricular filling pressures is to measure the pulmonary capillary wedge pressure (PCWP) with a Swan-Ganz catheter and to use this as a measure of LV filling pressure. Although this technique still has an important role it is not without problems (see Chapter 14), and in the majority of shocked patients the diagnosis can be achieved with a combination of ECG, chest x ray, and echocardiogram (Table 6.1). Central to this process is the provision of rapid echocardiography in all shocked patients.

The decision algorithm separates the diagnosis into primary cardiac and extracardiac aetiologies (Figure 6.1).

6.1.1 Excluding an extracardiac mechanism

Extracardiac mechanisms are admittedly rare but, as the prognosis of pump failure remains so poor, it is worth briefly considering the alternatives.

Table 6.1 Clinical patterns in the diagnosis of shock

	CVP	PCWP	ECG	CXR	Echo
LV failure	↑	↑	Extensive ST and/or Q waves	Pulmonary oedema	LV dysfunction or mechanical complication
RV failure	↑	↓	ST ↑ RV4	Clear	RV dysfunction
Pulmonary embolus	↑	↓	Sinus tachycardia	Clear	RV dysfunction ↑ PA pressure
Haemorrhage Drugs Sepsis	↑	↓	Sinus tachycardia	Clear*	Ventricular function better than expected

These patterns assume optimal filling pressure: hypovolaemia will mask any elevated pressure .

* In theory septic shock could co-exist with alveolar shadowing from ARDS but this would be unusual.

CVP=central venous pressure, PCWP=pulmonary capillary wedge pressure, PA=pulmonary artery pressure.

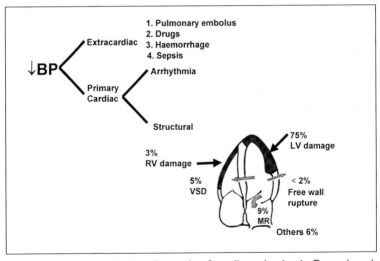

Figure 6.1 Algorithm for the diagnosis of cardiogenic shock. Reproduced with permission from Davies.[20]

Pulmonary embolism

With the increasing use of thrombolysis in the management of myocardial infarction this is rarer than the incidences quoted in most textbooks. Clues to the diagnosis include the absence of pulmonary oedema on CXR, disproportionately severe hypoxaemia for the degree of hypotension, and a disproportionately small initial infarction on the ECG. The abrupt onset of the deterioration and the possibility of pleuritic chest pain may provide further clues. Echocardiography will demonstrate relatively well preserved left ventricular function for the degree of hypotension. The RV will be dilated and hypokinetic; calculated pulmonary artery is usually (but not invariably) raised. Very occasionally the thrombus will be seen snaking its way through the right heart (an indication for thrombolysis).

The major diagnostic problem arises in differentiating pulmonary embolism from RV infarction as both may be associated with hypoxaemia, raised CVP, an absence of pulmonary oedema on the CXR, and occasionally a paradoxical rise in CVP with inspiration (Kussmaul's sign). The most useful differentiating features are the severity of the hypoxaemia (unusual and mild in RV infarction, invariable and severe in pulmonary embolus) and the absence of ST elevation in right sided ECG leads. Pulmonary artery pressure is usually (but not invariably) raised in pulmonary embolism but not usually elevated to the levels seen in chronic thromboembolic disease (the RV cannot acutely raise its systolic pressure to these levels).

Although radionucleotide ventilation perfusion scanning can differentiate between these two diagnoses this requires a relatively mobile patient and is rarely practicable. If genuine doubt persists, a pulmonary angiogram or spiral CT will resolve the issue but the contrast load associated with these is not without risk. Treatment of patients with pulmonary emboli is discussed in Chapter 5.

Drug induced/aggravated hypotension

Over-enthusiastic use of ACE inhibitors, ß-blockers, nitrates and occasionally diuretics may all result in hypotension none of which provide diagnostic difficulty. For a given blood pressure, patients tolerate drug induced hypotension better than pump failure. Always consider the possibility of whether ventricular damage has been underestimated and this has increased the patient's susceptibility to hypotension: unexpected nitrate induced intolerance may be the first clue to right ventricular infarction.

Haemorrhage

Massive haemorrhage is usually secondary to a combination of stress ulceration with thrombolysis/anticoagulation and can provoke genuine diagnostic uncertainty, particularly if the hypotension results in secondary cardiac ischaemia. The diagnostic clues in the absence of melena/haematemesis are a low JVP/CVP, the absence of pulmonary oedema either clinically or on CXR, and a disproportionate degree of hypotension for the magnitude of the original infarction. The haemaglobin level will have had insufficient time to fall but it is important to obtain a baseline value.

Blood loss secondary to a femoral haematoma following cardiac catheterisation is often underestimated due to blood tracking retrogradely into the abdominal cavity – an issue resolved by CT scanning.

Sepsis

Often omitted from the differential diagnosis, clues to the presence of septicaemia are early peripheral vasodilatation and a predisposing cause (usually an indwelling urinary catheter, sometimes infection of pulmonary oedema).

6.1.2 Defining a cardiac mechanism

The presence of ventricular tachycardia as a cause of hypotension will be obvious from the monitored ECG and is discussed further in Chapter 11. Atrial fibrillation is never a cause of shock in the absence of severe structural heart disease, any expectation that acute cardioversion in isolation will restore haemodynamic stability is ill founded.

The relative frequency of the structural mechanisms of cardiogenic shock in the SHOCK series are listed in Figure 6.1.[6]

Overwhelming LV damage

This is the mechanism in 75% of cases, either due to the proximal occlusion of a single coronary artery with a particularly large perfusion field, or to sequential occlusion of two coronary arteries (within a short space of time or with a history of a previous infarction). The typical patient has sustained an anterior myocardial infarct (MI) with a large enzyme rise (frequently with a protracted period of enzyme release) and did not receive thrombolysis.

The clinical diagnosis is usually straightforward with pulmonary oedema, a prominent third heart sound and an elevated JVP/CVP. The ECG confirms the presence of extensive infarction ST elevation in >80% of patients, whilst echocardiography confirms severely impaired left ventricular function. Problems arise in the absence of radiographic pulmonary oedema as this raises the possibility that LV underfilling (either from true hypovolaemia or secondary to damaged RV function) has occurred. Thus patients without evidence of radiographic pulmonary oedema and ECG evidence of an anterior MI should receive 250 ml of 0.9% saline over 15 minutes (Figure 6.2). If the BP fails to improve then insertion of a Swan-Ganz catheter is indicated (see below).

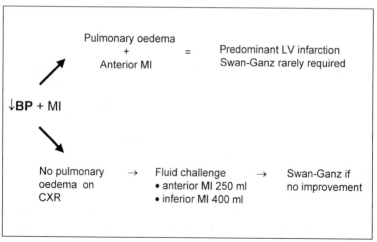

Figure 6.2 Algorithm for the treatment of cardiogenic shock.

Right ventricular infarction

Hypotension following an inferior infarction with a raised JVP and an absence of pulmonary oedema suggests right ventricular infarction. The significance of ST elevation in the right sided ECG leads is now well established[7] (ST elevation in RV4 has a sensitivity of 70% and a specificity of approaching 100%). This may be transient and this underscores the importance of performing right sided chest leads in all patients with inferior infarction on admission.

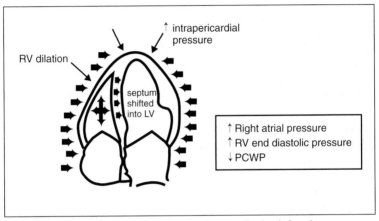

Figure 6.3 Diagram of the process of right ventricular infarction. Reproduced with permission from Davies.[20]

Right ventricular infarction produces characteristic haemodynamics,[8] in which dilatation of the thin walled ventricle is constrained by the pericardium (Figure 6.3). The subsequent rise in intrapericardial tension[9] produces a rise in diastolic pressures with impaired filling. The intraventricular septum then bulges into the left ventricular cavity producing a simultaneous impairment of left heart filling and equalisation of diastolic pressures in all four chambers.[10] Partial compensation for the impaired right ventricular contraction is obtained from the intraventricular septum being forced into the right ventricular cavity in systole[11] and from the contribution of right atrial systole.[12] Confusingly, hypoxaemia may occasionally be a feature of RV infarction as the elevated right sided pressures produce right–left shunting via a patent foramen ovale.[13]

The right ventricular dilatation and dysfunction is readily appreciated on echo from the apical four-chamber view. Unlike the majority of patients with acute pulmonary embolus, the pulmonary artery pressure calculated from the tricuspid regurgitation jet will not be elevated. Swan-Ganz catheterisation will demonstrate an unexpectedly low pulmonary capillary wedge pressure (PCWP), with equalisation of right atrial and RV end diastolic pressures.

Mechanical complications of infarction

These all represent myocardial rupture, the three clinical syndromes depending on the location (Table 6.2). Traditionally these occur 3–5 days following infarction at a time when neutrophil mediated resorption of infarcted myocardium is maximal and the strengthening effects of fibrosis had yet to occur. Thrombolysis has paradoxically increased the incidence of these complications[14] which now tend to occur earlier in the course of the illness. Echocardiography has displaced Swan-Ganz catheterisation in the diagnosis of these complications to a subsidiary role (for completeness, details of their haemodynamic profiles are listed in Chapter 14).

Table 6.2 Three clinical syndromes of myocardial rupture

	VSD	Free wall rupture	Papillary muscle rupture
Anterior MI	66%	50%	25%
Q waves	Most	Most	50%
New murmur	90%	25%	50%
Palpable thrill	Common	No	Rare
Echo	Hinge point	> 5 mm pericardial effusion	Suspiciously good LV function Flail mitral leaflet
Colour flow	L → R shunt		Severe mitral regurgitation

VSD: ventricular septal defect
Modified from Ryan et al.[15]

Ventricular septal defect (VSD)

Diagnosis is more straightforward than imagined with 90% of patients demonstrating a *harsh* murmur at the left sternal edge, and a palpable thrill is common. The ECG usually demonstrates an extensive Q wave infarction. Chest *x* ray shows alveolar shadowing (the fact that this is high flow within the vessels as opposed to pulmonary oedema is difficult to appreciate on portable films). Echocardiography demonstrates better LV function than expected, usually an extensive area of akinesis and often an abrupt "hinge point" between the normal and infarcted myocardium. The defect itself is not usually visualised but the colour flow of the left to right shunt is readily apparent. Severe impairment of left ventricular function in the presence of a VSD is an ominous sign requiring careful consideration before surgery is undertaken.

The moment of septal rupture is frequently accompanied by a recurrence of ST elevation and sometimes pain. This leads to a diagnosis of recurrent infarction and the repeat administration of thrombolytics. This softens the already friable myocardium, further reducing the chances of a successful repair. The clues to the diagnosis are that the ST elevation is usually at a site where there are established Q waves and secondly the presence of the characteristic murmur (emphasising the importance of clinical examination before contemplating rescue thrombolysis).

Mitral regurgitation due to papillary muscle infarction

This is associated with less extensive infarction than VSDs and in 50% of patients there is no associated Q wave.[16] Diagnosis is more problematic with a significant murmur developing in less than half. Conversely, almost 40% of patients develop functional mitral regurgitation at some point following an MI due to changes in ventricular geometry or transient papillary ischaemia. As with VSD the alerting feature of the echocardiogram is the relative preservation of left ventricular function in a patient who is shocked and in severe pulmonary oedema. Echocardiography usually demonstrates the presence of a flail mitral leaflet with colour Doppler demonstrating severe mitral regurgitation. Occasionally, the mechanism of mitral dysfunction cannot be demonstrated using transthoracic scanning and a transoesophageal echo is required.

Subacute rupture/tamponade

As discussed in Chapter 13 cardiac rupture usually presents as electromechanical dissociation. In some patients this is preceded by a prodromal phase of subacute rupture.[17,18] The subacute rupture syndrome has the following clinical features:

- Nausea
- Pleuritic chest pain
- Failure of ST resolution
- Upright T waves
- Transient hypotension and bradycardia

Subacute rupture is more common in elderly hypertensives with anterior infarctions. The raised JVP and absence of pulmonary oedema produced by tamponade may mimic the presentation of a right ventricular infarct, whilst the pleuritic chest pain misleadingly suggests pulmonary embolism. However, the unexplained hypotension will require echocardiography at which point the significant pericardial effusion will become apparent. It is important to appreciate that a small (< 5 mm) pericardial effusion is not uncommon during the course of many Q wave infarctions and does not, in isolation, represent pre-rupture.[18]

6.2 Management

6.2.1 Management of overwhelming left ventricular damage

Management is in three phases (Figure 6.4), optimisation of ventricular filling, followed by institution of supportive therapy, and lastly deciding on the appropriateness of revascularisation. As noted above the majority of patients with overwhelming left ventricular damage have radiographic evidence of pulmonary oedema and are assumed to have an excessive preload. In those without evidence of pulmonary oedema, it is essential to optimise left ventricular filling before contemplating inotrope therapy by raising the PCWP to 17 mmHg.[19]

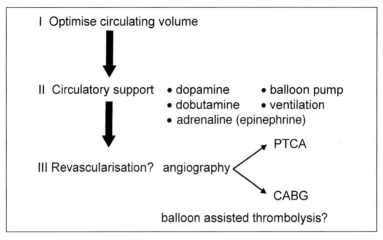

Figure 6.4 Three phases for the management of left ventricular damage.

Supportive therapy

Inotropic support

Standard management of cardiogenic shock involves the combinations of low dose dopamine (2.5–5 μg/kg/min) in an attempt to provide renal vasodilatation with dobutamine (5–20 μg/kg/min) providing inotropic support. If hypotension persists, adrenaline (epinephrine) can be substituted for dobutamine. The use of phosphodiesterase inhibitors such as milrinone offers no additional benefit. However, despite their widespread use there is little evidence to support either the use of inotropes in general in the setting of cardiogenic shock or the use of the dopamine/dobutamine combination in particular. Although the effect of inotropic support on survival in cardiogenic shock has never been formally evaluated there is strong clinical suspicion that it is largely ineffective. The static mortality figures for cardiogenic shock over the period of time when the use of inotropes in the UK became widespread supports this contention. The hope has always been that inotropes would raise blood pressure, improve myocardial perfusion and reverse the vicious spiral of decline that characterises cardiogenic shock. In reality, any benefits obtained through improvements in perfusion appear to be more than offset by the deleterious effects of infarct expansion and arrhythmias. Coupled with the failure to remedy the underlying problem of infarcted myocardium is the fact that the excessive catecholamine stimulation produces rapid β-adrenoceptor down-regulation with the development of tolerance necessitating a process of futile dose escalation. Despite the above, inotropes do have a role in transiently supporting patients undergoing investigation into the mechanism of shock and patients in whom a genuinely reversible cause of shock exists (septicaemial drug overdose postoperatively, etc.). However as a primary treatment for cardiogenic shock due to overwhelming left ventricular damage, they are essentially palliative. Once inotropes have been initiated, patients tend to pass through a phase of relative stability lasting 24–36 hours followed by a rapid decline. The small numbers of patients in whom successful weaning can be achieved rarely survive to leave hospital.

Intra-aortic balloon pumping

Similar problems exist with the use of intra-aortic balloon pumps. Early experience showed that although patients improved dramatically, they experienced an equally abrupt deterioration when support was withdrawn with no net increase in survival. Balloon pump support is invaluable to stabilise patients prior to revascularisation by angioplasty or bypass surgery.

Mechanical ventilation

Severe hypoxaemia contributes to myocardial dysfunction and the additional work of spontaneous ventilation is appreciable on the failing circulation. Mechanical ventilation would therefore seem a logical treatment in cardiogenic shock complicated by refractory pulmonary oedema and is advocated in some centres. Unfortunately as with inotropes and balloon pumping, patients rarely survive mechanical ventilation unless there is a reversible cause such as a mechanical complication of infarction or previously inadequate treatment of pulmonary oedema. For this reason it is not recommended. It should be stressed that this failure to recommend mechanical ventilation for patients with cardiogenic shock and pulmonary oedema does not extend to patients with fulminant pulmonary oedema and adequately maintained BP as discussed in Chapter 5.

Vasodilators

Although the failing ventricle is afterload dependent and vasodilators have been advocated as a treatment option, they are never a practical option in a shocked patient.

Assessing suitability for revascularisation

Intuitively, revascularisation using angioplasty/stenting (percutaneous transluminal coronary angioplasty, PTCA) or bypass surgery (coronary artery bypass graft, CABG) should offer a survival advantage in patients with overwhelming left ventricular damage. Although there are numerous uncontrolled series suggesting benefit,[20] all of these are seriously flawed by the fact that the patients selected for revascularisation tended to be those with a better than average prognosis at the outset. Of the two randomised trials, the first (SMASH)[21] was discontinued due to low recruitment without showing benefit whilst the second (SHOCK)[22] did not show any benefit at its primary 30 day end point. There was however a significant benefit of revascularisation on mortality at 6 and 12 months. The mechanisms underlying this failure to demonstrate benefit are complex[20] but, rightly or wrongly, the majority of interventional cardiologists consider the case for revascularisation proved[23] and no further trials are planned. This is clearly an unsatisfactory situation but with the prospect of improved long term survival we currently favour revascularisation in selected patients using criteria modified from the SHOCK trial itself but further restricting the time from infarction and introducing an age criterion (patients > 70 years did not benefit from revascularisation in SHOCK and this mirrors our clinical experience).

Time is the critical issue here; it is essential to consider whether a patient might be suitable for revascularisation as soon as hypotension manifests itself and not when they have been inotrope dependent for 24 hours (Box 6.1). One of the key changes in practice required before a strategy of active reperfusion can become a reality is the early recognition of the precursors of cardiogenic shock: large anterior infarctions which fail to reperfuse, early tachycardia, heart failure, and falls in BP. All too often, early signs of decompensation are ignored whilst false reassurance is derived from the transient improvements seen in the first few hours after inotropes are started.

Box 6.1 Selection criteria for revascularisation in cardiogenic shock

- ST elevation infarction
- Systolic BP < 90 mmHg for > 30 minutes
- Evidence of peripheral hypoperfusion
- Onset of shock < 36 hours post MI
- < 12 hours after the onset of shock
- Age < 70 years
- No prior CABG

Relative contraindications to consider are problems with femoral arterial access and abnormal renal function prior to the onset of shock.

The decision as to whether revascularisation is achieved by PTCA or CABG is beyond the scope of this book. The equivalent outcomes with either strategy in SHOCK almost certainly reflects selection bias. With the recent improvements in PTCA technology (stenting and abciximab) we strongly favour immediate revascularisation of the culprit vessel with PTCA coupled with IABP support followed by CABG several months later if required for multivessel disease.

6.2.2 Management of right ventricular infarction

Optimisation of ventricular filling pressures

The aim is to raise LV filling pressures to the point where cardiac output is maximal but not to exceed the point where the elevated left atrial pressure results in pulmonary oedema and this occurs at a PCWP of 17 mmHg.[19] To achieve this 200 ml of 0.9% saline should be administered over 15 minutes, followed by a further 200 ml over the next 30 minutes. At this point the patient's clinical condition should be reassessed. Most of these patients will require more fluid: on average a total of 1–2 litres over 4–5 hours. Unfortunately, the volumes required vary widely and if the patients have not improved after the initial 400 ml challenge then a Swan-Ganz catheter should be inserted. Contrary to accepted beliefs, optimisation of ventricular filling pressures results in clinical improvement in less than 50% of patients.[24]

Maintaining atrioventricular synchrony

Atrioventricular block complicates 50% of hypotensive RV infarctions[25] and atrial fibrillation in further 10%. With a non-functioning RV, right atrial contraction will be contributing almost all of the work of the right heart, and restoration of atrioventricular synchrony will produce important improvements in cardiac output. AV block under these circumstances is an indication for the insertion of a dual chamber temporary pacemaker (ventricular pacing to increase rate alone without restoration of AV synchrony is almost always insufficient[12]). For the same reasons atrial fibrillation should be managed aggressively with IV amiodarone loading (300 mg over 1 hour followed by 900 mg over the next 24 hours IV combined with 400 mg tds orally) and DC cardioversion under heparin cover after 6–8 hours. This is one of the few situations where acute cardioversion of atrial fibrillation is worthwhile.

Inotropes in RV infarction

Cardiogenic shock due to right ventricular infarction is regarded as a benign condition and although this might be true when compared to the 80% mortality of LV cardiogenic shock, mortality remains an appreciable 50% in large series. Patients who fail to improve following optimisation of filling and AV synchrony should receive the standard dopamine/dobutamine combination as outlined in the management of overwhelming LV damage. The encouraging feature of RV shock is that, even without reperfusion, RV function improves spontaneously over a 30 day period and thus in those patients who do survive, good functional recovery is the norm.[26]

Revascularisation

Indications for revascularisation in RV infarction are even less clear than for overwhelming LV damage and there will never be a randomised trial to clarify the issue. The risks of intervention must be balanced against the lower overall mortality and the potential for spontaneous improvement.

Recent studies have demonstrated the feasibility of undertaking PTCA and that RV function improves acutely.[26]

Revascularisation should be considered in those patients who are still hypotensive despite a dobutamine dose of >10 micrograms/kg/min. The time frame for intervention should be similar to that for LV infarction as, although the RV may recover despite prolonged hypoperfusion, the no-reflow phenomenon is likely to prevent patency of the distal right coronary artery if these times are exceeded.

6.2.3 Management of the mechanical complication of infarction

Ventricular septal rupture

Current opinion favours early closure rather than a protracted attempt to achieve stabilisation medically. Unfortunately, the encouraging results obtained from past surgical series were highly selected and probably do not reflect current practice. In particular there is a suspicion that thrombolysis has worsensed the outcome in these patients. The key factors in deciding whether surgery is appropriate are the presence of oliguria, and the degree of left ventricular impairment.[27] As two-thirds of patients have multivessel coronary disease coronary angiography is recommended prior to surgery. If calculation of the shunt magnitude is considered important then it can rapidly be performed at the time of cardiac catheterisation and Swan-Ganz catheterisation prior to this is unnecessary. Implantation of an intra-aortic balloon pump in the contralateral groin prior to cardiac catheterisation should be considered. Even with successful surgery, 30 day mortality remains high at 40–60%.

Mitral regurgitation due to papillary muscle infarction

As with septal rupture the current trend is towards earlier operations preceded by coronary angiography (with balloon pump support if needed). Vasodilators are also beneficial in the medical stabilisation of these patients prior to surgery if their BP is > 105 mmHg.

Subacute rupture

Subacute rupture frequently heralds acute rupture with fatal electromechanical dissociation and thus once diagnosed is an indication for urgent surgical repair. Again, despite encouraging literature,[18] a successful result is difficult to achieve in clinical practice.

6.3 Specific problems

6.3.1 Thrombolysis in cardiogenic shock

Although thrombolysis decreases the incidence of shock, it is ineffective once shock becomes established. As the severity of a patient's infarction increases so to does their likelihood of deriving benefit from thrombolysis. Thus patients with BP < 100 mmHg but > 90 mmHg achieved more than three times the average number of lives saved per 1000 in the FTT meta-analysis.[28] This underscores the vital importance of administering thrombolysis to high risk patients who are not yet shocked: it is common to see an inappropriate decision to withhold thrombolytics at the start of the notes of patients subsequently transferred with cardiogenic shock.

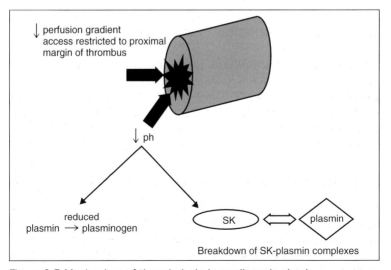

Figure 6.5 Mechanism of thrombolysis in cardiogenic shock.

However, patients with a BP < 90 mmHg do not appear to benefit from thrombolysis[29] and there are several mechanisms at work here. Firstly, thrombolytic agents normally gain access to the clot via pores in the fibrin mesh of the clot and, once the perfusion gradient along the artery drops below 80–90 mmHg, this mechanism ceases to operate. Secondly, the prevailing acidosis reduces the formation of plasmin from plasminogen and produces dissociation of the streptokinase-plasmin complexes.[30] (Figure 6.5). The use of a second or third generation thrombolytic such as alteplase or reteplase does not increase the effectiveness of thrombolysis in shock.[31]

One potential solution to this resistance is the combination of thrombolysis with an intra-aortic balloon pump (balloon assisted thrombolysis). The advantage of this approach is that it does not require immediate access to a cardiac catheter lab. The disadvantage (apart from the obvious risk of haemorrhage) is that few people besides invasive cardiologists feel comfortable with balloon pump insertion. To date there have been two encouraging retrospective series.[32,33] Unfortunately, the TACTICS trial was abandoned and so we will never have definite answers as to the validity of this approach. However, this is certainly an approach worth considering if the facilities are available (see below).

6.3.2 Fluid management in right ventricular infarction

Right ventricular infarction is misleadingly perceived as an essentially benign condition which rapidly responds to fluid loading. As noted above, the clinical reality is of a condition where mortality approaches 50%[34] and where volume loading fails to reverse shock in at least half.[24] Several points emerge from the literature, firstly that the fluid volumes required to optimise LV filling vary widely. Secondly, in animal experiments, although fluid loading initially augments fluid loading, the benefits of this may be subsequently offset by an increase in infarct size.[35] Raising right atrial pressure above 14 mmHg in clinical studies actually results in a decline in cardiac output.[36,37] In practical terms, this underscores the need for PCWP guidance if hypotension does not resolve following the initial 400 ml challenge and demonstrates the importance of not continuing to add fluid if hypotension does improve (not merely chasing the PCWP figure in isolation) and that inotropes should be added once right atrial pressure exceeds 14 mmHg.

6.3.3 Inotrope management in shock (Table 6.3)

Dopamine (2.5–15 micrograms/kg/min: At low doses (< 5 micrograms/kg/min) acts on specific dopamine[1] receptors to increase renal blood flow and antagonise the Na^+ symporter in the proximal tubule. At higher doses (> 5 micrograms/kg/min) it acts directly on β-adrenoceptors to increase cardiac output. Further dosage increments (> 10 micrograms/kg/min) result in the release of noradrenaline (norepinephrine) from pre-synaptic terminals to stimulate both α and β-adrenoceptors producing net vasoconstriction. In the UK, dopamine is now used solely in its capacity as a renal vasodilator, but owing to the unpredictability of the vasoconstrictor effects produced by a stimulation it must always be administered via a central line.

Dobutamine (5–20 micrograms/kg/min) is a synthetic agonist acting directly on $β_1$ and to a lesser extent $β_2$-receptors with some additional stimulation of α receptors. The α stimulation is offset by the more pronounced $β_2$ actions producing a net vasodilator effect and dobutamine may be administered peripherally: a useful option in elderly patients in whom the insertion of a central line is felt to be too invasive.

Adrenaline (epinephrine) (starting at 1–2 µg/min). Stimulates α in addition to β-receptors resulting in peripheral vasoconstriction which is potentially harmful in the afterload dependent circulation of heart failure but has a role in patients who are refractory to dobutamine.

Noradrenaline (norepinephrine) has pronounced α-adrenergic properties and is used in patients in whom a low peripheral vascular resistance is contributing to hypotension such as septicaemic shock.

Table 6.3 Inotropes used in the management of shock

Inotrope	Dose	Clinical use	Administration
Dopamine	2.5 μg/kg/min	renal vasodilator	central
Dobutamine	5.20 μg/kg/min	inotrope	central/peripheral
Adrenaline (epinephrine)	>0.1 μg/kg/min	inotrope+vasoconstrictor	central
Noradrenaline (norepinephrine)	1–10 μg/kg/min	vasoconstrictor+inotrope	central

6.3.4 Indications for Swan-Ganz insertion

In the past Swan-Ganz monitoring has undoubtedly been overused in the USA, but has arguably been underutilised in the UK. Measurement of PCWP is indicated in the presence of hypotension without radiographic evidence of pulmonary oedema if matters are not resolved following a fluid challenge (250 ml anterior infarction and 400 ml inferior infarction – Figure 6.2). Swan-Ganz insertion is recommended if the mechanism of shock remains uncertain after ECG, chest x ray, and echocardiography and may be particularly useful in achieving control of the peripheral circulation with co-existing sepsis. As discussed in the previous chapter, knowledge of the PCWP may be invaluable in the differential diagnosis of pulmonary oedema in the absence of hypotension. We usually recommend that the line be removed as soon as a diagnosis of the mechanism of shock has been made and optimal volume loading achieved – the additional information obtained from prolonged placement is not justified by the risks (See Chapter 14 for further details).

6.3.5 Communicating with patients, relatives and CCU staff

Successful management of a condition with such a high mortality requires a substantial commitment to communicating both with the patient, his/her relatives, and the CCU staff. Failure to warn relatives of the seriousness of the situation is a commonly cited cause of dissatisfaction, whilst failure to formulate a consistent management plan may leave nursing staff unsupported. Inexperienced physicians frequently initiate and then escalate inotrope therapy when there is little hope of a successful outcome and early consultation with experienced colleagues is recommended in the management of these patients.

Clinical cases

Case 6.1

A 75-year-old ex-marine presented 2 days following a substantial anterior MI (peak CK 4000 iu/l) which he had mistaken for indigestion, complicated by marked nausea and vomiting. Although initially haemodynamically stable his condition deteriorated over the following 48 hours. By this time his systolic BP had fallen to 80 mmHg and he had been oliguric for 12 hours. The regional centre was phoned to confirm that the outlook was hopeless and that neither inotropes or revascularisation were appropriate. On examination, there were several unusual features: he was bradycardic at 53/min, he was lying flat and his JVP was not raised. A CXR showed clear lung fields, whilst an ECG demonstrated a nodal rhythm with retrograde P waves. Cardiac ultrasound demonstrated severely impaired LV function with extensive anterior akinesis.

A temporary DDD pacemaker was inserted to restore atrioventricular (AV) synchrony with a short AV delay of 80 msec. Fluid replacement was undertaken guided by insertion of a Swan-Ganz catheter (initial PCWP was 10 mmHg). His condition improved over the following 24 hours and he was discharged 6 days later and was only mildly symptomatic on follow up 2 months later.

Be wary of clinical features that do not fit, in particular patients with "cardiogenic shock" and a clear CXR or the absence of tachycardia. Prominent vomiting predisposes to hypovolaemia. If pacing is indicated on haemodynamic criteria in MI then a dual chamber device is recommended.

Case 6.2

A 37-year-old man was referred with cardiogenic shock and ongoing ischaemic pain. Eight hours earlier he had presented with an anterior MI with widespread ST elevation and failure of ST segment resolution following tissue plasminogen activator (tPA) (peak CK subsequently 6500 iu/l). On arrival BP was 78/50, pulse 110/min and he was in pulmonary oedema. Cardiac ultrasound demonstrated severely impaired LV function both anteriorly and laterally. An intra-aortic balloon pump was inserted. Coronary angiography demonstrated chronic occlusion of the circumflex artery (clinically silent), a non-dominant right coronary artery and a critically stenosed LAD with TIMI 2 flow. Stenting of the LAD with administration of half dose abciximab restored TIMI 3 flow. He required ventilation for his pulmonary oedema and haemofilitration for anuria. A left ventricular assist device was inserted and his condition stabilised with a view to awaiting transplantation. He died 4 weeks following admission.

With ongoing ischaemic pain it may be worthwhile considering revascularisation outside the 18 hour SHOCK limit, however even using the most aggressive techniques (IABP, stenting, abciximab, LV assist devices) the outlook remains poor. The result of the TIMI 14 trial suggest that the doses of abciximab and tPA should both be halved when used simultaneously to prevent excessive risk of haemorrhage.

Case 6.3

A 52-year-old woman presented with a short history of severe chest pain complicated by three episodes of ventricular fibrillation. Her ECG showed widespread ST elevation in both anterior and lateral territories and her systolic BP fell to 70/50 mmHg. As the cardiac catheter lab was unavailable an intra-aortic balloon pump was inserted and front-loaded tPA was administered. Her condition stabilised and subsequent angiography demonstrated TIMI 3 flow in the LAD with recanalisation at the site of a non-occlusive LAD plaque. She was discharged home 7 days later with only moderately impaired LV function.

Balloon assisted thrombolysis remains an option in cardiogenic shock where PTCA is unavailable. Thrombolysis is not contraindicated if resuscitation has not been prolonged (< 5 minutes CPR).

Summary

Prognosis in all forms of cardiogenic shock remains poor

Prevention is important: do not deny patients thrombolysis (or PTCA) without good reason when they initially present with infarction

Thrombolysis is ineffective once shock becomes established

The mechanism of cardiogenic shock can be established in most patients with ECG, chest x ray, and echocardiography

Swan-Ganz insertion is usually only required for patients with shock and no radiographic evidence of pulmonary oedema

Consider patients with shock due to overwhelming left ventricular damage for revascularisation

Inotropes in isolation almost never cure cardiogenic shock due to overwhelming left ventricular damage

Fluid loading alone normalises arterial pressure in less than half of patients with shock due to right ventricular infarction

Single chamber pacing is inadequate in the management of patients with shock due to right ventricular infarction and heart block

Current outlook for patients with mechanical complications of infarction is not as good as imagined

References

1 Goldberg RJ, Samad NA, Yarzebski J, Gurwitz J, Bigelow, Gore JM. Temporal trends in cardiogenic shock complicating acute myocardial infarction. *N Engl J Med* 1999;**340**:1162–8.

2 Holmes DRJ, Bates ER, Kleiman NS, *et al.* Contemporary reperfusion therapy for cardiogenic shock: the GUSTO-I trial experience. The GUSTO-I Investigators. Global Utilization of Streptokinase and Tissue Plasminogen Activator for Occluded Coronary Arteries. *J Am Coll Cardiol* 1995;**26**:668–74.

3 Leor J, Goldbourt U, Reicher-Reiss H, Kaplinsky E, Behar. Cardiogenic shock complicating acute myocardial infarction in patients without heart failure on admission: incidence, risk factors, and outcome. SPRINT Study Group. *Am J Med* 1993;**94**:265-73.

4 Hands ME, Rutherford JD, Muller JE, *et al.* The in-hospital development of cardiogenic shock after myocardial infarction: incidence, predictors of occurrence, outcome and prognostic factors. *J Am Coll Cardiol* 1989;**14**: 40–6.

5 Hasdai D, Holmes DRJ, Califf RM, *et al.* Cardiogenic shock complicating acute myocardial infarction: predictors of death. GUSTO Investigators. Global Utilization of Streptokinase and Tissue-Plasminogen activator for Occluded Coronary Arteries. *Am Heart Journal* 1999;**138**:21–31.

6 Hochman JS, Boland J, Sleeper LA, *et al.* Current spectrum of cardiogenic shock and effect of early revascularization on mortality. Results of an International Registry. SHOCK Registry Investigators. *Circulation* 1995;**91**:873–81 .

7 Andersen HR, Falk E, Nielsen D. Right ventricular infarction: diagnostic accuracy of electrocardiographic right chest leads V3R to V7R investigated prospectively in 43 consecutive fatal cases from a coronary care unit. *Br Heart J* 1989;**61**:514–20.

8 Cohn JN, Guiha NH, Broder Ml, Limas CJ. Right ventricular infarction. Clinical and hemodynamic features. *Am J Cardiol* 1974;**33**:209–14.

9 Goldstein JA, Vlahakes GJ, Verrier ED, *et al.* Volume loading improves low cardiac output in experimental right ventricular infarction. *J Am Coll Cardiol* 1983;**2**:270–8.

10 Goldstein JA, Tweddell JS, Barzilai B, Yagi Y, Jaffe AS, Cox JL. Importance of left ventricular function and systolic ventricular interaction to right ventricular performance during acute right heart ischemia. *J Am Coll Cardiol* 1992;**19**:704–11

11 Goldstein JA, Barzilai B, Rosamond TL, Eisenberg PR1 Jaffe AS. Determinants of hemodynamic compromise with severe right ventricular

infarction. *Circulation* 1990;**82**:359–68.

12 Love JC, Haffajee CI, Gore JM, Alpert JS. Reversibility of hypotension and shock by atrial or atrioventricular sequential pacing in patients with right ventricular infarction. *Am Heart J* 1984;**108**:5–13.

13 Silver MT, Lieberman EH, Thibault GE. Refractory hypoxemia in inferior myocardial infarction from right-to-left shunting through a patent foramen ovale: a case report and review of the literature. *Clin Cardiol* 1994;**17**:627–30.

14 Kinn JW, O'Neill WW, Benzuly KH, Jones DE, Grines CL. Primary angioplasty reduces risk of myocardial rupture compared to thrombolysis for acute myocardial infarction. *Cath Cardiovasc Diag* 1997;**42**:151–7.

15 Ryan TJ, Anderson JL, Antman EM, *et al*. ACC/AHA guidelines for the management of patients with acute myocardial infarction: executive summary. A report of the American College of Cardiology/American Heart Association Task Force on Practice Guidelines (Committee on Management or Acute Myocardial Infarction). *Circulation* 1996;**94**: 2341–50.

16 Nishimura RA, Schaff HV, Shub C, Gersh BJ, Edwards WD, Tajik AJ. Papillary muscle rupture complicating acute myocardial infarction. analysis of 17 patients. *Am J Cardiol* 1983;**51**:373–7.

17 Oliva PB, Hammill SC, Edwards WD. Cardiac rupture, a clinically predictable complication of acute myocardial infarction: report of 70 cases with clinicopathologic correlations. *J Am Coll Cardiol* 1993;**22**: 720–6.

18 Lopez-Sendon J, Gonzalez, Lopez DS, *et al*. Diagnosis of subacute ventricular wall rupture after acute myocardial infarction: sensitivity and specificity of clinical, hemodynamic and echocardiographic criteria. *J Am Coll Cardiol* 1992;**19**:1145–53.

19 Crexells C, Chatterlee K, Forrester JS, Dikshit K, Swan, HJ. Optimal level of filling pressure in the left side of the heart in acute myocardial infarction. *N Engl J Med* 1973;**289**:1263–6.

20 Davies CH. Revascularisation for cardiogenic shock? *Quart J Med* 2001; in press.

21 Urban P, Stauffer JC, Bleed D, *et al*. A randomized evaluation of early revascularization to treat shock complicating acute myocardial infarction. The (Swiss) Multicenter Trial of Angioplasty for Shock-(S)MASH. *Eur Heart J* 1999;**20**:103–8.

22 Hochman JS, Sleeper LA, Webb JG, *et al*. Early revascularization in acute myocardial infarction complicated by cardiogenic shock. SHOCK Investigators. Should we emergently revascularize occluded coronaries for cardiogenic shock. *N Engl J Med* 1999;**341**:625–34.

23 de Belder MA, Hall JA. Infarct angioplasty. *Heart* 1999; **82**:399–401.

24 Edwards D, Whittaker S, Prior A. Cardiogenic shock without a critically raised left ventricular end diastolic pressure: management and outcome in eighteen patients. *Br Heart J* 1986;**55**:549–53.

25 Braat SH, de Zwaan C, Brugada P, Coenegracht JM, Wellens HJ. Right ventricular involvement with acute inferior wall myocardial infarction identifies high risk of developing atrioventricular nodal conduction disturbances. *Am Heart J* 1984;**107**:118–7.

26 Bowers TR, O'Neill WW, Grines C, Pica MC, Safian RD, Goldstein JA. Effect of reperfusion on biventricular function and survival after right ventricular infarction. *N Engl J Med* 1998; **338**:933–40.

27 Cummings RG, Califf RM, Jones RN, Reimer KA, Ng Y-H, We JE. Correlates of survival in patients with postinfarction ventricular septal defect. *Ann Thorac Surg* 1989;**47**:824–30.

28 FTT Collaborative Group. Indications for fibrinolytic therapy in

suspected acute myocardial infarction: collaborative overview of early mortality and major morbidity results from all randomised trials of more than 1000 patients. Fibrinolytic Therapy Trialists' (FTT) Collaborative Group. *Lancet* 1994;**343**:311–22.

29 White HD, Van de Werf FJ. Thrombolysis for acute myocardial infarction. *Circulation* 1998;**97**:1632–46.

30 Becker RC. Hemodynamic, mechanical, and metabolic determinants of thrombolytic efficacy: a theoretic framework for assessing the limitations of thrombolysis in patients with cardiogenic shock. *Am Heart J* 1993;**125**:919–29.

31 Hasdai D, Holmes DRJ, Topol EJ, *et al*. Frequency and clinical outcome of cardiogenic shock during acute myocardial infarction among patients receiving reteplase or alteplase. Results from GUSTO-III. Global Use of Strategies to Open Occluded Coronary Arteries. *Eur Heart J* 1999;**20**:128–35.

32 Bates ER, Stomel RJ, Hochman JS, Ohman EM. The use of intraaortic balloon counterpulsation as an adjunct to reperfusion therapy in cardiogenic shock. *Int J Cardiol* 1998;**65**(Suppl 1):S37–42.

33 Kovack PJ, Rasak MA, Bates ER, Ohman EM, Stomel RJ. Thrombolysis plus aortic counterpulsation: improved survival in patients who present to community hospitals with cardiogenic shock. *J Am Coll Cardiol* 1997;**29**:1454–8.

34 Hochman JS, Buller CE, Dzavik V, *et al*. Cardiogenic shock (CS) complicating acute MI-etiologies, management and outcome; overall findings of the Shock trial registry. *Circulation* 1998; **778**(Abstract).

35 Johnston WE, Lin CY, Feerick AE, Spray B, Vinten-Johansen J. Volume expansion increases right ventricular infarct size in dogs by reducing collateral perfusion. *Chest* 1996;**109**:494–503.

36 Berisha S, Kastrati A, Goda A, Popa Y. Optimal value of filling pressure in the right side of the heart in acute right ventricular infarction. *Br Heart J* 1990;**63**:98–102.

37 Dell 'Italia LJ, Starling MR, Blumhardt R, Lasher JC, O'Rourke RA. Comparative effects of volume loading, dobutamine, and nitroprusside in patients with predominant right ventricular infarction. *Circulation* 1985;**72**:1327–35.

7: Aortic dissection and related syndromes

CH DAVIES

The principal cause of aortic pain is aortic dissection, although other, rarer conditions can occasionally produce similar symptoms:[1]

- Aortic dissection.
- Intramural haematoma (IMH).
- Rupture of thoracic aortic aneurysm.
- Penetrating aortic ulcer.

These conditions are thankfully uncommon as they pose substantial problems in both diagnosis and management to both generalists and specialists. Dissection in particular is a perennial source of anxiety: generalists are hampered by lack of familiarity and the absence of a reliable screening test, whilst specialists struggle with inconclusive imaging results and technically demanding surgery.

7.1 Pathology

"Dissecting aortic aneurysm" is a misnomer as dissection does not usually occur at the site of pre-existing aneurysms. The basic pathological feature is the presence of blood in the aortic media for which there are two potential mechanisms. Most commonly, a defective aortic media is exposed to systolic blood pressure via a tear in the intima (Figure 7.1a). Blood then extends through the aorta by splitting ("dissecting") the media, forming a false lumen separated from the true aortic lumen by an intimal flap. The clinical features depend on the extent and direction of this medial expansion and the pattern of subsequent side branch involvement. Obstruction to flow in these vessels is either due to direct extension of the false lumen into the branch or from obstruction of the aorta itself prior to the origin of the branch. Blood may eventually track back into the true lumen via an exit tear or occasionally ruptures out through the adventitia. In 15% of cases no entry/exit site is detected and the initiating event is considered to be primary haemorrhage into the media (Figure 7.1b). This haemorrhage may rupture into the aorta producing an appearance indistinguishable from classical dissection, or remain localised within the media, a condition now termed intramural haematoma (IMH). Most dissections occur in

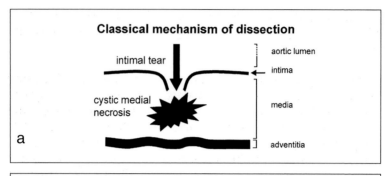

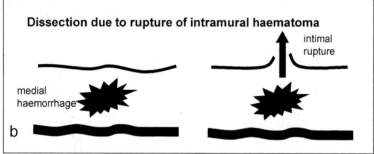

Figure 7.1 Mechanisms in aortic dissection. Modified from Lindsay *et al*.[13]

individuals predisposed to degeneration of the elastic components of the aortic media:

- Hypertension (>80% of cases).
- Bicuspid aortic valve (10%).
- Marfan's syndrome.
- Turner's syndrome.
- Ehlers–Danlos syndrome.
- Pregnancy.
- Cocaine use.
- Prior cardiac surgery.
- Trauma.

The Stanford classification remains the most clinically relevant as it relates most closely to the management decisions required. Type A (proximal) dissections involve the ascending aorta, confusingly defined as the origin of the left subclavian, whilst type B (distal) dissections occur beyond this point

(Figure 7.2, Box 7.1). Further confusion occurs as a type B dissection may occasionally rupture retrogradely into the ascending aorta.

Penetrating atherosclerotic ulcers occur when an ulcerating plaque penetrates the internal elastic lamina with subsequent secondary haemorrhage, almost exclusively in the descending aorta. In contrast to dissection and IMH there is little longitudinal extension of this haemorrhage, although perforation through the adventitia does occur producing a pseudoaneurysm and the potential for aortic rupture. As would be expected, this is a disease of the elderly with widespread atherosclerotic disease and an accompanying risk profile.

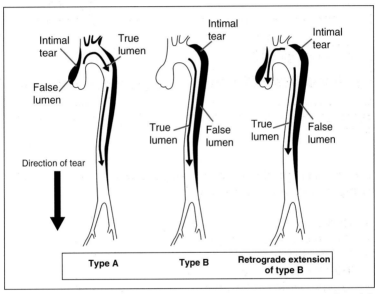

Figure 7.2 Stanford Classification of aortic dissection into types A and B with the variant picture produced by retrograde extension of a type B into the aortic root.

7.2 Clinical features

Over three-quarters of patients present with severe chest pain, which is classically described as "tearing", "ripping", or "stabbing".[2-4] Many patients additionally describe the pain as migrating along the path of the dissection. Involvement of aortic branches may produce confusing presentations such as stroke, abdominal or limb ischaemia, and syncope. On examination hypertension is common, although hypotension (usually due to tamponade[5] or intrapleural rupture) occurs in 20% of cases. The combination of a patient who appears shocked but is found to be *hypertensive* is very suggestive of dissection. Pulse defects are present in half of patients with proximal aortic involvement but only 15% of those with distal involvement. Careful documentation of these is important as they are frequently transient. Aortic regurgitation complicates two-thirds of proximal dissections, but as this is frequently acute the physical signs may not be particularly impressive. Less common signs include reactive left sided pleural effusions, signs of abdominal ischaemia, and Horner's syndrome.

Patients with intramural haemorrhage have an almost identical presentation to those with classical dissection (including the possibility of a pericardial effusion and side branch compromise), in contrast to those with penetrating atherosclerotic ulcers who tend to experience pain in isolation. Patients with rupture or prerupture of thoracic aortic aneurysms present with severe pain and hypotension, occasionally accompanied by signs of aortic regurgitation due to root dilatation. In dissection, the pattern of clinical features may provide some indication as to the site.

Box 7.1 Clinical presentations of type A and type B dissections

Proximal (type A)	Distal (type B)
Initial pain in the anterior chest	Interscapular pain
Aortic regurgitation	Hypertension
Reduced pulses in right neck and arm	Left sided pleural effusion
Marfan's syndrome	
Bicuspid aortic valve	
Syncope	

7.3 Initial investigations

7.3.1 ECG

This demonstrates evidence of electrical left ventricular hypertrophy (LVH) in 30% of patients but the important point is that the vast majority (>98%) do not show ST elevation in a patient who is clearly experiencing severe chest pain. As noted in Chapter 4, it is important to differentiate between ST segment shift in the presence of marked electrical LVH from patients with planar ST depression occurring in the context of an unstable coronary syndrome. If the sum of the R wave in V5 and the S wave in V2 exceeds 35 mm, interpretation of ST depression is inherently unreliable. Failure to appreciate this results in the misdiagnosis of an acute coronary syndrome and the inappropriate administration of anticoagulants, with disastrous results.

7.3.2 Chest x ray

Widening of the aortic silhouette occurs in 80–90% of cases of dissection, whilst there may be an associated pleural effusion (more commonly left sided). However mediastinal widening is virtually universal on the poorly positioned antero-posterior portable x rays produced in emergency departments and these signs are of little practical use in diagnosing dissection. By contrast, the majority of thoracic aortic aneurysms are readily apparent.

7.3.3 Biochemistry and haematology

Plasma levels of lactate dehydrogenase (LDH) may be elevated due to haemolysis of thrombus within the false lumen, but creatine phosphokinase (CPK) levels are normal. Occasionally the presence of thrombus may provoke a low grade coagulopathy or an elevated platelet count, particularly in distal dissections where the total volume of thrombus is larger.

7.4 Specialised imaging

All of the currently available techniques have disadvantages and to some extent the choice depends on local availability and expertise.[6-9] It is important to accept that some patients require the use of multiple imaging modalities to achieve a diagnosis (Table 7.1).

Table 7.1 Summary of specialised imaging techniques

	Angio	CT	MRI	TOE
Sensitivity	Poor	Average	Excellent	Excellent
Specificity	Good	Good	Excellent	Good
Site of tear	Good	Poor	Excellent	Good
Aortic regurgitation	Excellent	Useless	Excellent	Excellent
Pericardial effusion	Useless	Poor	Excellent	Good
Coronaries	Excellent	Useless	Good	Average

Modified from Cigarroa JE et al.[6]

7.4.1 CT scanning

Visualisation depends on demonstrating dual aortic lumens in dissection or the presence of asymmetrical thickening of the aortic wall in IMH. Its principle advantage is one of almost universal availability. The disadvantages are that the sensitivity is relatively low (80%) and that it provides no information about left ventricular function, coronary anatomy, or aortic regurgitation. In addition, the entry tear is only rarely identified. The availability of ultrafast electron beam scanners is likely to improve the diagnostic accuracy of CT within the near future.

7.4.2 Transthoracic echocardiography

The low sensitivity of this technique (60–85%) makes it of little value for detecting dissection in isolation. However, it remains useful in the management of hypotensive patients for detecting tamponade, regional wall motion abnormalities, and aortic regurgitation.

7.4.3 Transoesophageal echocardiography (TOE)

This has excellent sensitivity (99%) and is usually able to detect the exit and entry sites, although the specificity is less impressive, particularly with less experienced operators. It provides information about the proximal coronaries in addition to regional wall motion disturbances and the presence of aortic regurgitation. Its principle attraction is that it can be performed at the bedside of acutely ill patients or in the anaesthetic room prior to surgery (Figure 7.3).

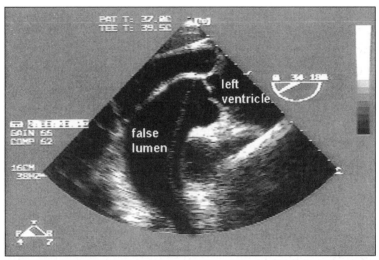

Figure 7.3 Transoesophageal echo demonstrating dual aortic lumens. It should be noted that the presence of differential flow in the two aortic lumens and ideally the presence of entry and exit sites should also be demonstrated.

7.4.4 Magnetic resonance imaging (MRI)

Although this represents the current "gold standard" technique it is not readily available in the UK and is simply impracticable for the majority of acutely ill patients. With an appropriate scanner, information on aortic regurgitation and coronary anatomy is also available but for the moment it has no place in acute management.

7.4.5 Angiography

This is now rarely used; it lacks sensitivity (<80%) and is unable to detect intramural haematomas as these do not result in a dual lumen. In addition, it tends to be difficult to organise out of hours and carries small but significant risks. Its sole advantage remains its ability to delineate coronary anatomy, but this is only occasionally required (see below, under "Specific problems" – is coronary angiography necessary prior to surgery?).

Our current policy is to employ CT scanning as the screening technique in district hospitals due to its wide availability. If this demonstrates dissection the patient is transferred to the surgical centre where shocked patients are taken directly to the operating suite. In non-shocked patients a TOE is performed after induction of anaesthesia to identify entry/exit sites and guide the surgical approach. Patients in whom there is diagnostic uncertainty after CT scanning are transferred to the surgical centre where combined transthoracic and transoesophageal echocardiography is performed on the coronary care unit (CCU). MRI is reserved for patients in whom uncertainty persists despite a TOE.

7.5 Medical management

The outlook for untreated aortic dissection and intramural haematoma is probably equally bleak and at the present time these cases should be managed identically: over 25% of patients die within the first 24 hours and up to 50% by 48 hours.[9-11] The prognosis of a rupturing thoracic aneurysm is even worse with over 75% of patients dead at 24 hours. By contrast, the natural history of penetrating atherosclerotic ulcer appears more benign although further studies are needed to clarify this.

The fundamental principle of management is that patients with dissection or haematoma involving the ascending aorta require surgery to prevent the medial extension reaching the pericardium and producing fatal tamponade. Patients with type B dissections do not benefit from the routine use of surgery. Unfortunately this "A=surgery, B=medical" divide ignores the fact that all non-shocked patients require medical management prior to surgery and that a significant minority of type B patients will not settle with optimal medical management. In addition, it produces confusion over management of dissections limited to the aortic arch where initial management should be medical. The aim of medical management is to reduce both the absolute pressure on the damaged aortic media and the rate of rise of that pressure (dP/dT). Its goals can be summarised as:

- Systolic BP < 100 mmHg.
- Pain free.
- Adequate renal perfusion (urine output > 30 ml/hr).
- No evidence of cerebral hypoperfusion.
- Minimised shear stress (β blocked to < 55/min).

Achieving these goals requires that the patient be admitted to a coronary or intensive care unit. Large bore venous access should be obtained and a urinary catheter inserted. Blood pressure should be measured in the arm with the highest reading and a radial pressure line is recommended for this. Opioid analgesia combined with an anti-emetic is required. It should be noted that the doses needed are often in excess of those used in the management of myocardial infarction and that repeat administration may be required.

The combination of reduced dP/dT and hypotension is most conveniently achieved with the combined α- and β-blocker labetalol administered iv at a rate 2–20 mg/min. Failure to control the blood pressure with labetalol may necessitate the use of nitroprusside 0.5–10 micrograms/kg/min or GTN (1–10 mg/min initially). Patients who are normotensive still require β-blockade to reduce dP/dT. Operative intervention should be considered for patients with type B dissections under certain circumstances (Box 7.2) although it should be emphasised that surgery is indicated only after failure of optimal medical management, not as a replacement for it.

Box 7.2 Indications for operation in distal dissection

- Ongoing pain/progression of dissection
- Retrograde extension into the ascending aorta
- Rupture or impending rupture
- Ischaemia due to occlusion of a major branch artery

Aortic regurgitation is frequently cited as an indication for operation in the management of distal dissections but this is only the case for regurgitation producing heart failure refractory to medical management: a very rare scenario. Having acutely controlled the blood pressure in distal dissections the patient should be transferred to an oral regimen without a loss of BP control; this will almost always require multiple anti-hypertensive agents.

7.6 Surgical management

A detailed discussion of the available surgical options in dissection and IMH is beyond the scope of this book. However, an understanding of the principles involved is helpful. The traditional operation for type A dissections aimed to isolate the dissecting media from the pericardium to prevent the fatal complication of tamponade. This was achieved by interposing a dacron graft into the ascending aorta, if this did not extend to the exit site, the distal dissection was left to heal by thrombosis. More recently the distal dissection has been sealed using tissue glue. Severe aortic regurgitation requires simultaneous aortic valve replacement, although resuspension of the native valve is an alternative. For distal dissections a dacron graft is interposed over the diseased aorta although in the near future, percutaneous stenting may provide an alternative.[12]

Rupture of a thoracic aortic aneurysm requires immediate surgery with excision followed by replacement with a dacron graft.

7.7 Specific problems

7.7.1 Differentiating dissection from infarction

Involvement of a coronary ostium by the dissection flap may produce myocardial infarction in 1–2% of patients. This generates considerable anxiety as the administration of thrombolytics to these patients usually results in fatal tamponade. Unfortunately, the routine use of chest x rays has been shown to be unhelpful in resolving this dilemma. In the vast majority of cases it is the right coronary ostium that is involved as acute left main occlusion results in sudden death, and thus the question only arises for inferior infarctions. The pain of dissection is characteristically worst at the moment it starts (in contrast to ischaemic pain which tends to intensify over several minutes) and does not have the migratory component that occurs in 70% of dissections. In addition, many of the patients who incorrectly received thrombolysis during dissection in the past had ECGs with non-specific changes which failed to meet current criteria for thrombolytic or anticoagulant administration. For these reasons the dissection/infarction dilemma is only rarely a problem in clinical practice, but if there is genuine doubt then thrombolysis should be withheld whilst specialised imaging is undertaken.

7.7.2 Differential arm blood pressures

A 5–10 mmHg difference in systolic blood pressure between the right and left arms is not uncommon and the significance of minor changes overinterpreted. Significant differences are usually in the excess of 15–20 mmHg. Conversely, not all patients with differential arm blood pressures turn out to have dissection as localised deposits of atheroma may produce subclavian stenosis.

7.7.3 Minimising delay

Probably because of its relative rarity it may be difficult to impress the vital importance of urgency when managing aortic syndromes onto the natural inertia of hospital systems. The fact that in over a third of patients with dissection this was not the initial diagnosis serves as a reminder that we need to consider the possibility of an aortic syndrome more frequently in the differential diagnosis of chest pain. In an audit of 100 patients transferred to the Oxford Cardiothoracic Centre with acute dissection it took an average of over 6 hours for the initial diagnosis to be made. Appropriate medical therapy was not instituted for a further 2 hours and, on average, adequate blood pressure control was not achieved for another 4 hours (Figure 7.4). Personal involvement of a senior physician at an early stage of management is strongly recommended for these difficult problems.

7.7.4 Patients with Marfan's syndrome

Particular care is needed in dealing with patients with Marfan's syndrome, pregnancy, or both, who present with chest pain as the risk of dissection is especially high in these groups. These are very definite exceptions to the Goldman principle of a normal ECG equating to a low risk situation.

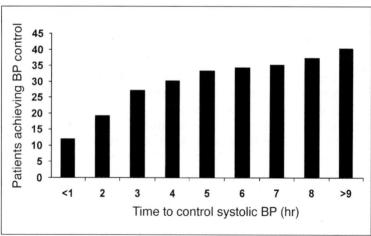

Figure 7.4 Number of patients achieving satisfactory blood pressure control in a series of 100 patients subsequently transferred to the Oxford Cardiothoracic Centre. (Figure courtesy of Percy Joki.)

7.7.5 Inadequate blood pressure control

Failure to adequately control the blood pressure is the most common management problem encountered; in the Oxford audit, only 50% of patients had achieved satisfactory control on arrival. The critical importance of reducing both pressure and shear force on the damaged aortic wall cannot be overemphasised. The aim should be a systolic BP of 100 mmHg titrated against renal and cerebral perfusion. Clearly there is a risk of cerebral ischaemia with systolic BP reductions in excess of 30%, but these risks must be weighed against the prohibitive mortality of inadequate treatment of the dissection.

The usual problem is a failure to administer a sufficient dose of labetalol: the infusion is started and the BP faithfully recorded but no further action is taken. The labetalol dose should be increased to a dose of 20–400 micrograms/kg/min and if control has not been achieved at this point second line therapy instituted; this requires analysis of which portion of labetalol's actions are proving insufficient (α- or β-blockade). The commonest scenario is one of adequate β-blockade but poor blood pressure control and under these circumstances sodium nitroprusside should be added at a dose of 20–400 micrograms/kg/min. Nitroprusside is not particularly easy to use (see Appendix) and reluctance to use it may be responsible for some of the poor hypertensive control that occurs. The mixed arterial and venous dilatation of GTN (1–10 mg/hr) is a less logical but acceptable alternative in this situation and has the advantage of familiarity. One problem with this approach is that nitrate tolerance is often troublesome, particularly in the more protracted treatment required in type B dissections.

Inadequate β-blockade should be managed by discontinuing the labetalol and using metoprolol 5 mg iv repeated every 5 minutes to a maximum of 15 mg whilst at the same time starting sodium nitroprusside or GTN. The ultra short acting β-blocker esmolol (1 mg/kg IV bolus then 150–300 micrograms/kg/min) might appear to be an attractive option, particularly in combination with sodium nitroprusside as both could be swiftly discontinued if haemodynamic deterioration occurred. Unfortunately, in our experience, adequate β-blockade is difficult to achieve within the recommended dose range.

There is insufficient use of simultaneous oral and parental medication in resistant patients who do not require immediate surgery; adding an oral calcium antagonist or ACE inhibitor often improves the acute situation and can pave the way for a gradual transition to oral medication. In general, the risks of inadequate BP control outweigh the risks of using longer acting medications, particularly after the initial 24 hours.

There is a tendency for BP to initially fall with treatment only to subsequently rise during transfer to the surgical centre. As a result these are one of the few patient groups who require transfer with a doctor as opposed to the usually excellent nurse/paramedic combination.

7.7.6 Inadequate β-blockade

Patients whose systolic BP is between 105 and 120 mmHg still require β-blockade to minimise aortic shear strain yet only rarely receive treatment. It is important to appreciate that the use of a vasodilator in isolation will actually increase aortic shear stress by widening the pulse pressure and the dP/dT of left ventricular ejection. As with the use of β-blockade in acute myocardial infarction spurious contraindications are frequently generated: in the Oxford dissection audit, only 65% of patients eligible for β-blockade received it and of these only 45% attained a pulse < 55/min. If there is genuine doubt about a patient's suitability then esmolol has a potential role in this situation but this caution is rarely justified. Alternatively, in patients with normal left ventricular function then negatively chronotropic calcium antagonists such as diltiazem (60 mg tds) or verapamil (5–10 mg IV followed as an oral dose of 40 mg tds) should be substituted.

7.7.7 Problems with pain control

Episodes of recurrent pain usually reflect inadequate control of blood pressure resulting in further cleavage of the aortic media. In the Oxford dissection audit, almost 40% of patients transferred with a diagnosis of dissection were in pain on arrival. A vicious cycle of pain $\rightarrow$ hypertension $\rightarrow$ medial damage, then becomes established. The occurrence of pain in the presence of good control of blood pressure and heart rate is an indication to expedite surgery.

7.7.8 Blood pressure control during transoesophageal echocardiography

As oesophageal intubation is uncomfortable and associated with significant BP rises, it is essential that adequate BP control is obtained before the procedure and that pressure is carefully monitored throughout. In patients in whom the diagnosis of dissection has been established but a TOE is required prior to surgery, this should be performed in the anaesthetic room following induction. This approach is sometimes advocated for all dissections but is clearly inappropriate in those in whom the diagnosis is uncertain. In these, intensive sedation is important and our preference is for midazolam (2.5–10 mg and occasionally more in 2.5 mg increments) with fentanyl (50–100 micrograms) if required. At this level of sedation skilled nursing or anaesthetic assistance is essential and in view of the fact that recovery may be protracted our policy is to consent the patient for operation at the same time as the TOE consent. This will require the participation of a member of the surgical team but this only emphasises the fact that the management of this difficult condition necessitates a collaborative approach.

7.7.9 Interpretation of transoesophageal echocardiography

Of the commonly used imaging techniques, TOE is the most operator dependent. Although the appearances of dissection are usually clear cut this is not always the case – reverberation artefacts may mimic dissection flaps, the aortic arch may be difficult to visualise and the entry tear may be elusive. Occasionally a dilated azygous vein can produce the appearances of a double aortic lumen. As a rule it is important to see the flap in two orthogonal planes, and not to rely on the presence of a flap in isolation – the critical test is the presence of differential colour flow in the two lumens. In summary, this is a difficult scan to perform and not one for the inexperienced operator to attempt single handed in the middle of the night.

7.7.10 Is coronary angiography necessary prior to surgery?

The advent of TOE has relegated angiography to a fourth place position. TOE frequently provides views of the left main stem and proximal right coronary arteries whilst the presence of segmental contraction abnormalities permits some inference as to the state of the more distal coronary anatomy. Despite this some surgeons still feel happier if a coronary angiogram is performed. However, most patients who die from aortic dissection do so from the effects of dissection itself and not co-existent coronary disease and for this reason the current trend does not favour performing coronary angiography prior to surgery.

7.7.11 Management of pericardial effusions

As noted above, the presence of a pericardial effusion is a grave prognostic sign and an indication for immediate surgery. No attempt should normally be made to tap these effusions as decompression usually results in torrential bleeding, fed from the false lumen via the pericardium.[5] The only exception to this is in patients who arrest prior to surgery or who develop profound shock. In these, the insertion of a wide bore needle into the pericardial space may permit their immediate transfer to the operating theatre, although the prognosis at this point remains very poor.

7.7.12 Failing to recognise mesenteric ischaemia

Mesenteric ischaemia is a feared complication of distal dissections. It tends to present with non-specific abdominal discomfort with few accompanying signs (although a declining plasma bicarbonate level may provide a clue). By the time the problem has become clinically apparent the situation is usually irretrievable. Cyanide poisoning due to excess sodium nitroprusside administration may occasionally present as abdominal discomfort.

7.7.13 Postoperative care

It is not uncommon for physicians who diligently performed the pre-operative imaging to neglect to see the patient with a type A dissection postoperatively (they have, after all, "been cured" by the operation). In reality these patients' blood pressure still requires meticulous control (systolic BP < 130 mmHg), both in the immediate postoperative phase and following hospital discharge. Particular difficulty may be encountered in patients who have undergone arch repairs due to the removal of aortic baroreceptors.

7.7.14 Anticoagulation in aortic dissection

Thrombosis of the intimal flap is central to the resolution of all medically managed dissections and in those postoperative patients in whom the distal flap has not been glued. For this reason all anticoagulation must be aggressively reversed, however compelling the original indication.

7.7.15 Failure to settle with distal dissections

Distal dissection is frequently perceived as a relatively benign disease, which it is not. Although it lacks the early risk of sudden death due to tamponade, controlling the blood pressure often proves to be a protracted battle in an elderly population with significant co-morbidity. It is important to initiate oral anti-hypertensive agents as soon as possible and aim to have discontinued all IV drugs by 24–36 hours as this tends to produce more consistent BP control.

7.7.16 Uncertainties in the management of intramural haematoma

The concept of intramural haematoma is a relatively recent one and the belief that it should be managed in a similar fashion to dissection is only based on very small numbers of patients.[8, 11] As more experience is gained it may be possible to define a subgroup of patients with ascending aortic haematomas in whom conservative management is appropriate. Similarly, there is currently uncertainty concerning the management of patients with aortic tears but no evidence of haematoma which will hopefully be clarified by future work.

Clinical cases

Case 7.1

A 42-year-old man with a six month history of hypertension presented to the on-call surgical team with pain and numbness in his left leg which was noted to be pulseless. Direct questioning revealed an episode of severe chest pain some hours earlier and he was referred for a medical opinion. Clinical examination confirmed a pulseless left leg, a BP of 180/105 mmHg, and aortic regurgitation. Pulses were reduced in his left arm and were accompanied by a 40 mmHg reduction in his systolic BP. Chest x ray and ECG were both unremarkable and a thoracic CT with contrast was reported as being normal. Transthoracic echocardiography demonstrated mild dilatation of his aortic root with left ventricular hypertrophy and moderate aortic regurgitation but no evidence of dissection. The aortic regurgitation was attributed to his hypertension and as a dissection was felt to have been excluded he was admitted overnight for observation. Eight hours later he developed further chest pain swiftly followed by cardiac arrest with pulseless electrical activity. Post mortem confirmed a type A dissection with pre-terminal rupture into the pericardium.

Negative transthoracic echocardiography and CT scans do not exclude dissection. A TOE or MRI is essential in patients where the index of suspicion is high and no diagnosis has been made. A subgroup of patients with aortic tears but little in the way of medial haemorrhage may cause particular difficulty.

Case 7.2

A 60-year-old man with poorly controlled hypertension who was receiving haemodialysis presented with severe chest pain radiating to his back. A TOE demonstrated an intramural haematoma in his descending aorta with no flow within the haematoma or visible entry/exit points. His hypertension and pain initially settled with intensification of his medical management but six days later he experienced further pain and TOE was repeated. This revealed flow within the media with well defined entry and exit points. His pain and BP again settled with medical management and as there was no vascular compromise associated with the dissection he was successfully managed medically.

An intra-aortic haematoma can progress to true dissection, supporting the contention that in some patients the initiating event is one of medial haemorrhage as opposed to an intimal tear. Management is the same as it would be for a classical dissection at the same site.

Further reading

Spittell PC, Aortic dissection, diagnosis and management. In: Brown DL, ed. *Cardiac Intensive Care*. WB Saunders, Philadelphia, 1998.

References

1 Eagle KA, Quertermous T, Kritzer GA, *et al*. Spectrum of conditions initially suggesting acute aortic dissection but with negative aortograms. *Am J Cardiol* 1986;**57**:322–26.
2 Rosman HS, Patel S, Borzak S, Paone G, Retter K. Quality of history taking in patients with aortic dissection. *Chest* 1998;**114**:793–5.
3 Spittell PC, Spittell JAJ, Joyce JW, *et al*. Clinical features and differential diagnosis of aortic dissection: experience with 236 cases (1980 through 1990). *Mayo Clinic Proceedings* 1993;**68**:642–51.
4 O'Gara PT, DeSanctis RW. Acute aortic dissection and its variants. Toward a common diagnostic and therapeutic approach. *Circulation* 1995;**92**:1376–8.
5 Isselbacher EM, Cigarroa JE, Eagle KA. Cardiac tamponade complicating proximal aortic dissection. Is pericardiocentesis harmful? *Circulation* 1994;**90**:2375–8.
6 Cigarroa JE, Isselbacher EM, DeSanctis RW, Eagle KA. Diagnostic imaging in the evaluation of suspected aortic dissection. Old standards and new directions. *N Engl J Med* 1993;**328**:35–43.
7 Svensson LG, Labib SB, Eisenhauer AC, Butterly JR. Intimal tear without hematoma: an important variant of aortic dissection that can elude current imaging techniques. *Circulation* 1999;**99**:1331–6.
8 Kodolitsch Y, Krause N, Spielmann R, Nienaber CA. Diagnostic potential of combined transthoracic echocardiography and x ray computed tomography in suspected aortic dissection. *Clin Cardiol* 1999;**22**:345–52.

9 Kang DH, Song JK, Song MG, *et al*. Clinical and echocardiographic outcomes of aortic intramural hemorrhage compared with acute aortic dissection. *Am J Cardiol* 1998;**81**:202–6.
10 Glower DD, Fann JI, Speier RH, *et al*. Comparison of medical and surgical therapy for uncomplicated descending aortic dissection. *Circulation* 1990;**82**: IV39–46.
11 Nienaber CA, von Kodolitsch Y, Petersen B, *et al*. Intramural hemorrhage of the thoracic aorta. Diagnostic and therapeutic implications. *Circulation* 1995;**92**:1465–72.
12 Nienaber CA, Fattori R, Lund G, *et al*. Nonsurgical reconstruction of thoracic aortic dissection by stent-graft placement. *N Engl J Med* 1999; **340**:1539–45.
13 Linsday J, *et al*. Aortic dissection. *Heart Dis Stroke* 1992;**1**:69.

8: Pulmonary embolism

KM CHANNON, Y BASHIR

8.1 Background

Pulmonary embolism (PE) is an important and potentially life-threatening condition which needs to be considered in the differential diagnosis of a wide range of acute cardiorespiratory syndromes (dyspnoea, chest pain, haemodynamic collapse, etc.). It is common but also commonly misdiagnosed. Recent clinicopathological surveys have shown that PE was not suspected on clinical grounds in up to 70% of patients in whom it was subsequently shown to be a major cause of death.[1] Conversely, post mortem studies have also failed to confirm a clinical diagnosis of PE in a significant proportion of cases.[2] Thus, PE is both underdiagnosed (patients fail to receive treatment for a life-threatening condition) and overdiagnosed (patients unnecessarily hospitalised and exposed to the hazard of inappropriate anticoagulant therapy). The problem stems partly from over-reliance on ventilation-perfusion (V/Q) isotope scanning to diagnose or exclude PE, and too little use of pulmonary angiography in cases where the diagnosis is uncertain. Recent research including the PIOPED study have clarified the role and limitations of traditional diagnostic tests for PE. However, this is an evolving field and there may be a growing role for new imaging modalities such as spiral CT scanning and MRI, as well as for measurement of plasma D-dimer levels to rule out thromboembolic disease. The need for prompt, accurate diagnosis has never been greater as high-risk patients are being increasingly considered for thrombolytic therapy.

Although the situation has undoubtedly improved over the last few decades, many of the clinical challenges in the diagnosis and treatment of PE remain unchanged.[3] A high degree of clinical suspicion, appropriate use of investigations and awareness of the immediate aims of therapy remain central to the management of this important medical emergency.[4]

8.2 Diagnosis

Diagnosis is based on initial clinical assessment of the likelihood of PE, combined with the results of investigations. Bedside assessment of the patient requires awareness of the disparate clinical presentations of PE, and of the predisposing conditions or risk factors for venous thromboembolism generally. Numerous modalities have been used for investigation of patients with suspected PE, but not all of these will be accessible or appropriate for each individual case. In particular, gold standard tests such as pulmonary angiography may not be immediately available. Accurate diagnosis of PE often depends on understanding the limitations of particular investigations in the specific clinical context, rather than relying on any single test.

8.2.1 Clinical features

The disparate clinical presentations of PE reflect variability in the size and time course of the embolic episode(s), and the cardiovascular status of the patient in which they occur. A small PE may cause no haemodynamic compromise, be asymptomatic, or result in pleuritic pain, breathlessness, and haemoptysis. Larger PE causes increasing haemodynamic compromise, hypoxia, tachycardia, and ultimately profound hypoxia, hypotension, collapse, and death. A smaller PE may cause a marked clinical deterioration in a patient with existing cardiorespiratory compromise. In contrast to these acute presentations, multiple chronic PE may be asymptomatic until symptoms of chronic pulmonary hypertension develop: exertional breathlessness and right heart failure.

The key to the diagnosis and treatment of PE is recognition that while the range of clinical presentations is wide, PE *commonly* presents as distinct clinical syndromes:

- *Pleurisy ± haemoptysis*: small or moderate PE causing peripheral rather than central pulmonary artery occlusion, with segmental pulmonary infarction. Patients may not exhibit hypoxia or signs of cardiopulmonary disturbance. Localising clinical or radiographic signs are more common.
- *Dyspnoea and hypoxia* in the absence of other causes suggests PE: usually moderate or large, with signs of cardiopulmonary disturbance (tachycardia, tachypnoea, elevated JVP).
- *Circulatory collapse*: a common presentation in hospitalised patients with large or massive PE. Typically a high risk patient (often postoperative) with unheralded collapse or unexplained clinical deterioration, with hypotension, tachycardia, and hypoxia. In patients with coexisting pulmonary or cardiac disease, their lack of reserve may result in this presentation even with small or moderate PE.

Overall, the most common symptoms and signs in PE are (in order of decreasing frequency): dyspnoea, tachypnoea, pleuritic pain, tachycardia, cough, haemoptysis, and features of deep vein thrombosis (DVT). These findings have either low sensitivity or low specificity for PE, so that clinical features alone are inadequate for diagnosis. However, the clinical features are of crucial importance as they provide the context for the interpretation of diagnostic tests (see below). Furthermore, whilst clinical features alone cannot be used to make a positive diagnosis of PE, their absence may be very useful in helping to rule out PE from the differential diagnosis.

Tachypnoea (respiratory rate >20/min) emerges in several studies as the most useful clinical sign, and one that can be objectively measured and recorded. Less than 10% of patients with confirmed PE are not tachypnoeic, only 3% have neither tachypnoea nor pleuritic pain, and the additional findings of a normal CXR and blood gases virtually exclude PE (see below).[5-7] In particular, young patients, often women using oral contraceptives, are often referred with isolated pleuritic pain. However the absence of other risk factors, age < 40, respiratory rate < 20/min and a normal CXR makes PE extremely unlikely.

8.2.2 Clinical risk factors

In accordance with Virchow's triad, venous thrombosis and subsequent PE depend principally on abnormalities of blood flow and/or coagulability in the deep veins of the lower limb. Predisposing factors are found in 90% of patients with PE in most studies, so the identification of risk factors is an important aid to the diagnosis or PE.

Recent surgery is a strong risk factor. In minor surgery, the risk of PE is very low, but in major abdominal, gynaecological or lower limb surgery, especially for malignancy or fracture, the risk of PE is at least 5%. In non-surgical patients, immobility due to stroke or other neurological injury, and intensive care admissions for >3 days indicate high risk. Other cardiorespiratory disorders, notably recent myocardial infarction (MI) and heart failure, and any malignancy (but particularly uterus, pancreas, breast, and stomach) are also important risk factors. Box 8.1 shows the specific risk factors with most predictive value in a large prospective study of 1200 patients with suspected PE.[5,6] Of note, the significance of oral contraception as a predisposing factor in young women (< 40 years) tends to be overestimated in clinical practice. PE is frequently suspected if such patients present with isolated pleuritic chest pain but is almost never confirmed unless there are associated features such as tachypnoea, hypoxia, or abormalities on the chest x ray.

Box 8.1 Specific risk factors for PE

- Surgery within 12 weeks
- Immobilisation for > 3 days in last 4 weeks, or paralysis
- Previous DVT or PE
- Lower limb fracture
- Family history of DVT or PE
- Malignancy in last 6 months
- Postpartum

Always consider PE in the setting of **unexplained collapse, hypotension, or hypoxia** in hospitalised patients, especially if postoperative or those with cancer or heart failure, even in the apparent absence of "classical" features

8.2.3 Investigations

Chest x ray

Whilst mandatory in a patient with an acute cardiorespiratory syndrome, the value of a chest x ray (CXR) in the diagnosis of PE lies as much in its ability to diagnose other conditions that may be confused with PE, such as pulmonary oedema or pneumonia. Several radiographic features of PE on the CXR are described, including hypoperfusion of one lung or lobe, and features of infarction (segmental shadows, pleural effusion, loss of volume). Often, the most useful aspect of a chest film in acute PE is that the lung fields appear relatively normal, or that any abnormalities appear minor in relation to the degree of clinical cardiorespiratory compromise.

Blood gases

Haemodynamically significant PE causes ventilation-perfusion mismatching and results in hypoxia. Compensatory hyperventilation results in a reduced Pa_{CO_2}, so that the calculated A–a gradient is increased.[a] In PIOPED patients with PE (see "V/Q scanning", below), 15–38% had Pa_{O_2} > 11 kPa, Pa_{CO_2} > 5 kPa and/or A–a gradient < 3 kPa, suggesting that blood gas determination alone is of little individual use in either confirming or excluding PE.[8] However, the finding of hypoxia and/or an increased A–a gradient in a patient without known pulmonary disease clearly increases clinical suspicion and identifies significant V/Q mismatch that demands diagnosis. More recent studies than PIOPED, possibly including more patients with a high pre-test probability of PE, found that a Pao_2 >11 kPa is valuable in excluding PE, especially if combined with other factors.[7]

ECG

ECG changes are very common in PE (80–90%), but are usually non-specific, e.g. sinus tachycardia, or minor ST and T wave abnormalities, which are of little use in either diagnosing or excluding PE. In large or massive PE, the more classical ECG features of acute right ventricular strain (S1, Q3, T3) right bundle branch block (RBBB) or atrial fibrillation (AF) are more common. The value of ECG in the assessment of PE lies as much in the exclusion of other cardiorespiratory emergencies such as acute myocardial infarction with right ventricular involvement.

D-dimer

Endogenous lysis of cross-linked fibrin clot leads to the release of cross-linked fibrin degradation products or D-dimers. The availability of convenient latex agglutination tests and rapid ELISA tests to measure D-dimer levels in plasma has resulted in its widespread use in the evaluation of suspected thromboembolism. Unfortunately, D-dimer levels are elevated in a wide range of conditions including recent surgery, malignancy, and inflammatory states, and 60–75% of patients with suspected PE will have high D-dimer levels due to the high incidence of these and other conditions in this patient group. However, the value of D-dimer testing lies in its ability to exclude PE if D-dimer levels are not elevated. Several studies suggest that the negative predictive value of D-dimer levels < 500 ng/ml for excluding PE is as high as 99%,[9] and that this diagnostic power is increased even further in combination

---

[a]The alveolar-arterial (A–a) oxygen difference is estimated by subtracting the sum of the arterial Po_2 and the arterial Pco_2/R (R = gas exchange ratio, approximates to 0.8) from the inspired Po_2. Inspired Po_2 is Fio_2 (in %) x 100 kPa. Room air is Fio_2 21%, inspired Po_2 21 kPa. With Pao_2 11 kPa whilst breathing room air, $Paco_2$ should be approximately 5.6 kPa if A–a gradient is 3 kPa.

with clinical features and blood gas estimation[6,7,10] The principal limitations to this approach are: (i) D-dimer will only be useful in a minority of patients with suspected PE; (ii) D-dimer tests are not always available urgently; and (iii) there is concern about reproducibility between the different types of latex and ELISA tests in use by different centres.

> Elevated D-dimers are not useful in diagnosing PE. However, a normal D-dimer level (< 500 ng/ml) excludes PE with 95–99% certainty; combined with $Pao_2 > 11$ kPa and respiratory rate < 20/min excludes PE with almost 100% certainty.[6]

Echocardiography

Echocardiography is of little value for the diagnosis of PE in haemodynamically stable patients presenting with isolated dyspnoea or pleuritic chest pain. In patients with large or massive PE, transthoracic echocardiography may occasionally detect large thrombi in the pulmonary artery or right heart chambers.[11] More commonly the findings reflect the haemodynamic effects of acute right heart strain: dilatation and hypokinesia of the RA and RV, flattening or bulging of the interventricular septum, and raised pulmonary artery (PA) pressure (calculated from the velocity of the tricuspid regurgitation (TR) jet) may all be useful indicators. However, the overall sensitivity and specificity of echocardiography for diagnosis of PE are low.[12] Rather, the principal utility of echocardiography is the evaluation of haemodynamically compromised patients with suspected massive PE to exclude alternative cardiac diagnoses such as tamponade, right ventricular infarction, or aortic dissection, rather than making the diagnosis of PE itself. Echocardiography may also be useful in assessing the acute haemodynamic response to treatment such as thrombolysis.

Transoesophageal echocardiography (TOE) may be more sensitive for detecting PE in the pulmonary arteries, but no data support its use as a first line diagnostic investigation. However, TOE may be useful in individual cases, for example in ventilated patients on the intensive therapy unit (ITU), when TOE is more readily performed than other diagnostic modalities.

V/Q scanning (Figure 8.1b)

Isotope ventilation-perfusion scanning has gained widespread popularity for the assessment of possible PE due to its ease and safety. It relies on the fact that a significant PE will result in regional hypoperfusion of a segment or lobe without a corresponding defect in ventilation (Figure 8.1a). To simplify the procedure, a normal CXR is sometimes used as a surrogate to imply normal ventilation.

However, V/Q scans have low sensitivity and specificity, especially in the patients who are at risk from PE and most difficult to diagnose clinically, e.g. coexistent pulmonary disease, postoperative atelectasis, and heart failure, that all cause abnormalities of ventilation and or perfusion. The transient nature of PE, delay before scanning and the early response to treatment may result in loss of detectable V/Q mismatch (Box 8.2).

The PIOPED Study (Prospective Investigation of Pulmonary Embolism Diagnosis) is the largest study of V/Q scanning in PE, carried out in six centres in the USA between 1985 and 1986, and published in 1990.[13] Approximately 950 patients had V/Q scanning, of whom 750 also underwent pulmonary angiography, enabling a direct evaluation of the sensitivity and specificity of V/Q scanning in the diagnosis of PE, compared with the "gold standard" of pulmonary angiography. The results are summarised in Tables 8.1 and 8.2.

Only 25% had normal or high probability scans; all others had low or intermediate scans. The true incidence of PE by angiography was 33%; 64% had no evidence of PE on angiography and in only 3% was the angiogram uncertain.

Table 8.1 PIOPED Study: main results.

Diagnostic category	% total scans (N=931)	% total angiograms (N=755)	Sensitivity of VQ scan for PE	Specificity of VQ scan for PE	Positive predictive value of V/Q scan	Negative predictive value of V/Q scan
High	13	33	0.41	0.97	0.88	
Intermediate	39	3			0.30	
Low	34	0				0.84–0.88
Normal	14	64				0.91–0.96

Table 8.2 Proportion of patients with proven PE according to initial clinical assessment and V/Q scan results in the PIOPED Study.

	Clinical probability of PE		
V/Q scan result	Highly likely	Uncertain	Unlikely
High probability	96%	88%	56%
Intermediate probability	66%	28%	16%
Low probability	40%	16%	4%
Normal	0%	6%	2%

The PIOPED study also required clinicians to assess the clinical likelihood of PE before V/Q scan and angiography. A high clinical likelihood of PE in combination with a high probability V/Q scan increased the positive predictive value to 0.96, whereas a low clinical suspicion in combination with a low probability or normal V/Q scan increased the negative predictive value to 0.96. Importantly, if PE was considered likely on clinical grounds, the diagnosis was subsequently confirmed in 40% of patients with a low probability V/Q scan.

Box 8.2 V/Q scanning: advantages and disadvantages

V/Q scanning: good points

A **high probability scan** or a **normal scan** are diagnostically powerful (>95%), especially in the setting of high or low clinical suspicion.

V/Q scanning: limitations

More than 75% of scans will be in the low or intermediate category which are less useful in either confirming or excluding the diagnosis.

Less than half of the patients with a proven diagnosis of PE will have a high probability V/Q scan.

The PIOPED study had significant limitations, not least that only 931 out of 5600 eligible patients underwent V/Q scanning, and only 81% of these underwent pulmonary angiography. Nevertheless, the important message from the PIOPED study is that V/Q scanning is helpful in the diagnosis of PE, but needs to be interpreted in the context of the clinical likelihood of PE. In particular, the large majority of scans that are intermediate probability for PE should not be used to either confirm or refute the diagnosis. In the PISA-PED study,[14] only perfusion scans were performed, and a normal CXR substituted for a normal ventilation scan, without any apparent loss of diagnostic accuracy.

Detection of deep venous thrombosis

Pulmonary embolism is almost always a consequence of thrombosis in the deep veins of the thigh, although in most cases of PE this is asymptomatic. Thus, detection of deep venous thrombosis (DVT) in the setting of suspected pulmonary embolism may guide diagnosis and management decisions. Imaging of femoral veins is indicated in patients who either have symptoms suggestive of DVT, since confirmation of this diagnosis alone warrants anticoagulation even if embolisation has not definitely occurred; or when investigations for suspected PE, in particular V/Q scanning, are indeterminate.

Contrast venography
This is highly sensitive and specific for detection of DVT. Although considered the "gold standard', contrast venography is modestly invasive and time-consuming.

Ultrasound techniques
These have emerged as safe, non-invasive and highly accurate alternatives to contrast venography for the assessment of DVT.[10,15] Techniques usually involve B-mode (brightness modulation) and Doppler (the combination is duplex ultrasonography) to produce real-time images of the venous lumen and blood flow, in the femoral and popliteal veins. The critical test is compressibility of the venous lumen: complete *compression* excludes thrombus, whereas failure to compress with gentle pressure from the probe suggests thrombus, especially in combination with reduced blood flow and intraluminal echoes.

Ultrasound detects first episodes of thigh DVT with a sensitivity and specificity of more than 95%, giving positive and negative predictive values for the diagnosis or exclusion of DVT of 95–100%,[15,16] although this diagnostic accuracy is

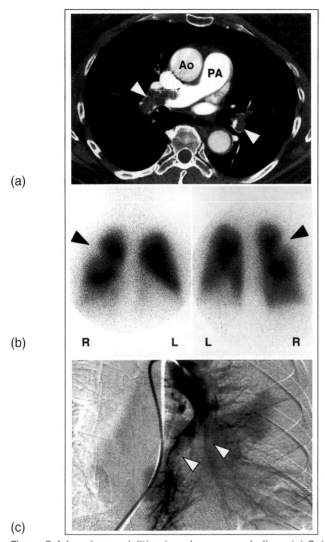

(a)

(b)

(c)

Figure 8.1 Imaging modalities in pulmonary embolism. (a) Spiral CT. White arrowheads show large embolus in main right pulmonary artery, and emboli in left lobar pulmonary artery. PA=pulmonary artery, Ao=aorta. (b) Isotope perfusion scans show anterior (left panel) and posterior (right panel) projections. Segmental defect in right upper lobe (black arrowheads) is highly suggestive of pulmonary embolism. (c) Pulmonary angiography shows selective injection of left main pulmonary artery. A large filling defect, caused by an embolus, is visible in a major branch of the left lower lobe pulmonary artery, and another branch is virtually occluded (white arrowheads).

compromised by previous episodes of DVT, or in technically difficult patients (e.g. post-orthopaedic surgery). Ultrasonography does not detect below knee thrombosis, but the risk of significant thromboembolism from these small veins is low.

In patients with suspected PE but a non-diagnostic V/Q scan, the finding of DVT on venous ultrasound makes PE very likely and mandates anticoagulation. If no DVT is found in this setting, previous PE is not excluded (the thrombus may have already embolised), but the risk of subsequent episodes of significant DVT or PE is low: approximately 2% over 6 months, allowing deferment of anticoagulation and completion of other investigations.[15] In patients with previous DVT or continued diagnostic uncertainty, serial venous ultrasonography increases diagnostic yield further by excluding progressive DVT.

Pulmonary angiography (Figure 8.1c)

Contrast angiography of the pulmonary arteries, via a catheter inserted through the right heart, has been regarded as the "gold standard" investigation for the diagnosis of PE. Unfortunately, this modality is greatly underused in the UK. Despite recommendations that pulmonary angiography should be considered in up to one-third of patients with suspected PE,[16,17] the majority of hospitals do not have a pulmonary angiography service, and those that do perform very few angiograms so that expertise is limited. Pulmonary angiography is perceived as costly and risky, although the incidence of serious complications or death, even in unstable patients is only 0.3–1.0 % in most studies.

Pulmonary angiography should be considered in patients with suspected PE who are haemodynamically unstable, when thrombolysis should be given if the diagnosis is confirmed, or when other investigations have failed to provide a diagnosis. Evidence strongly supports the wider use of pulmonary angiography in UK patients with suspected PE.

New CT and MRI modalities

Recent developments in CT and MRI technology allow imaging of the pulmonary arteries to detect thrombi[18,19]. Spiral CT scanning involves movement of the patient through a rotating scanner. Rapid, continuous scans can be obtained during a single breath hold. Spiral CT detects thrombi in the main, lobar, and segmental pulmonary arteries, with sensitivities of 73–97% and specificities of 86–98% when compared with pulmonary angiography (Figure 8.1a).[18] Electron beam CT has a very rapid acquisition time, making breath-holding unnecessary.

Magnetic resonance angiography using gadolinium enhancement offers a new non-invasive approach to PE diagnosis. Thrombi in segmental and subsegmental arteries can be detected with sensitivities and specificities of 75 to 100% and 95 to 100%, respectively.[20] In addition, MRI has the potential to detect pulmonary artery and leg vein thrombi at the same time, and to differentiate new from old thrombi.[18]

In centres with spiral CT facilities, this modality is becoming the non-invasive investigation of choice for diagnosis of PE. However, electron beam CT and MR angiography are only available in specialist centres, and experience with these techniques is still limited. While these modalities are promising for the future, at present they have limited potential in the management of most patients with possible PE in district hospitals in the UK.

Summary: diagnostic approach to PE (Figure 8.2)

An assessment of the likelihood of PE, based on specific risk factors plus the clinical parameters, arterial blood gases and CXR remains central to the diagnosis of PE, and directs early therapy. V/Q scanning is a useful non-invasive tool which may add to the diagnostic certainty, but must be interpreted within the clinical context. Pulmonary angiography should be considered when rapid and accurate diagnosis is required; spiral CT is an alternative in an increasing number of centres.

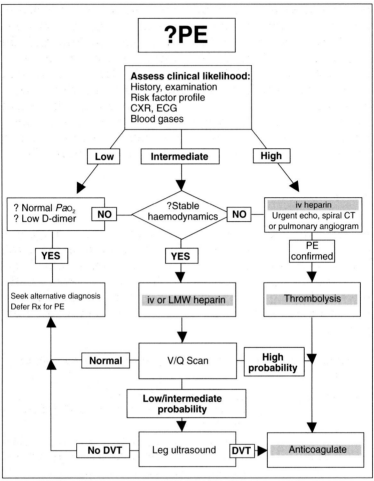

Figure 8.2 Diagnostic approach in patients with suspected pulmonary embolism.

8.3 Treatment of pulmonary embolism: acute management

The treatment of PE depends on the clinical syndrome: the management of the acutely ill patient with massive PE differs greatly from the management of a patient with a small, haemodynamically insignificant PE. Overall, treatment of PE involves measures for circulatory compromise or collapse, prevention of further thromboembolic events, and long-term prophylaxis against continued thromboembolism and the associated complications. In contrast to acute MI, however, the treatment of PE is hampered by lack of large-scale randomised controlled trials, and the inadequacies of rapid diagnostic tests. For these reasons, treatment is usually instituted whilst the diagnosis is still being confirmed; immediate measures being used to stabilise the patient until further diagnostic information can be obtained (Box 8.3).

8.3.1 Oxygen

All patients with suspected PE should receive oxygen; if oxygen is given at a known percentage via a venturi mask, this will not compromise the utility of arterial blood gas estimation. Hypoxic patients with acute PE, even in the presence of chronic obstructive pulmonary disease, have a strong respiratory drive, so CO_2 retention is not a significant concern.

Box 8.3 Management of pulmonary embolism according to presentation

? Small PE	S/C heparin if PE suspected Warfarin following confirmation of diagnosis with V/Q scan
? Large or massive PE	Immediate maximal O_2; IV heparin and IV fluids if CXR and ECG exclude MI/pulmonary oedema
	Consider echocardiography, spiral CT or pulmonary angiography if clinical conditions and local availability allow
	If haemodynamic compromise or deterioration, thrombolysis with tPA 100 mg over 2 hours, then continued IV heparin
	For massive PE, alternative is surgical embolectomy if available immediately
Multiple chronic PE	Warfarin. Refer for outpatient cardiological assessment

8.3.2 Intravenous fluids

Intravenous colloid should be given in patients with suspected PE and hypotension, in order to maintain a high central venous pressure and increase right heart filling pressures. Diuretics and/or vasodilators, including opiates, are contraindicated.

8.3.3 Heparin

Immediate heparin remains the cornerstone of treatment for acute PE. Heparin should be administered when there is intermediate or high clinical suspicion of PE, whilst investigations are completed. Unfractioned intravenous heparin should be given as an initial bolus of 5000–10000 U, followed by a weight-adjusted infusion to prolong the APTT to 2–2.5 times the control value. Bolus IV heparin remains preferable in large or massive PE, on account of its immediate effect. However, evidence suggests that subcutaneous low molecular weight (LMW) heparin is at least as effective as unfractionated IV heparin in patients with small or moderate PE. The THESEE Study[21] compared dose-adjusted unfractionated IV heparin with a single daily sc dose of 175 lU/kg tinzaparin in 612 patients with PE proven on angiography or V/Q scan, but stable enough not to justify thrombolysis or embolectomy. There were no differences in mortality, haemodynamic end points, or in major bleeding between the study groups at 8 or 90 days.

> Heparin should be given to all patients with suspected PE unless there are contraindications. For large PE, bolus IV heparin is indicated; for other patients, sc LMW heparin is an equally effective convenient alternative

8.3.4 Thrombolytics

Following the success of thrombolysis in acute myocardial infarction, a large number of studies have evaluated the use of urokinase (UK), streptokinase (SK) or tissue plasminogen activator (tPA) in acute pulmonary embolism.[22] Compared with anticoagulation, thrombolysis results in more rapid clot lysis, faster restoration of pulmonary blood flow, and improved right heart haemodynamics.[23] Thrombolysis may produce dramatic improvement in some patients with massive PE and shock. All of these studies, however, even in randomised trials such as PAIMS 2,[24] have tended to include small numbers of patients, have used surrogate end points of haemodynamic improvement, and have not been powered to detect effects on mortality. Conversely, the German registry study,[23] whilst not randomised, included >1000 patients, and found that thrombolysis was associated with significantly improved 30 day survival in patients without shock but with evidence of haemodynamic compromise and/or right ventricular dysfunction, compared with heparin alone.

All of the thrombolytic agents approved for the treatment of PE appear to be equally effective, although tPA may result in more rapid clot lysis in the first 2 hours. Major haemorrhage may be more common with UK. Bolus therapy with tPA appears no more effective than a 2 hour infusion, nor does direct infusion into the pulmonary artery confer additional benefit over systemic administration.

Concern over bleeding complications has continued to limit the use of thrombolytics in PE. Major bleeding, notably from puncture sites, GI tract, or retroperitoneum, is a significant risk and may occur in up to half of PE patients treated with thrombolytic drugs. However, the incidence of intracranial haemorrhage (ICH) in a total of nearly 900 patients in randomised studies was only 1.2%, and fatal ICH 0.6%.[22]

Current evidence supports the use of thrombolytics in patients with PE presenting with systemic hypotension or systemic hypoperfusion, where the risks of bleeding are outweighed by the potential benefit of rapid clot dissolution and haemodynamic improvement. Their use in patients with "softer" evidence of haemodynamic compromise, such as echocardiographic evidence of right ventricular strain, remains controversial.

Thrombolysis with TPA should be first line treatment for patients with PE in the presence of hypotension, severe hypoxia, or other evidence of marked haemodynamic compromise

8.3.5 Surgical embolectomy

Immediate surgical embolectomy, with or without cardiopulmonary bypass, provides an option to rapidly restore the circulation and oxygenation in patients with massive PE and circulatory collapse. Comparisons of surgical embolectomy have been performed, but these are very small studies, often non-randomised and have shown that the mortality of patients undergoing surgical embolectomy is substantial (> 30%), as expected in this high-risk group.[25] The requirement for preoperative cardiopulmonary resuscitation (CPR) is an indicator of poor outcome (> 70% mortality), and whilst immediate embolectomy in the setting of circulatory arrest may occasionally be life saving, rapid institution of cardiopulmonary bypass allows embolectomy under more controlled conditions.[26] Embolectomy may offer an alternative to patients with PE and severe circulatory compromise in whom thrombolytics are contraindicated or have been ineffective.[26] However, the principal limitation of surgical embolectomy as a treatment strategy for massive PE lies in the fact that specialised cardiothoracic units are not immediately available to the majority of patients sick enough to justify this approach.

8.4 Treatment of pulmonary embolism: long-term issues

8.4.1 Long-term anticoagulation

Initial treatment with heparin should be followed by commencement of oral anticoagulation with warfarin as soon as the diagnosis of PE is confirmed, aiming for a INR of 2.0–3.0. For PE in the setting of a remediable underlying cause (e.g. surgery, immobility), anticoagulation for 6 weeks is adequate. Other patients in whom predisposing factors might be considered to continue (e.g. heart failure), the incidence of recurrent PE is significant, and anticoagulation should be continued for longer: usually 3 or 6 months. Some studies show no benefit of continuing warfarin for 6 months compared with 6 weeks,[27] although after a second episode of confirmed venous thromboembolism, long term warfarin significantly reduces further recurrences.[28] However, recent data indicate that even after a first episode of thromboembolism, the risk of recurrence after completing 3 months anticoagulation is high: 35% in the following 2 years. The recurrence rate can be reduced to < 5% by continuing warfarin treatment throughout this time,[29] although with no apparent mortality benefit.

8.4.2 IVC filters

The use of filter devices, inserted percutaneously into the IVC, aims to limit embolisation of deep vein thrombosis to the lungs. The original Greenfield filter is a wire "umbrella" that is deployed by self expansion from a catheter sheath, and held in place with small hooks on the ends of the wire struts. However, this device is generally not removable, and complications include filter embolisation, occlusion, or continued embolism of thrombus originating from the filter itself or through venous collaterals that develop when the filter occludes. Newer filter designs may be inserted temporarily and removed percutaneously.

IVC filters should be considered in patients with PE and confirmed leg vein thrombosis in whom anticoagulation is contraindicated, or when embolism continues despite adequate anticoagulation. The wider use of IVC filters, however, is not supported by any clinical trial evidence.

8.4.3 Screening for thrombophilia

Recognition of genetic and systemic disorders that predispose to a prothrombotic state has received considerable attention.[30] Routine screening for thrombophilia is not justified, but in selected groups of patients, the diagnostic yield is high (Box 8.4). Exhaustive screening for anticoagulant deficiency and/or genetic variants in clotting factors reveals one or more defects in 75% of patients with recurrent thromboembolism. Conversely, there is no need for screening for thrombophilia in patients in whom an isolated PE occurs in the setting of a temporary high-risk setting, e.g. postoperative. Also consider other pro-thrombotic conditions such as malignancy, Bechet's disease, or paroxysmal nocturnal haemoglobinuria.

Box 8.4 When to screen for thrombophilia

A thrombophilia should be considered in patients presenting with PE when:

- *Age <40 with no other risk factor*
- *First degree relative with a history of venous thromboembolism*
- *Previous episodes of venous thromboembolism*

If a thrombophilia screen is to be undertaken, **blood samples must be taken before commencing warfarin therapy** for tests of proteins S and C, antithrombin III, and lupus anticoagulant (Table 8.3). Tests for anticardiolipin antibodies and for genetic polymorphisms are not affected by warfarin.

Table 8.3 Thrombotic variants to be tested for before undertaking warfarin therapy

Thrombotic variant	How common?	Recurrent VTE risk	Comments
Antithrombin III deficiency	5% in recurrent VTE [31]	High (20–30 × controls); 2%/ year; 70–100% cumulative risk of VTE by age 50	
Protein S deficiency	5% in recurrent VTE [31]		
Protein C deficiency	0.5% in patients with VTE [27], 3-5% in recurrent VTE [31]		

Table 8.3 Thrombotic variants to be tested for before undertaking warfarin therapy (continued)

Thrombotic variant	How common?	Recurrent VTE risk	Comments
Factor V Leiden	25–40% of VTE patients 3–13% of Caucasians Rare in Japanese, Africans	Moderate (5–10 × controls) Larger effect in combination with other factors	Common polymorphism in factor V gene, related to higher incidence of VTE, but not a strong predictor of recurrent PE after 3 months anticoagulation [29]
Anticardiolipin antibodies	5% of VTE patients	High	
Lupus anticoagulant	5% of VTE patients	Very high[29]	
Combined defects	?15 20% of VTE patients	May act synergistically to greatly increase risk	

VTE=venous thromboembolism

The following websites have the respective statements/ guidelines for the diagnosis and management of venous thromboembolism:

British Thoracic Society: www.brit-thoracic.org.uk

American Thoracic Society: www.thoracic.org

American Heart Association: www.americanheart.org

Clinical cases

Case 8.1

A 64-year-old man is making a poor postoperative recovery 4 days after an anterior resection of a colonic carcinoma. He has a low grade fever, moderate tachycardia and is persistently hypoxic, requiring 40% O_2 by mask to maintain oxygen saturations above 95%. Portable CXR shows patchy shadows in both lower zones, interpreted as postoperative atelectasis. V/Q scan is reported as low probability of PE.

PE should be considered as a very likely diagnosis, based on high risk (postoperative cancer, immobility) and suggestive clinical features, particularly unexplained hypoxia which on blood gas measurement may be more marked than saturations alone may indicate. The CXR appearances are entirely consistent with PE, and the "low probability" V/Q scan (not normal) is of no value in excluding PE in this setting. Should be treated with iv heparin.

Case 8.2

A 76-year-old woman is recovering from inpatient therapy for a probable urinary tract infection on the medical ward. The cardiac arrest team is called when she collapses after returning from the bathroom during the night. She is cyanosed with a barely recordable blood pressure. The cardiac monitor shows a sinus tachycardia at 120/min, and an urgent blood gas, taken after institution of maximal O_2 by rebreathing mask, reveals Pao_2 9 kPa.

Sudden hypoxic collapse should always suggest PE. Immediate iv heparin should be given. 12 lead ECG and possibly echocardiography would be useful to exclude other causes of cardiopulmonary collapse such as MI. If no contraindications, consider thrombolysis with tPA if hypoxia and hypotension do not improve immediately.

Case 8.3

A 22-year-old woman presents to the A & E Department with acute severe pleuritic chest pain and a feeling of breathlessness. She takes, the combined oral contraceptive pill. She has a mild fever (37.7°C), is clearly in pain and finds it difficult to take deep breaths. Respiratory rate is 16/min. Blood gases show Pao_2 14 kPa and Pco_2 4.1 kPa.

Respiratory rate <20/min and normal gases make PE unlikely. A normal D-dimer would virtually exclude PE in this situation.

How to send home a patient referred with ?PE

Patients are commonly referred as an emergency with possible PE. The practical issue for the admitting doctor is whether to admit all of these patients and treat with heparin until other investigations (usually V/Q scan) can be completed, or whether patients can be safely discharged for outpatient investigation if necessary.

Isolated pleuritic chest pain in a well young patient (often woman on OCP)

If no other risk factors for PE other than OCP, patient is age < 40, has respiratory rate of < 20/min and a normal CXR, the risk of PE is extremely small.

Chest pain and/or breathlessness

If no pleuritic pain, respiratory rate < 20/min, and Pao_2 > 11 kPa on air, PE is very unlikely (< 3%). If D-dimer level <500 ng/ml, respiratory rate < 20/min, and Pao_2 >11 kPa on air, PE excluded (> 99% certainty).

Summary

The clinical presentation of PE is extremely broad, but is commonly one of three clinical syndromes: dyspnoea with hypoxia, cardiovascular collapse, or pleurisy.

All diagnostic tests for PE have limited sensitivity and specificity, and **must** be interpreted in the context of the clinical likelihood of PE, based on risk factor profile and clinical features.

V/Q scanning is only useful if the scan is **normal** or **high probability**. Most patients have intermediate scans that are of little diagnostic use in either confirming or refuting the diagnosis.

Pulmonary angiography or spiral CT scanning have the highest diagnostic power for PE. Echocardiography is useful to **exclude** other causes of serious cardiovascular compromise.

D-dimers are very useful to **exclude** PE if not elevated.

All patients with PE should receive heparin. Thrombolysis with tPA should be considered if there is hypotension and/or severe hypoxia.

References

1 Stein PD, Henry JW. Prevalence of acute pulmonary embolism among patients in a general hospital and at autopsy. *Chest* 1995;**108**:978–81.
2 Modan B, Sharon E, Jelin N. Factors contributing to the incorrect diagnosis of pulmonary embolic disease. *Chest* 1972;**62**:388–93.
3 Oakley CM. Diagnosis of pulmonary embolism. *BMJ* 1970;**2**:773–7.
4 Goldhaber SZ. Pulmonary embolism. *N Engl J Med* 1998;**339**:93–104.
5 Wells PS, Ginsberg JS, Anderson DR, *et al*. Use of a clinical model for safe management of patients with suspected pulmonary embolism. *Ann Intern Med* 1998;**129**:997–1005.
6 Lennox AF, Nicolaides AN. Rapid D-dimer testing as an adjunct to clinical findings in excluding pulmonary embolism. *Thorax* 1999;**54** Suppl 2:S33–6.

7 Egermayer P, Town GI, Turner JG, Heaton DC, Mee AL, Beard ME. Usefulness of D-dimer, blood gas, and respiratory rate measurements for excluding pulmonary embolism. *Thorax* 1998;**53**:830–4.

8 Stein PD, Goldhaber SZ, Henry JW, Miller AC. Arterial blood gas analysis in the assessment of suspected acute pulmonary embolism. *Chest* 1996;**109**:78–81.

9 Ginsberg JS, Wells PS, Kearon C, *et al.* Sensitivity and specificity of a rapid whole-blood assay for D-dimer in the diagnosis of pulmonary embolism. *Ann Intern Med* 1998;**129**:1006–11.

10 Perrier A, Desmarais S, Miron MJ, *et al.* Non-invasive diagnosis of venous thromboembolism in outpatients. *Lancet* 1999;**353**:190–5.

11 Conraads VM, Rademakers FE, Jorens PG, Boeckxstaens CJ, Snoeck JP. Importance of transthoracic two-dimensional echocardiography for the diagnosis and management of pulmonary embolism. *Eur Heart J* 1994;**15**:404–6.

12 Perrier A, Tamm C, Unger PF, Lerch R, Sztajzel J. Diagnostic accuracy of Doppler echocardiography in unselected patients with suspected pulmonary embolism. *Int J Cardiol* 1998;**65**:101–9.

13 PIOPED Investigators. Value of the ventilation/perfusion scan in acute pulmonary embolism. Results of the prospective investigation of pulmonary embolism diagnosis (PIOPED). *JAMA* 1990;**263**:2753–9.

14 Miniati M, Pistolesi M, Marini C, *et al.* Value of perfusion lung scan in the diagnosis of pulmonary embolism: results of the Prospective Investigative Study of Acute Pulmonary Embolism Diagnosis (PISA-PED). *Am J Resp Crit Care Med* 1996;**154**:1387–93.

15 Kearon C, Ginsberg JS, Hirsh J. The role of venous ultrasonography in the diagnosis of suspected deep venous thrombosis and pulmonary embolism. *Ann Intern Med* 1998;**129**:1044–9.

16 Tapson VF, Carroll BA, Davidson BL, *et al.* The diagnostic approach to acute venous thromboembolism. Clinical practice guideline. American Thoracic Society. *Am J Resp Crit Care Med* 1999;**160**:1043–66.

17 British Thoracic Society. Suspected pulmonary embolism: a practical approach. *Thorax* 1997;**52**:S3–15.

18 Tapson VF. Pulmonary embolism – new diagnostic approaches. *N Engl J Med* 1997;**336**:1449–51.

19 Woodard PK, Yusen RD. Diagnosis of pulmonary embolism with spiral computed tomography and magnetic resonance angiography. *Curr Opin Cardiol* 1999;**14**:442–7.

20 Meaney JF, Weg JG, Chenevert TL, Stafford-Johnson D, Hamilton BH, Prince MR. Diagnosis of pulmonary embolism with magnetic resonance angiography. *N Engl J Med* 1997;**336**:1422–7.

21 Simonneau G, Sors H, Charbonnier B, *et al.* A comparison of low-molecular-weight heparin with unfractionated heparin for acute pulmonary embolism. The THESEE Study Group. Tinzaparine ou Heparine Standard: Evaluations dans l'Embolie Pulmonaire. *N Engl J Med* 1997;**337**:663–9.

22 Arcasoy SM, Kreit JW. Thrombolytic therapy of pulmonary embolism: a comprehensive review of current evidence. *Chest* 1999;**115**:1695–707.

23 Konstantinides S, Geibel A, Olschewski M, *et al.* Association between thrombolytic treatment and the prognosis of hemodynamically stable patients with major pulmonary embolism: results of a multicenter registry. *Circulation* 1997;**96**:882–8.

24 Dalla-Volta S, Palla A, Santolicandro A, *et al.* PAIMS 2: alteplase combined with heparin versus heparin in the treatment of acute pulmonary embolism. Plasminogen activator Italian multicenter study 2. *J Am Coll Cardiol* 1992;**20**:520–6.

25 Gulba DC, Schmid C, Borst HG, Lichtlen P, Dietz R, Luft FC. Medical compared with surgical treatment for massive pulmonary embolism. *Lancet* 1994;**343**:576–7.

26 Doerge HC, Schoendube FA, Loeser H, Walter M, Messmer BJ. Pulmonary embolectomy: review of a 15-year experience and role in the age of thrombolytic therapy. *Eur J Cardiothorac Surg* 1996;**10**:952–7.

27 Schulman S, Rhedin AS, Lindmarker P, *et al.* A comparison of six weeks with six months of oral anticoagulant therapy after a first episode of venous thromboembolism. Duration of Anticoagulation Trial Study Group. *N Engl J Med* 1995;**332**:1661–5.

28 Schulman S, Granqvist S, Holmstrom M, *et al.* The duration of oral anticoagulant therapy after a second episode of venous thromboembolism. The Duration of Anticoagulation Trial Study Group. *N Engl J Med* 1997;**336**:393–8.

29 Kearon C, Gent M, Hirsh J, *et al.* A comparison of three months of anticoagulation with extended anticoagulation for a first episode of idiopathic venous thromboembolism. *N Engl J Med* 1999;**340**:901–7.

30 Laffan M. Genetics and pulmonary medicine: pulmonary embolism. *Thorax* 1998;**53**:698–702.

31 Salomon O, Steinberg DM, Zivelin A, *et al.* Single and combined prothrombotic factors in patients with idiopathic venous thromboembolism: prevalence and risk assessment. *Arterioscler Thromb Vasc Biol* 1999;**19**:511–18

9: Acute atrial fibrillation

I MIRZA, Y BASHIR

9.1 Introduction

Atrial fibrillation (AF) is the most common arrhythmia encountered in acute medical practice, occurring in approximately 7% of emergency admissions.[1] In some of these cases, AF is longstanding and/or incidental to clinical management, but more often AF has developed acutely as either the primary clinical problem or as a complication of another acute medical condition (pneumonia, myocardial infarction, septicaemia, etc). However, it may not be possible to differentiate between a self-limiting attack of "paroxysmal AF" (expected to convert spontaneously to sinus rhythm), or the onset of "persistent AF" (sinus rhythm will only be restored by electrical or pharmacological cardioversion) if this is the patient's first episode. There is a trend towards active management of AF in the acute setting, but comparatively few randomised trials or other sources of hard evidence on which to base strategy. The major goals of treatment are:

- To alleviate the associated symptoms and/or haemodynamic disturbance.
- To reduce the risk of systemic thromboembolism.
- To shorten or avoid hospitalisation.

The third aim relates to resource utilisation/health economics rather than primary clinical considerations, but is important because acute AF is such a common problem and can often be successfully managed on an outpatient basis. The emergency medical services could be swamped if, for example, every patient with an attack of paroxysmal AF were admitted and offered (possibly unnecessary) interventions. For clinicians, determining management in individual cases can appear complex and confusing because the available therapeutic options include:

- Electrical cardioversion (immediate or interval) with or without maintenance antiarrhythmic drugs.
- Pharmacological cardioversion with intravenous or oral agents.
- Pharmacological rate-control.
- Anticoagulation (parenteral or oral).

Moreover, these can be used in various permutations and combinations. The most appropriate selection depends on factors such as the duration of the acute episode, the severity of symptoms/haemodynamic disturbance, and the presence of structural heart disease. Not surprisingly the management of acute AF is littered with "grey areas". In the current state of knowledge, it is not possible to offer rigid guidelines but in this chapter we will attempt to illustrate some of the key issues and suggest an overall approach for handling these patients.

9.2 Thromboembolic risk in acute AF: role of left atrial mechanical function

The possibility of systemic thromboembolism provides an additional, unique dimension to the management of acute AF compared to other tachyarrhythmias. Cardioversion (electrical or pharmacological) of patients with AF of over 48 hours duration is associated with a 5–7% risk of embolic events without prior anticoagulation, which can be reduced to 0–1.6% risk with 3–4 weeks of warfarin therapy beforehand.[2] The underlying pathophysiological mechanisms have been clarified by transoesophageal echocardiography (TOE). In most cases, pre-existing intracardiac thrombi have formed within the fibrillating left atrium due to relative stasis, and become dislodged following restoration of atrial systole and organised contraction (Figure 9.1). However, thromboembolism can still occur even if left atrial thrombi have been carefully excluded by TOE prior to cardioversion. This is because restoration of sinus rhythm seems to be associated with a transient, paradoxical worsening of mechanical dysfunction of the left atrium (particularly the left atrial appendage), so called "atrial stunning", during which *de novo* intracardiac thrombus formation may occur.[3] The stunning is probably related to the duration of AF rather than the mode of cardioversion. Thus, if patients present with AF of > 48 hours duration, whenever possible, cardioversion should be deferred to allow 3–4 weeks of oral anticoagulation beforehand, followed by at least 4 weeks afterwards to cover resumption of mechanical atrial function. If early cardioversion is mandated on haemodynamic grounds, TOE should be performed beforehand to exclude left atrial thrombi and the patient should then be fully anticoagulated with heparin to cover the initial period of stunning, followed by warfarin for a month.[4]

For patients presenting within 48 hours of the onset of acute AF, the risk of clinical thromboembolism with conversion of sinus rhythm appears to be much lower, probably < 1%,[5] even though some TOE studies have shown that it is possible to form left atrial thrombi within this time frame. The absence of subsequent "atrial stunning" may be an important protective factor. It is generally agreed that these patients can undergo electrical or pharmacological cardioversion without the need for systemic anticoagulation, provided that it is performed within the 48 hour "window of opportunity".

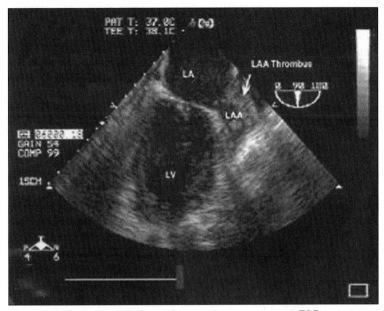

Figure 9.1 Thrombus in left atrial appendage as seen on TOE.

Summary: Acute AF, thromboembolism and left atrial mechanical function

Cardioversion may be carried out without anticoagulation for an episode of acute atrial fibrillation within 48 hours of onset.

Cardioversion of atrial fibrillation more than 48 hours after onset is associated with 5–7% risk of embolic events.

Anticoagulation for 3–4 weeks prior to cardioversion will reduce this risk to 0–1.6%.

The risk of thromboembolism is due to both pre-cardioversion left atrial thrombi and "atrial stunning" following restoration of sinus rhythm.

Early cardioversion may be performed if TOE has excluded left atrial thrombus but must be followed by full anticoagulation for 4 weeks to prevent *de novo* thrombus formation due to atrial stunning.

9.3 Management: initial assessment

In addition to the history and examination, the initial evaluation must include a 12-lead ECG to confirm the clinical diagnosis of AF (Figure 9.2). A chest *x* ray, renal function/electrolytes and thyroid function are other useful investigations. The clinician should address the following key issues.

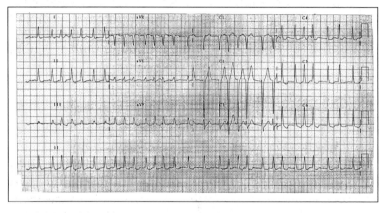

Figure 9.2 ECG of AF.

9.3.1 Duration of AF

The time since onset of the arrhythmia must be ascertained as closely as possible. In most cases this will be obvious from the history, but if the presenting symptoms are mild or non-specific, the time of onset of AF may be uncertain. It is an important determinant of management because patients with AF of < 48 hours duration can be considered for immediate cardioversion without anticoagulation, otherwise pre-treatment with warfarin for 3–4 weeks or "TOE guidance" are required (see above). If the duration of the acute episode is uncertain, it is safer to treat the patient as for AF of > 48 hours duration.

9.3.2 Classification of AF

Paroxysmal AF will revert to sinus rhythm spontaneously, whereas persistent AF will only do so as a result of electrical or pharmacological cardioversion. If there is a prior history of self-limiting attacks, diagnosing paroxysmal AF is straightforward but if the patient is presenting with AF for the first time, classification may be impossible. The time since onset of the arrhythmia (if known) offers a further clue. Paroxysmal AF accounts for 60–70% of acute episodes of < 48 hours duration, but is much less common if AF has already persisted for > 48 hours, and rare if the arrhythmia continues for longer than 7 days.

9.3.3 Severity of symptoms/haemodynamic disturbance

This can usually be gauged from clinical assessment plus a chest *x* ray (to check for pulmonary congestion) and is another important determinant of immediate management and the need for hospitalisation. The clinical presentation of acute AF depends on a number of factors, particularly ventricular rate, loss of AV synchrony, cycle length irregularity, and the presence of underlying cardiac disease. The resulting spectrum of symptomatology is broad. Some patients are completely asymptomatic. More often they complain of palpitation, dyspnoea, or lassitude, possibly associated with chest discomfort or lightheadedness, but the attack is still reasonably well tolerated. In a minority of cases AF is poorly tolerated due to severe angina or haemodynamic decompensation, i.e. pulmonary oedema, hypotension, or rarely, circulatory collapse with syncope. It would be unusual for acute AF to cause significant haemodynamic disturbance in the absence of structural heart disease, particularly impaired LV function and/or abnormal compliance (e.g. left ventricular hypertrophy (LVH), acute myocardial infarction, etc.), or valvular problems such as mitral stenosis or aortic stenosis.

9.3.4 Presence of underlying cardiac disease

Structural heart disease is present in a significant proportion of patients presenting with acute AF. Apart from the fact that specific investigation and treatment may be required, in due course, for conditions such as coronary artery disease, heart failure, mitral stenosis, etc., their presence may influence the options for immediate management. In particular, ischaemic heart disease and/or impaired LV function are relative contraindications to the use of class I antiarrhythmic drugs such as flecainide or propafenone for pharmacological cardioversion. Clues to the presence of heart disease may be obtained from the history (angina, previous myocardial infarction (MI), hypertension, etc.), examination (signs of heart failure or valvular disease), 12-lead ECG (recent or old MI, LVH, etc.) and chest x ray (cardiomegaly + pulmonary congestion). Echocardiography is arguably the most useful non-invasive tool for investigating cardiac structure and function. In an ideal world, this would be performed as part of the initial assessment but in practice echocardiography is seldom available at the time of presentation and has to be deferred (usually until outpatient review). Thus, if patients present with reasonably well tolerated AF, no prior history of cardiovascular disease and no abnormality on clinical examination, ECG (apart from AF), or chest x ray, it is reasonable to manage them as cases of "lone AF" arising in a structurally normal heart.

9.3.5 Acute precipitants

In some cases the AF has been clearly triggered by another condition, most commonly respiratory tract infection or other sepsis, general anaesthesia, or myocardial infarction/ischaemia. Sometimes the precipitant (e.g. pneumonia) may require treatment in its own right and if possible cardioversion should be deferred until after it has resolved to reduce the risk of recurrent AF.

Summary: Initial assessment

History, examination, 12-lead ECG plus chest x ray. Renal function/electrolytes, glucose and thyroid function.

Duration of AF: 0–48 hours or >48 hours since onset *but* If uncertain assume >48 hours since onset.

Classification of AF: paroxysmal or persistent?

Severity of symptoms/haemodynamic disturbance.

Presence of underlying cardiac disease.

Acute precipitants.

9.4 Management: AF duration less than 48 hours (Figure 9.3)

Patients presenting within 48 hours of the onset of AF can be offered immediate pharmacological or electrical cardioversion *without* anticoagulation (see above). The arguments in favour of early intervention are: (i) prompt relief of symptoms; (ii) it may allow the patient to be discharged directly from the emergency department; (iii) it may avoid the inconvenience of prolonged oral anticoagulation for elective DC cardioversion which would be required if the attack persisted for over 48 hours. On the other hand, at least 50–60% patients in this group have paroxysmal AF and will revert to sinus rhythm spontaneously without the need for general anaesthesia or exposure to the proarrhythmic effects of drug therapy.

9.4.1 To cardiovert or wait?

We use a pragmatic approach to avoid unnecessary intervention without sacrificing the benefits of early restoration of sinus rhythm as follows:

- Patients with reasonably well tolerated AF of 0–24 hours duration and/or a prior history of self-limiting episodes can be discharged without treatment but advised to return to the emergency department 24 hours later for cardioversion if the attack has not abated by then (see below). The rationale is that most of these patients have paroxysmal AF and will return to sinus rhythm spontaneously, and perhaps only 20–30% will require active intervention (i.e. cardioversion) 24 hours later but this can still be performed inside the 48 hours "window of opportunity".

- Patients presenting from 24–48 hours of onset *or* with poorly tolerated AF should undergo immediate cardioversion. If cardioversion is successful, they can usually be discharged directly from the emergency department. However, some patients will need to be admitted, particularly if acute AF precipitated haemodynamic deterioration (high probability of underlying heart disease and early recurrence of AF) or there is an intercurrent medical problem such as myocardial infarction.

If admission to hospital is not required, arrangements should be made for outpatient review (usually by a cardiologist) plus echocardiography at a later date unless the patient has already been evaluated in this way. Low-dose aspirin is often prescribed as an interim measure.

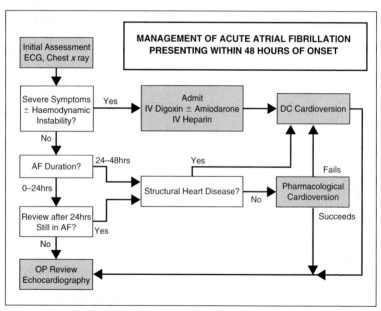

Figure 9.3 Algorithm for management of AF within 48 hours of onset.

9.4.2 Electrical or pharmacological cardioversion?

Electrical cardioversion using synchronised DC shocks is highly effective and can be used whether or not the patient has underlying heart disease or is haemodynamically compromised. It will not prevent reversion to AF and requires general anaesthesia. Pharmacological cardioversion avoids the inconvenience and potential delay of general anaesthesia but is subject to several disadvantages: (i) it is not 100% effective; (ii) all antiarrhythmic agents are negatively inotropic to a greater or lesser extent and may precipitate or worsen haemodynamic disturbance; (iii) there is a risk of proarrhythmia (including organising AF into atrial flutter with paradoxical acceleration of the ventricular rate). Class I agents including flecainide and propafenone are relatively contraindicated in the presence of structural cardiac disease (particularly ischaemic heart disease and impaired LV function) because of increased susceptibility to life-threatening proarrhythmias. A suitable strategy is as follows:

- Electrical cardioversion is the treatment of choice in patients with known or suspected structural heart disease, particularly those with haemodynamic disturbance. Most studies suggest that energies < 200 J are unlikely to succeed and therefore our recommended protocol is 200 J, followed by 360 J, followed by 360 J with anteroposterior paddle positions. Success may be limited by improper electrode placement or poor paddle contact. As these individuals are often at high risk of early relapse into AF, consideration should be given to adjunctive antiarrhythmic therapy, usually intravenous or oral amiodarone (1.2 g/day) (Table 9.1).
- Pharmacological cardioversion may be attempted in patients with well tolerated AF and no evidence of heart disease (see above). The selection of antiarrhythmic agent and route of administration are discussed below. If this proves unsuccessful, patients should normally be offered electrical cardioversion.

The protocol for DC cardioversion is given in Chapter 13.

9.4.3 Which antiarrhythmic agent for pharmacological cardioversion? (Table 9.1)

Various antiarrhythmic drugs have been evaluated for conversion of acute AF, traditionally using intravenous administration for rapidity of action. These include class IC agents (flecainide and propafenone), class IA drugs (e.g. disopyramide, digoxin, amiodarone, sotalol), and novel class III agents such as ibutilide and dofetilide. It is difficult to judge their relative efficacy and safety because there have been so few direct comparisons. Moreover, published studies are often difficult to compare because of important differences in the entry criteria and endpoints. For example, the rate of "successful" pharmacological cardioversion using a particular drug will invariably be lower if a study includes cases with AF of greater than 7 days duration, than would have been obtained if recruitment were restricted to patients within 48 hours of onset of the arrhythmia. Accepting these limitations, pooled analysis of the available data[6] suggests the following conclusions.

- Class IC agents such as flecainide and propafenone are the most effective agents for achieving rapid restoration of sinus rhythm. In AF of less than 72 hours duration, IV flecainide 2 mg/kg (maximum 150 mg) will produce acute conversion rates of 70–80% within 0–3 hours of administration.
- Digoxin slows the ventricular rate but does *not* enhance conversion of acute AF.
- Intravenous amiodarone is associated with a lower conversion rate than class IC agents, delayed onset of action (12–24 hours), and ideally should be administered via central venous access. However, it can be used with reasonable safety in patients with structural heart disease/impaired LV function, it slows the ventricular rate during AF, and it reduces the propensity to recurrent AF. These properties make amiodarone a useful adjunct to electrical cardioversion in patients presenting with poorly tolerated AF and haemodynamic instability, who are often at high risk of early relapse to AF.
- The novel class III agents such as ibutilide and dofetilide (not currently available in the UK) appear to be associated

with a lower acute conversion rate than class IC agents and a higher overall incidence of serious proarrhythmia (usually in the form of torsade de pointes). However, these agents are probably safer than class IC drugs in patients with structural heart disease and may offer an alternative to electrical cardioversion for such cases. At present, they should only be used with continuous ECG monitoring for at least 12 hours afterwards.

Thus, we consider intravenous flecainide to be the drug of choice for pharmacological cardioversion provided that there is no evidence of major structural heart disease. Patients should be kept on ECG monitoring for up to 2–3 hours following IV administration in case of proarrhythmia but can usually then be discharged. If AF persists, an early decision should be reached with regard to electrical cardioversion (Figure 9.4).

9.4.4 Intravenous or oral administration?

Recently, several groups have investigated the use of single oral doses of flecainide (200–300 mg stat) or propafenone (450–600 mg stat) in acute AF and reported comparable conversion rates (70–80%) to intravenous administration although these are achieved over 4–8 hours rather than 0–3 hours. Oral administration has been proposed as a simple alternative for pharmacological cardioversion: the patient is given a single dose of flecainide or propafenone and asked to return 24 hours later if still in AF. However, we would still favour intravenous administration for patients presenting with acute AF for the first time because it is quicker, and it can be given under direct supervision with ECG monitoring in the emergency department. Oral administration may have a valuable role in patients presenting with recurrent AF who have already been fully evaluated for underlying heart disease. Indeed, in many such cases the treatment could be prescribed in the community (by the general practitioner or self-medication) and perhaps avoid the need for hospital attendance altogether.

9.4.5 Maintenance antiarrhythmic drug therapy?

In most cases, maintenance antiarrhythmic drug treatment does not need to be started following a first episode of acute AF and a decision about this can be deferred until the patient has been fully evaluated in the clinic. However, treatment should be considered if there is a recent history of frequent attacks or if the patient returns to the emergency department with recurrence of AF soon after cardioversion (pharmacological or electrical). If there are no contraindications, a standard β-blocker or sotalol should be used initially. Sotalol acts almost exclusively as a β-blocker at doses of 40–120 mg bd, but exerts additional class III antiarrhythmic activity at 160 mg bd or above. Class I drugs such flecainide are best avoided until the patient has been fully evaluated. If β-blockers are contraindicated and there is a background of known cardiac problems such as ischaemic heart disease or chronic heart failure, it may be appropriate to start amiodarone.

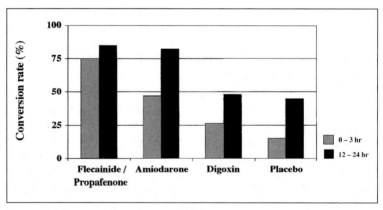

Figure 9.4 Comparative efficacy of intravenous antiarrhythmic agents for pharmacological cardioversion of acute AF at 0–3 hours (grey bars) and 12–24 hours (black bars) after treatment.

Summary: Management of acute AF within 48 hours of onset (Figure 9.3)

Patients with severe symptoms/haemodynamic disturbance should be admitted to undergo immediate DC cardioversion, evaluation for underlying heart disease (including echocardiography), and treatment for intercurrent medical problems. Most are at high risk of early recurrence and should be considered for adjunctive treatment with amiodarone (intravenous and/or oral) *and* anticoagulation.

Patients with reasonably well tolerated AF presenting within 0–24 hours can be discharged without treatment. If the arrhythmia is self-limiting they can be referred for further cardiac evaluation on an outpatient basis, otherwise they should return to the emergency department for cardioversion 24 hours later.

Patients who are still in AF at 24–48 hours can normally undergo attempted pharmacological cardioversion with IV flecainide. However, DC cardioversion should be used if there is evidence of structural heart disease, or if flecainide fails to restore sinus rhythm. Most of these cases can be discharged directly from the emergency department and further evaluation delayed until clinic review.

Patients with previous attacks of AF who have been fully evaluated may be considered for single dose oral flecainide.

9.5 Management: AF duration over 48 hours or uncertain (Figure 9.5)

The management issues are very different for patients presenting more than 48 hours after the onset of AF. Most episodes of paroxysmal AF do not persist for that long, and so spontaneous conversion to sinus rhythm is unusual in this subgroup. Furthermore, because of the increased thromboembolic risk, early cardioversion is only considered for the few cases in which the patient is severely haemodynamically compromised. Otherwise, the immediate issues for the clinician are pharmacological rate-control, antithrombotic therapy, and whether the patient needs emergency admission. At some stage, a decision also has to be made about interval DC cardioversion, with or without adjunctive antiarrhythmic drug therapy, but often this can be deferred until outpatient review.

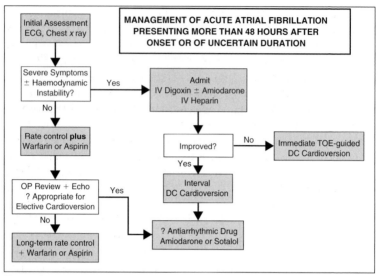

Figure 9.5 Algorithm for management of AF of more than 48 hours after onset *or* uncertain duration.

9.5.1 Emergency admission or outpatient management?

Admission should only be required if acute AF has precipitated severe symptoms/ haemodynamic disturbance, or treatment is required for some associated medical problem such as myocardial infarction, pneumonia, etc. Most patients can be discharged from the emergency department on appropriate medication for rate-control and antithrombotic prophylaxis (see below), with follow-up arrangements in the outpatient clinic to carry out further evaluation/echocardiography, and to decide about subsequent management, particularly whether to undertake interval cardioversion.

9.5.2 Early cardioversion

Most cases of acute AF presenting after 48 hours with signs of haemodynamic compromise should be managed by pharmacological rate-control in the first instance (see below). Very rarely the patient is admitted *in extremis* and requires immediate DC cardioversion. A more common situation is that early restoration of sinus rhythm within the next few days would be desirable because of continuing symptomatic and haemodynamic problems despite slowing of the ventricular rate, rather than waiting for interval cardioversion in 3–4 weeks time. The advent of transoesophageal echocardiography (now available in most district hospitals as well as regional centres) has greatly expanded the scope for early cardioversion in this situation; provided that there is no evidence of left atrial thrombus *and* the patient receives full systemic anticoagulation (heparin followed by warfarin) for 4 weeks afterwards to cover atrial stunning, the risk of systemic thromboembolism appears to be very low. Because these individuals are at relatively high risk of early recurrence of AF, adjunctive antiarrhythmic treatment usually with intravenous or oral amiodarone (1.2 g/d for 7–10 days, then 200 mg/d) should always be considered. It is preferable, if the cardioversion can be delayed for a few days, to allow amiodarone preloading.

9.5.3 Pharmacological rate-control (Table 9.1)

If the resting heart rate during acute AF exceeds 100 bpm, AV nodal blocking drugs may be used to slow the ventricular rate and ameliorate symptoms and improve haemodynamic function. The most commonly used agents are digoxin, calcium-channel antagonists (diltiazem or verapamil), and β-blockers, all of which can be administered by the intravenous route if necessary to achieve a rapid therapeutic effect. In haemodynamically stable patients, there is little to choose between these agents. Intravenous digoxin remains the preferred treatment if acute AF is associated with haemodynamic compromise because of its positive inotropic effects, whereas β-blockers, diltiazem and verapamil can cause further depression of myocardial contractility. The value of IV digoxin in this setting has been reaffirmed by the recent DAAF Trial.[7] Intravenous amiodarone has also been shown to produce rapid slowing of the ventricular rate and may be a useful adjunct or alternative to IV digoxin in haemodynamically unstable patients if early DC cardioversion is being considered (see above).

Table 9.1 Pharmacological treatments in acute AF.

Drug	Administration
Pharmacological cardioversion	
Flecainide	2 mg/kg IV over 10 min (max 150 mg) *or* 200–300 mg PO stat.
Amiodarone*	300 mg IV over 60 min, then 1200 mg/24 hours *or* 400 mg tds PO for 7–10 days.
Propafenone	2 mg/kg IV over 5–10 min *or* 450–600 mg PO stat.
Sotalol	20–100 mg IV slow injection.
Rate-control	
Digoxin	0.5–1 mg IV in 50 ml saline over 1 hour *or* 0.5 mg PO 12 hourly (2–3 doses) then 0.0625-0.25 mg daily.
Metoprolol	5–15 mg slowly IV *or* 25–100 mg tds PO.
Verapamil	5 mg IV over 2 min repeated every 5 min up to 20 mg *or* 40–120 mg tds PO.

* IV amiodarone is effective for rate-control as well as cardioversion.

9.5.4 Antithrombotic therapy

Anticoagulation may be required in acute AF for two separate reasons: (i) to reduce the specific risk of thromboembolism associated with immediate or interval cardioversion; (ii) as prophylaxis against the background, long-term risk of systemic embolisation associated with AF per se, particularly if the patient is to be left in AF for a prolonged period of time or permanently. The following guidance may be offered.

- Patients who are being considered for early TOE-guided cardioversion (see above) should all be started on heparin followed by warfarin for 4 weeks.
- Patients in whom a definite decision is made to undertake interval DC cardioversion (see below) should be started on warfarin (target INR 2.0–3.0) as a minimum of 3–4 weeks anticoagulation is required beforehand.
- If a decision about cardioversion is being deferred until the time of outpatient follow-up, antithrombotic therapy

(aspirin or warfarin) should be prescribed during the interim to protect the patient against the background risk of systemic embolisation from AF. It is beyond the scope of this book to consider the indications and risks/benefits of long-term anticoagulation versus antiplatelet agents in persistent/permanent AF. However, there are considerable differences in susceptibility among individual patients, and warfarin should be started immediately if acute AF is associated with high-risk features such as heart failure/poor LV function, mitral stenosis, untreated thyrotoxicosis, previous history of ischaemic stroke, transient ischaemic attack (TIA), or other systemic emboli.

9.5.5 Interval DC cardioversion

In patients who are haemodynamically stable, a decision about interval DC cardioversion can be made at the time of presentation or deferred until clinic review. Either way, there are three separate issues to resolve.

Is cardioversion feasible?

The chances of restoring and maintaining sinus rhythm are inversely related to the duration of AF. Cardioversion should not usually be attempted if patients have been in persistent AF for more than 1–2 years. The other major predictor of failure is relapse to AF following previous cardioversions, particularly if this has occurred despite maintenance antiarrhythmic drug therapy. By contrast, advanced age and structural heart disease are often said to be relative contraindications to cardioversion, although there is little objective evidence to suggest that the chances of success are markedly reduced by either. On the other side of the equation, the chances of success are better with AF of short duration and particularly if there has been an acute precipitant that has resolved (e.g. pneumonia, general anaesthesia, etc.).

Is cardioversion indicated?

The main and only definite indication for cardioversion is persistent symptoms (palpitation, reduced functional capacity, lassitude, etc.) despite adequate ventricular rate-control. However, it is often performed in minimally symptomatic patients in the hope of avoiding the need for long-term warfarin, particularly if there are relative contraindications to anticoagulants. It must be emphasised that there is at present no evidence to support the concept that restoration of sinus rhythm confers comparable protection against ischaemic stroke to anticoagulation, although this issue is being examined in ongoing multicentre trials (AFFIRM, RACE, etc.).

Should adjunctive antiarrhythmic drugs be used?

Overall, 70–80% of patients revert to AF within 12 months of successful cardioversion if no antiarrhythmic treatment is prescribed. The chances of relapse can be reduced by drug treatment. Sotalol at class III dosage (at least 160 mg bd) and amiodarone are the most commonly used drugs. However, even amiodarone only reduces the chance of recurrent AF to 20–30% by 1 year. Class I agents (flecainide, propafenone, disopyramide, etc.) are seldom prescribed for this purpose in the light of mounting evidence that they increase cardiac mortality, particularly among patients with ischaemic heart disease.

In many cases, these decisions can be made at the time of presentation to the emergency department and the appropriate treatment plan set in motion without waiting for an outpatient appointment.

Clinical cases

Case 9.1

A 45-year-old man attended the casualty department complaining of rapid palpitation with no associated symptoms, which had come on abruptly 2 hours beforehand. An ECG showed AF 120 bpm and no other abnormality. He had experienced several similar episodes over the last 3 months, but all of these had resolved spontaneously within a few minutes. Clinical examination and chest x ray were unremarkable. In view of the prior history of self-limiting episodes, a presumptive diagnosis of paroxysmal AF was made. He duly reverted to sinus rhythm spontaneously after 30 minutes. He was started on aspirin and arrangements were made for further evaluation as an outpatient.

The prior history of self-limiting episodes of palpitation made it likely that this patient was suffering from paroxysmal AF and would revert to sinus rhythm spontaneously.

Case 9.2

A 65-year-old man was seen in the casualty department having been awoken from sleep with acute onset of breathlessness. Over the preceding 6 weeks he had noticed increasing dyspnoea and orthopnoea, with palpitation (awareness of irregular heartbeat) for 3–4 months. He had a past history of hypertension and an MI ten years previously. Examination revealed AF 120–130 bpm, BP 160/90, with signs of mitral reflux and congestive heart failure. ECG confirmed AF 130 bpm with old anterior Q waves. Chest x ray showed cardiomegaly and pulmonary congestion. He was admitted and treated with oxygen, diuretics and an ACE inhibitor, IV digoxin for rate-control, and IV heparin. Echocardiography showed globally reduced LV function, mild mitral incompetence and left atrial enlargement (4.4 cm). His condition improved and he was converted to oral treatment with enalapril, frusemide, digoxin, and warfarin. Prior to discharge, amiodarone was started with a view to interval DC cardioversion after 4 weeks. This was successful and restoration of sinus rhythm was associated with further symptomatic benefit.

This patient required admission because of acute haemodynamic decompensation. He had almost certainly been in AF for several months and so was managed by rate-control, anticoagulation, and standard heart failure treatment pending interval cardioversion.

Case 9.3

A previously fit 55-year-old lady attended the emergency department with mild breathlessness and rapid palpitation for 6 hours. She denied any previous episodes or other cardiac symptoms. An ECG confirmed AF 130–140 bpm with no other abnormality. Examination revealed the tachycardia but was otherwise unremarkable with no signs of haemodynamic compromise or heart failure. Chest x ray showed a normal sized heart with no pulmonary congestion. She was discharged but asked to return for review 24 hours later, and prescribed aspirin and digoxin (0.5 mg stat, 0.5 mg at 6 hrs and 0.25 mg at 12 hrs). At follow-up, she remained in AF although the ventricular rate had slowed to 110 bpm and she was only minimally symptomatic. As it was now 30 hours since the onset of the episode, pharmacological cardioversion was attempted with IV flecainide 2 mg/kg. She reverted to sinus rhythm 30 minutes later and was discharged taking aspirin alone with arrangement for review in the cardiology clinic.

As this patient presented within a few hours of onset of acute AF and was tolerating the arrhythmia well, it was reasonable to wait for 24 hours before intervening in the hope that she would revert to sinus rhythm spontaneously. She remained in AF at follow-up but was still inside the 48 hour "window of opportunity" for cardioversion without anticoagulation. Because there was no evidence of structural heart disease, it was considered safe to use intravenous flecainide for this purpose.

Case 9.4

A 69-year-old man with known chronic stable angina was admitted with a 36-hour history of irregular palpitation and lassitude. His medications included atenolol, aspirin, and pravastatin. There was no clinical or radiological evidence of heart failure. ECG showed AF 80–90 bpm with old inferior Q waves but no acute changes. As he had recently eaten, DC cardioversion was performed under GA four hours later and he was successfully converted to sinus rhythm with a 360 J shock. Atenolol was switched to sotalol 160 mg bd and he was discharged directly from the emergency department later that day with arrangements for follow-up in the cardiac clinic.

This patient presented with well tolerated AF within 24–48 hours of onset but was unsuitable for pharmacological cardioversion because of the associated ischaemic heart disease. If there had been no history of angina and a normal ECG he could have been considered for IV flecainide.

Case 9.5

A 73-year-old man with longstanding hypertension, diabetes mellitus and chronic obstructive pulmonary disease (ex-smoker) was admitted with a history of worsening dyspnoea for several days but no awareness of palpitation. He was taking enalapril, bendrofluazide, and glibenclamide. He was found to be hypotensive BP 80/55, in rapid AF 160–180 bpm with signs of heart failure and the chest x ray showed cardiomegaly and pulmonary congestion. He was admitted and treated with IV frusemide and started on IV digoxin (0.5 mg stat and at 6 hours, followed by 0.25 mg/d) and IV heparin. By the following day, there had been some improvement with BP 100/60, heart rate 120 bpm and a reasonable diuresis, but he remained very weak and dyspnoeic. Transthoracic echocardiography showed concentric LVH with severe, globally impaired systolic function and normal valves with functional mitral regurgitation. IV amiodarone 1.2 g/d was added but there was little improvement over the next 36 hours despite further slowing of the heart rate to 100 bpm. Accordingly, successful DC cardioversion was performed after transoesophageal echocardiography showed no evidence of left atrial thrombus (just spontaneous contrast echoes). He was loaded with amiodarone (400 mg tds po for 1 week, followed by 200 mg od) and anticoagulated with warfarin. He thereafter made steady progress. He was discharged several days later on amiodarone, digoxin, warfarin, furosemide (frusemide), and enalapril. At 4-week follow-up, he remained in sinus rhythm and felt back to normal. Transthoracic echocardiography showed substantial improvement in LV function.

This patient had been in AF for an indeterminate period but remained haemodynamically compromised despite rate-control and so underwent early TOE guided DC cardioversion (rather than interval cardioversion). The subsequent improvement in LV function suggests a rate-related cardiomyopathy superimposed on pre-existing hypertensive heart disease.

Summary: Management of AF more than 48 hours after onset or uncertain duration (Figure 9.5)

Most patients can be managed initially with drugs to control the ventricular rate plus warfarin or aspirin and discharged from the emergency department with outpatient follow-up to determine strategy (cardioversion, rate-control plus long-term anticoagulation, etc.).

Patients at high risk of systemic emboli (heart failure, previous TIA or ischaemic stroke, untreated thyrotoxicosis) should be started on anticoagulants immediately. Warfarin should also be started if interval DC cardioversion is definitely planned. Otherwise the decision can be deferred until the time of follow-up.

Patients with severe symptoms and/or haemodynamic instability should be admitted and initially treated with iv digoxin plus heparin. Early DC cardioversion can be considered if they fail to improve with rate-control provided that TOE shows no evidence of left atrial thrombus. Ideally they should be preloaded with iv or oral amiodarone for a few days to reduce the risk of relapse to AF. Full anticoagulation must be continued for at least 4 weeks post-cardioversion.

Interval DC cardioversion is primarily indicated for persistent symptoms despite rate-control. It can be offered to minimally symptomatic patients to avoid long-term anticoagulation but this is an unproven strategy. Most will require adjunctive antiarrhythmic drugs (sotalol or amiodarone) to maintain sinus rhythm. The chances of success are best with AF of short duration and/or an acute precipitant.

References

1 Lip GY, Tean KN, Dunn FG. Treatment of atrial fibrillation in a district general hospital. *Br Heart J* 1994;**71**:92–95.
2 Bjerkelund CJ, Ornin OM. The efficacy of anticoagulant therapy in preventing embolism related to DC electrical cardioversion of atrial fibrillation. *Am J Cardiol* 1969;**23**:208–16.
3 Fatkin D, Kuchar DL, Thorburn CW, Feneley MP. Transoesophageal echocardiography before and during direct current cardioversion of atrial

fibrillation: evidence for "Atrial Stunning" as a mechanism of thromboembolic complications. *J Am Coll Cardiol* 1994;**23**:307–16.

4 Cheitlin MD, Alport JS, Armstrong WF, *et al*. ACC/AHA guidelines for the clinical application of echocardiography: a report of the American College of Cardiology/American Heart Association Task Force on Practice Guidelines (Committee on Clinical Application of Echocardiography). *Circulation* 1997;**95**:1686–744.

5 Weigner MJ, Caulfield TA, Danias PG, Silverman DI, Manning WJ. Risk for clinical thromboembolism associated with conversion to sinus rhythm in patients with atrial fibrillation lasting less than 48 hours. *Ann Intern Med* 1997;**126**:615–20.

6 Mortara A, Davies C, Bashir Y. Comparative efficacy and safety of intravenous antiarrhythmic agents for conversion of recent onset atrial fibrillation. *Eur Heart J* 1999;**20**:351.

7 The Digitalis in Acute Atrial Fibrillation (DAAF) Trial Group. Intravenous digoxin in acute atrial fibrillation. Results of a randomised, placebo-controlled multicentre trial in 239 patients. *Eur Heart J* 1997;**18**:649–54.

10: Narrow complex tachycardia

Y BASHIR, N LEVER

10.1 Introduction

"Narrow complex tachycardia" is one of the three common presentations of tachyarrhythmias in emergency medicine, the others being "broad complex tachycardia" (see Chapter 11) and acute atrial fibrillation (AF) (see Chapter 9). By convention the term refers to *tachyarrhythmias, with normal QRS duration (<120 ms) and regular cycle length*. Thus AF and atrial flutter with variable block are excluded, but the differential diagnosis includes atrial flutter with regular 2:1 block. Because QRS complexes of normal width and morphology can only result from rapid depolarisation of the entire ventricular muscle mass through the atrioventricular (AV) junction and specialised His-Purkinje network, *narrow complex tachycardia is always supraventricular in origin* and never due to ventricular tachycardia. However, an arrhythmia should only be classified as "narrow complex tachycardia" on the basis of a full 12-lead ECG recording wherever possible. In some cases of broad complex tachycardia, the QRS complexes may appear of normal width in one or more individual ECG leads if a single-channel rhythm strip is examined in isolation (Figure 10.1). Most cases of narrow complex tachycardia are not associated with structural heart disease and the prognosis is benign unless the patient also has Wolff–Parkinson–White syndrome or the arrhythmia becomes incessant leading to rate-related cardiomyopathy (see below). Only a few patients require hospitalisation, and the majority can be managed in the emergency department and discharged directly.

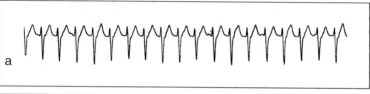

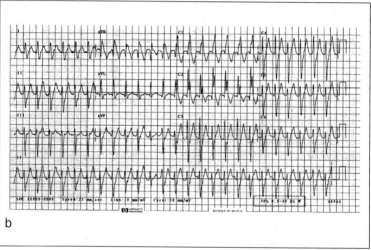

Figure 10.1 Example of a broad complex tachycardia mistaken for narrow complex tachycardia on the basis of a single-lead rhythm strip (a). The full 12-lead ECG (b) clearly shows broad complex tachycardia with ventriculo-atrial (VA) dissociation, indicating that the correct diagnosis was ventricular tachycardia.

The emergence of curative catheter ablation techniques over the past decade has revolutionised long-term treatment of supraventricular tachyarrhythmias[1] but has been largely irrelevant to the emergency setting. Important developments in the acute management of narrow complex tachycardia include the emergence of a modern, clinically relevant classification based on the underlying electrophysiological mechanism.[2] The two major categories are (i) *junctional tachyarrhythmias* in which the AV junction is an obligatory part of the arrhythmia circuit, and (ii) *intra-atrial tachyarrhythmias* in which the arrhythmia arises entirely within the atria and the AV junction is an incidental bystander. The other key change has been the introduction of intravenous adenosine for diagnosis and treatment of narrow complex tachycardia.[3] These issues are also explored in more detail below.

10.2 Differential diagnosis, classification and electrophysiological mechanisms

The differential diagnosis of narrow complex tachycardia is shown in Box 10.1. Traditional medical textbooks are often vague about the mechanisms and classification of narrow complex tachycardias. The modern approach is to subdivide these into two major categories: "junctional tachycardias" in which the arrhythmia is dependent upon the AV junction usually as part of a re-entrant circuit, and "atrial tachyarrhythmias" in which the arrhythmia arises entirely within the atria and the AV junction acts merely as a bystander.[2] In general, vagal manoeuvres, intravenous adenosine and other AV nodal blocking drugs (verapamil, digoxin etc.) will tend to terminate a junctional tachycardia but will only slow the ventricular response to an atrial tachyarrhythmia.

Box 10.1 Differential diagnosis of narrow complex tachycardia

Junctional tachyarrhythmias

- Atrioventricular nodal re-entrant tachycardia (AVNRT)
- Atrioventricular re-entrant tachycardia (AVRT) ±
  Wolff–Parkinson–White syndrome
- Junctional ectopic tachycardia (rare)

Intra-atrial tachyarrhythmias

- Atrial flutter
- Atrial tachycardia
- Sinus node re-entrant tachycardia (SNRT)
- Sinus tachycardia

10.2.1 Junctional tachyarrhythmias

Atrioventricular nodal re-entrant tachycardia (AVNRT)

This is the commonest cause of paroxysmal SVT in adulthood. AVNRT is due to re-entrant activation of a circuit within the AV node itself consisting of distinct longitudinal routes of conduction that are also referred to as "pathways" (Figure 10.2a). Two or more AV nodal pathways can be demonstrated in a majority of the population, but the electrical properties are only suitable for re-entrant tachycardia in a small proportion of these (otherwise SVT would be almost universal!). In the commonest or "typical" form of AVNRT, the antegrade limb is a "slow pathway" located posteriorly (near the coronary sinus) and the retrograde limb is a "fast pathway" located more anterosuperiorly near the His bundle. This results in near simultaneous activation of the atria and ventricles during tachycardia (1:1 relationship but with the retrograde P waves buried into QRS complexes; Figure 10.2a). In "atypical" cases the retrograde limb either conducts relatively slowly (P waves fall after the QRS complexes) or the sequence is effectively reversed with the slow pathway forming the retrograde limb (P wave delayed until late diastole to produce a "long RP" tachycardia; Figure 10.3). These ECG appearances are discussed in more detail below. Like AVRT, AVNRT is dependent on the AV junction for its perpetuation and may also be terminated by vagal manoeuvres or by AV nodal blocking drugs such as adenosine and verapamil.

Atrioventricular re-entrant tachycardia (AVRT)

This arrhythmia occurs because of re-entrant electrical activation using a circuit formed by the AV junction in the antegrade direction and an "accessory pathway" in the retrograde (VA) direction to allow electrical impulses to return to the atria (Figures 10.2b, 10.5). Accessory pathways are congenital extra-nodal connections between the atria and ventricle which are present in up to 0.2% of the population. Re-entry is most often initiated either by appropriately timed spontaneous ectopic beats or sinus tachycardia. AVRT is the commonest arrhythmia in patients with Wolff–Parkinson–White syndrome: in sinus rhythm the ECG shows a delta wave because the pathway is conducting in the AV direction to pre-excite the ventricles but during AVRT the delta wave disappears because the pathway is conducting exclusively the retrograde VA direction, and hence a narrow complex tachycardia is produced (see Chapter 11, Figures 11.4, 11.5). AVRT can also occur in patients with "concealed" accessory pathways which are only capable of unidirectional conduction in the retrograde VA direction: these individuals will suffer attacks of narrow complex tachycardia but will not exhibit pre-excitation (i.e. a delta wave) during sinus rhythm. As indicated above, AVRT may be terminated by vagal manoeuvres, adenosine and verapamil.

Junctional ectopic tachycardia (JET)

This uncommon arrhythmia is due to an automatic focus arising in the His-bundle region, generating a narrow complex tachyarrhythmia often with retrograde block to the atria and thus VA dissociation. It is most commonly encountered in children (particularly after cardiac surgery) but rare adult cases are seen.

Narrow complex tachycardia

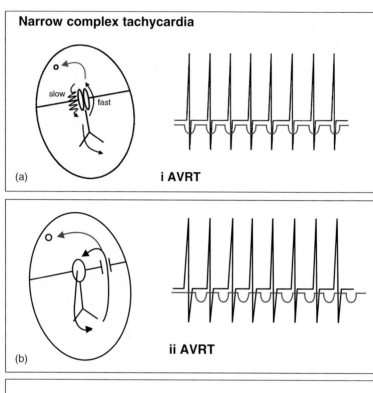

(a) **i AVRT**

(b) **ii AVRT**

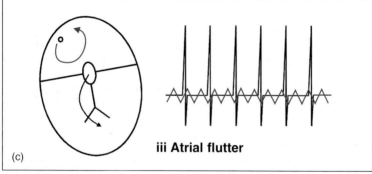

(c) **iii Atrial flutter**

Figure 10.2(a) Atrioventricular nodal re-entrant tachycardia (AVNRT). Re-entry using dual AV nodal pathways with near simultaneous activation of atria and ventricles, therefore the retrograde P waves are typically hidden in the QRS complexes. (b) Atrioventricular re-entrant tachycardia (AVRT). Re-entry using AV node (antegrade) and accessory pathway (retrograde) therefore retrograde P waves inscribed after the QRS complexes (may be visible in the inferior leads). (c) Atrial flutter with 2:1 block. Macroreentrant excitation of right atrium producing a continuous "sawtooth" baseline with no isoelectric phase.

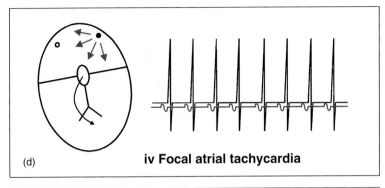

(d)   **iv Focal atrial tachycardia**

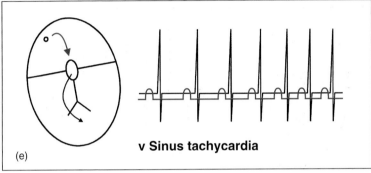

(e)   **v Sinus tachycardia**

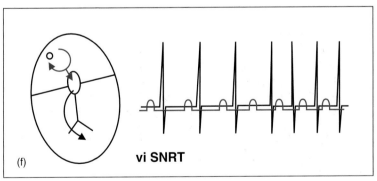

(f)   **vi SNRT**

Figure 10.2(d) Atrial tachycardia with 1:1 conduction. Discrete P waves of abnormal morphology with an isoelectric phase, reflecting activation of the atria from a focal source. (e) Sinus node re-entrant tachycardia (SNRT). Re-entrant activation within high right atrium involving sinus node tissue generating P waves of normal morphology with abrupt change in heart rate at onset or offset. (f) Sinus tachycardia. Physiological acceleration of sinus rate, resulting in P waves of normal morphology but no abrupt onset or offset (unlike SNRT).

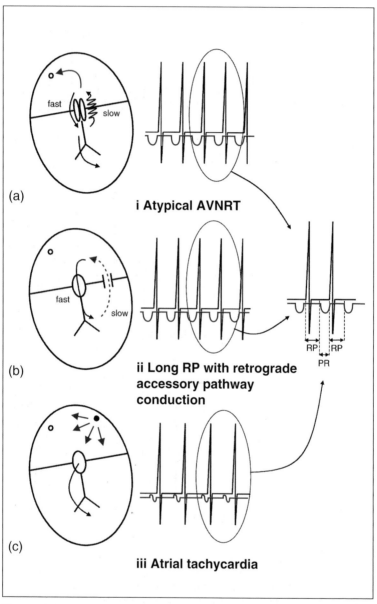

i Atypical AVNRT

ii Long RP with retrograde accessory pathway conduction

iii Atrial tachycardia

Figure 10.3 Long RP tachycardia. Narrow complex tachycardia with 1:1 atrioventricular relationship but P waves late during diastole such that RP interval >PR interval. This may arise from: (a), atypical AVNRT (reversed slow and fast pathway activation); (b) AVRT with slow-conducting accessory pathway; (c) or atrial tachycardia.

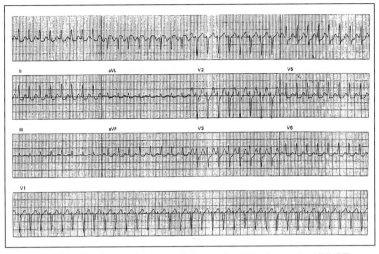

Fig.10.4 ECG of atrioventricular nodal re-entrant tachycardia (AVNRT). Narrow complex tachycardia with no discernible P waves.

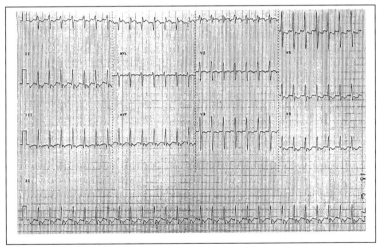

Figure 10.5 ECG of atrioventricular re-entrant tachycardia (AVRT). Narrow complex tachycardia with retrograde (inverted) P waves visible in the inferior leads 80 ms after QRS offset. This patient subsequently underwent ablation of a left lateral accessory pathway (concealed).

10.2.2 Intra-atrial tachyarrhythmias

Atrial flutter

This arrhythmia is caused by "macroreentrant" excitation of the right atrium. In the common or typical form (sometimes referred to as "type I" flutter) the circuit involves counterclockwise activation via the floor of the right atrium, the interatrial septum and the lateral right atrial wall, traversing the isthmus between the tricuspid annulus and the inferior vena cava where the arrhythmia can be interrupted by catheter ablation. Continuous electrical activation of the right atrium at 250–350 bpm by this macoreentrant process is responsible for the classical "sawtooth" baseline with no isoelectric phase between each cycle (unlike atrial tachycardia) (Figures 10.2c, 10.6). Atypical forms of atrial flutter involve variants of the circuit described above. Atrial flutter is not dependent on the AV junction, and so vagal manoeuvres, adenosine, etc., will usually just produce transient slowing of the ventricular rate to reveal the underlying atrial rhythm (Figure 10.2c). Pharmacological termination or suppression requires drugs which alter the electrophysiological properties of atrial myocardium. Flutter is closely related to AF, and it is not unusual for both arrhythmias to occur in the same patient. Like AF, flutter is most commonly found in association with structural heart disease although a proportion of patients seem to have morphologically normal hearts.

Atrial tachycardia

This is sometimes referred to as "ectopic atrial tachycardia". In contrast to atrial flutter, the arrhythmia is caused by a discrete focus of electrical activity firing more rapidly than the sinus node, and activating the atria centrifugally. As a result, the ECG shows a series of P waves usually of abnormal morphology, separated by an isoelectric baseline corresponding to the diastolic phase (Figures 10.2d, 10.7). Atrial tachycardia may be due to either microreentry or an automatic focus. In children and young adults it often occurs in the context of a normal heart, but in older patients atrial tachycardia is more likely to be associated with structural heart disease. As with flutter, manoeuvres to block the AV node will usually just slow the ventricular rate to reveal the underlying atrial rhythm. However, some forms of atrial tachycardia (particularly sinus node re-entrant tachycardia) are adenosine-sensitive and may be terminated by IV adenosine.

Sinus node re-entrant tachycardia (SNRT)

This is a specific form of re-entrant atrial tachycardia exiting from the vicinity of the sinus node in the high lateral wall of the right atrium. Thus, the ECG appearance is identical to sinus tachycardia but the characteristic feature is abrupt offset and onset (Figures 10.2e, 10.8). These sudden changes in heart rate differentiate SNRT from physiological sinus tachychardia (see below). SNRT is also terminated by adenosine because the re-entrant circuit invariably involves some sinus node tissue. This arrhythmia is probably very common as a cause of mild symptomatic tachcardia and often co-exists with other SVT mechanisms. However, SNRT is the primary or dominant arrhythmia in less than 5% of SVT cases.

Sinus tachycardia

Physiological sinus tachycardia can be difficult to differentiate from other forms of narrow complex tachycardia if each P wave becomes buried in the preceding T wave or QRS complex, particularly at heart rates exceeding 140 bpm (Figure 10.1f). This situation is most commonly encountered with sick patients on intensive care units who may be haemodynamically compromised and receiving adrenaline (epinephrine) or other catecholamine infusions. Adenosine provocation will produce gradual deceleration of the sinus rate followed by acceleration (often to a faster rate than at baseline), with or without AV block, in contrast to the abrupt termination seen in SNRT.

10.3 Management (step 1): initial assessment

The initial evaluation of a patient presenting with narrow complex tachycardia should always include: (i) 12-lead ECG, and (ii) assessment of haemodynamic status. As indicated previously, the 12-lead ECG is essential because some cases of broad complex tachycardia can be mistaken for narrow complex tachycardia if a single-lead rhythm strip is recorded in isolation. As ventricular tachycardia is the most common cause of broad complex tachycardia, such a misdiagnosis could have serious consequences. ECG interpretation can also provide clues to the underlying arrhythmia (see below).

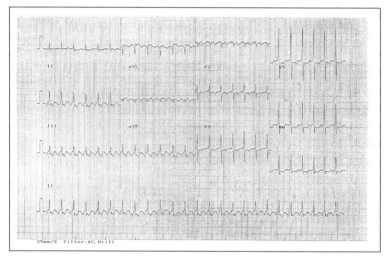

Figure 10.6 ECG of atrial flutter with 2:1 conduction. Narrow complex tachycardia with classical "sawtooth" baseline due to continuous, macroreentrant activation of the atria.

Unlike broad complex tachycardia, most cases of narrow complex tachycardia occur in healthy individuals with structurally normal hearts with the exception of atrial flutter. Although patients frequently complain of symptoms such as dyspnoea, lightheadedness, anginal-type chest discomfort, etc., it is rare for narrow complex tachycardia to be associated with objective evidence of haemodynamic disturbance such as pulmonary oedema, profound hypotension, or shock, and such adverse findings are highly suggestive of underlying cardiac disease.

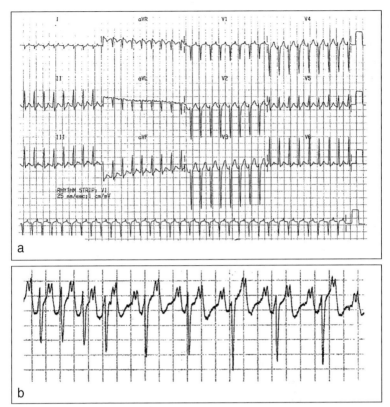

Figure 10.7 ECG of atrial tachycardia with 1:1 conduction. (a) Narrow complex tachycardia at 200 bpm with abnormal P wave morphology (positive in V1). This patient subsequently underwent catheter ablation of a left atrial focus. (b) Transient 2:1 conduction of the atrial tachycardia revealed following administration of IV adenosine 18 mg.

10.4 Management (step 2): determining the mechanism of narrow complex tachycardia

The modern approach to cases of narrow complex tachycardia should include an attempt to identify the underlying electrophysiological mechanism, particularly whether the. arrhythmia is atrial or junctional in origin. ECG interpretation in narrow complex tachycardia depends on identifying subtle variations in underlying P wave (atrial) activity, and the findings are often not sufficiently specific to determine the

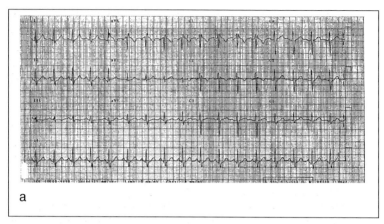

a

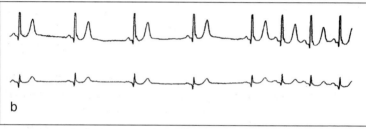

b

Figure 10.8(a) Sinus node reentrant tachycardia (SNRT). Narrow complex tachycardia at 120 bpm with normal P wave morphology, equally consistent with physiological sinus tachycardia. (b) Rhythm strip demonstrates abrupt onset of tachycardia (heart rate jumps from 75 to 120 bpm) with no change in P wave morphology.

mechanism with certainty (see below). In such cases it is necessary to resort to further testing with reflex vagal manoeuvres and/or adenosine administration. The rationale behind both techniques is to produce transient AV block which will:

- Terminate a junctional tachycardia, because the AV node is an obligatory part of the re-entrant circuit.
- Temporarily slow the ventricular rate of intra-atrial tachyarrhythmias to unmask the underlying atrial electrical activity.

The distinction between atrial and junctional tachyarrhythmias is of clinical importance with respect to several issues.

- *Immediate treatment.* Junctional tachyarrhythmias can be terminated either by vagal manoeuvres or AV nodal blocking drugs (adenosine, verapamil, etc.) with almost 100% success. Most atrial tachyarrhythmias will only respond to antiarrhythmic agents with electrophysiological actions on atrial muscle (flecainide, procainamide, amiodarone, etc.). Furthermore, as pharmacological conversion is much less successful than for junctional tachyarrhythmias, electrical cardioversion can be required. In some cases, rate-control with digoxin or other AV nodal blocking drugs may be more appropriate than attempts to restore sinus rhythm.
- *Thromboembolic risk.* If the diagnosis is of an atrial tachyarrhythmia (particularly flutter) which has persisted for >48 hours, attempts to restore sinus rhythm immediately will be associated with some risk of systemic thromboembolism as also applies to acute AF (see Chapter 9).
- *Subsequent management.* As with acute treatment, the electrophysiological mechanism also influences selection of maintenance antiarrhythmic drug therapy.
- *Associated cardiac disease.* Atrial tachyarrhythmias (particularly flutter) are more likely to be associated with underlying structural heart disease.

10.4.1 ECG interpretation

By definition, all cases of narrow complex tachycardia exhibit both normal QRS morphology and regular cycle length (thus, arrhythmias such as SVT with bundle branch block aberration, atrial flutter with variable block, and AF do not enter the differential diagnosis). Differences in the ECG appearance of narrow complex tachycardia may arise due to variations in atrioventricular ratio, P wave morphology and timing of the P waves relative to the QRS complexes and these are discussed in more detail below. Interpretation of these comparatively subtle ECG signs is not always straightforward (even for arrhythmia experts), especially as the P waves are frequently obscured by ventricular electrical activity (i.e. QRS complexes, ST segments, or T waves). Furthermore, the ECG appearances in themselves may not be sufficiently specific to determine the underlying mechanism of the tachycardia without resorting to vagal manoeuvres and/or adenosine provocation. It is important to stress that a detailed knowledge of the ECG variants in narrow complex tachycardia is not a prerequisite for successful diagnosis and acute management.

Atrioventricular ratio

All junctional tachyarrhythmias and many cases of atrial tachycardia (including SNRT) exhibit a 1:1 atrioventricular relationship. Rapid atrial tachycardia and most cases of atrial flutter may conduct to the ventricles with a 2:1 ratio. However, ventricular activity may make it difficult to detect such a 2:1 relationship without vagal manoeuvres or adenosine to transiently increase AV block (see Figure).

Morphology of the P wave

P wave morphology is often obscured by ventricular activity but, if apparent, may yield important information. With junctional tachycardias there is reverse activation of the atria from the AV junction upwards (compared to the normal activation from the sinus node downwards) resulting in inverted P waves in the inferior leads. Atrial tachycardia will result in normal P wave morphology if arising from the high right atrium (including SNRT), otherwise the appearance depends on location of the ectopic focus. For example, left atrial tachycardia classically produces positive P waves in V1 and/or negative P waves in aVL (Figure 10.7). In atrial flutter, there is continuous atrial activation (due to macroreentrant excitation of the right atrium) with no isoelectric phase producing the classical sawtooth baseline. In many cases of narrow complex tachycardia, the underlying atrial activity can only be properly scrutinised during transient AV block produced with vagal manoeuvres or adenosme.

Timing of P waves relative to the QRS complexes

In typical AVNRT, there is almost simultaneous activation of atria and ventricles and the P waves are usually "lost" in the QRS complexes (Figure 10.4) or may be just visible as a notch (r') on the end of the QRS complex in V1. In AVRT, ventricular activation precedes atrial activation and the retrograde P waves may be visible within the early part of the ST segment clear of the QRS complexes, particularly in the inferior leads (Figure 10.5). In atrial tachycardia with 1:1 conduction, each P wave is conducted antegradely and followed by a QRS complex. However, if the "PR" interval is close to the cycle length of the tachycardia, the P wave may become buried into the preceding QRS complex simulating the timing of typical AVNRT. Similarly, if the "PR" interval is slightly shorter than the atrial tachycardia cycle length, the P waves may fall within the ST segment and resemble AVRT. Thus, the relative timing of P waves and QRS complexes may not allow the mechanism of tachycardia to be determined without further testing.

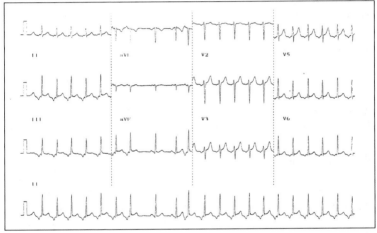

Figure 10.9 Long RP tachycardia. Narrow complex tachycardia at 140 bpm with retrograde (inverted) P waves visible in the inferior leads and RP interval >PR interval. Tachycardia terminates to reveal two beats of sinus rhythm with normal P wave morphology, then reinitiates. This patient was suffering from incessant tachycardia with rate-related cardiomyopathy and subsequently underwent catheter ablation for an atypical AVNRT.

Long RP tachycardias

A specific subset of narrow complex tachycardia is formed by the so-called "long RP" tachycardias, in which atrial activation occurs late in diastole such that the "RP" interval is greater than the "PR" interval to the next QRS complex (Figures 10.3,

10.9). This relatively uncommon appearance may be generated by a variety of mechanisms: atypical forms of AVNRT (in which the typical slow-fast pattern is reversed), unusual forms of AVRT using slow conducting bypass tracts, 1:1 atrial tachycardia with a relatively short "PR" interval, and 2:1 atrial tachycardia if every other P wave is lost in the QRS complexes. Once again, it may not be possible to differentiate junctional and atrial forms of long RP tachycardia without vagal manoeuvres ± adenosine testing.

10.4.2 Vagal manoeuvres

The use of physical manoeuvres to elicit reflex vagal efferent stimulation of the AV node for termination of SVT, or to increase AV block during atrial tachyarrhythmias, has been part of standard clinical practice for many years. The most commonly employed techniques are carotid sinus massage, Valsalva manoeuvre, and the diving reflex (face immersion in cold water). Whichever method is used, an ECG rhythm strip must be recorded continuously during testing to document the response for later scrutiny. Ideally a simultaneous 3- or 6-channel recording should be used, as a single-lead strip may not reveal the underlying atrial activity so clearly.

Some studies have suggested that vagal manoeuvres can terminate over 50% of junctional tachycardias, but these were performed in patients undergoing intracardiac electrophysiological testing and within 5 minutes of arrhythmia induction.[4] The true "efficacy" of physical manoeuvres is probably much lower in spontaneous cases of narrow complex tachycardia presenting to the emergency department, often after a delay of several hours. The most effective technique appears to be the Valsalva manoeuvre (ideally forced expiration into an aneroid manometer at 30–40 mmHg for 15 seconds without taking a deep inspiration beforehand). All vagal manoeuvres are more successful if performed with the patient supine rather than erect to minimise sympathetic drive. They are also more likely to work in young adults and children who exhibit proportionately greater increases in efferent parasympathetic response (because baroreflex sensitivity is age-related).

10.4.3 Adenosine

Adenosine is an endogenous purine nucleotide which is rapidly metabolised and produces transient atrioventricular nodal block following bolus intravenous administration.[3,5] The brief duration of action (circulatory half-life of approximately 10 seconds) makes it an extremely safe agent to use in the emergency management of tachyarrhythmias unlike longer-acting AV nodal blocking drugs such as verapamil.[6] However, it is essential to be aware of the following points.

- There is a 10-fold variation in the minimum effective dose between patients, and up to 20% of patients may require more than 12 mg of adenosine to achieve termination or AV block. Accordingly, our suggested incremental dosing schedule is 6 mg → 12 mg → 18 mg → 24 mg. An ECG rhythm strip (preferably multi-channel) must be recorded continuously during testing to document the response.
- Adenosine also exerts profound electrophysiological effects on the atrium and sinus node; some forms of atrial tachycardia, particularly sinus node re-entrant tachycardia, are "adenosine-sensitive" and may also be terminated following bolus administration. By contrast, adenosine administration in physiological sinus tachycardia should produce gradual deceleration of the sinus rate (with or without AV block) followed by gradual acceleration.
- Dose-titration may be limited by intolerable side-effects (chest pain, dyspnoea, or flushing). The patient should always be warned about these in advance and discouraged from hyperventilating which tends to disrupt the ECG recording.
- Adenosine has an excellent safety record in the emergency management of arrhythmias. Although asthma is often listed as a relative contraindication, because of the ultrashort circulatory half-life, adenosine can be used with reasonable safety except in patients with acute asthmatic attacks.
- A few patients are at increased risk of severe bradycardia, in particular cardiac transplant recipients (denervation hypersensitivity to adenosine), those receiving concomitant dipyridamole treatment (potentiation of adenosine),and those with sino-atrial disease but no

pacemaker, particularly in the so-called tachy-brady syndrome. In these cases, it is advisable to use 3 mg dose increments and to ensure the availability of transcutaneous pacing facilities for back up (see Chapter 12).

10.5 Management (step 3): treatment of junctional tachycardias

The immediate treatment of junctional tachycardia (AVNRT or AVRT) should always be to restore sinus rhythm. This is usually straightforward and can be achieved in almost 100% of cases. Subsequent management depends on several factors, in particular whether the patient has Wolff–Parkinson–White syndrome, and the frequency/severity of attacks. The available options for acute termination are as follows.

10.5.1 Vagal manoeuvres and adenosine

It will be apparent that in patients with junctional tachycardia, these serve a combined diagnostic and therapeutic function (see Table 10.1 for details). Vagal manoeuvres avoid the need for intravenous cannulation and hence are the preferred treatment for children.

10.5.2 Verapamil

Intravenous verapamil (5–15 mg by slow injection) was the traditional first-line treatment for junctional tachycardia until the introduction of adenosine. Comparative studies have shown that the efficacy of these two agents is very similar,[3,6] although adenosine may have to be given at doses exceeding 12 mg in a significant minority of cases. The potential disadvantages of verapamil are that it cannot be administered to patients already taking a β-blocker or those exhibiting signs of haemodynamic compromise or instability (heart failure or hypotension). Apart from these few exceptions, it remains a useful treatment for junctional tachycardia and should always be tried if adenosine fails. Verapamil may be the drug of choice if adenosine is not tolerated due to side-effects or is relatively contra-indicated due to acute asthma, dipyridamole treatment, or prior cardiac transplantation.

Table 10.1 Effects of vagal manoeuvres, adenosine, and verapamil in narrow complex tachycardia.

	Vagal manoeuvres	IV adenosine	IV verapamil
AVNRT	Terminates (+)	Terminates (++)	Terminates (++)
AVRT	Terminates (+)	Terminates (++)	Terminates (++)
Atrial flutter	Slows (+)	Slows (++) Terminates (±)	Slows (++)
Atrial tachycardia	Slows (+)	Slows (++) Terminates (±)	Slows (++)
SNRT	Terminates (±)	Terminates (++)	No effect
Sinus tachycardia	Slows (±)	Slows (+)	No effect

10.5.3 Other antiarrhythmic agents

Although a variety of other drugs such as intravenous flecainide (2 mg/kg maximum 150 mg) or intravenous sotalol (60–120 mg) can be used to restore sinus rhythm with moderate efficacy, these are rarely needed because of the very high conversion rates achieved with vagal manoeuvres or adenosine/verapamil. Occasional patients with known Wolff–Parkinson–White syndrome and AVRT may receive flecainide if they are known to be at high risk of pre-excited AF.

10.5.4 DC cardioversion

This is seldom required but may be indicated in patients exhibiting haemodynamic instability who have not responded to adenosine at adequate dosage.

Following restoration of sinus rhythm, the 12-lead ECG must be repeated specifically to check for the presence of pre-excitation. All patients with Wolff–Parkinson–White syndrome should be referred for full evaluation by a cardiologist because there is a small risk of sudden cardiac death from degeneration of rapid pre-excited AF to VF (see Chapter 11, Figures 11.3, 11.4). Thus, in some of these cases, curative catheter ablation of the accessory pathway will be recommended on prognostic grounds irrespective of symptomatology.[1] As an interim measure, it may be advisable to start an antiarrhythmic agent that will prolong the antegrade refractory period of the pathway and thus offer some protection during an episode of AF. Flecainide 100–150 mg bd is our first choice drug (or another class IC agent). A β-blocker would be a suitable alternative.

If the ECG back in sinus rhythm shows no evidence of pre-excitation, subsequent management depends principally on the frequency and severity of the attacks. Following a first ever episode of paroxysmal SVT, the patient can be reassured and given instruction in how to perform vagal manoeuvres but there is no automatic indication to start antiarrhythmic drugs. If the attacks have been occurring on a regular basis and/or have been poorly tolerated, patients should be offered pharmacological treatment. The most commonly used agents are verapamil 80 mg tds (or 240 mg od as a slow-release preparation), β-blockers, or occasionally digoxin. Sotalol acts purely as a β-blocker at lower doses (40–80 mg bd) but with additional class III activity at higher doses (120–160 mg bd). If medical therapy has failed to control the arrhythmias or the patient is reluctant to take long-term medication, referral for catheter ablation on symptomatic grounds is appropriate.[1]

Most patients presenting with a junctional tachycardia (including those with Wolff–Parkinson–White syndrome) can be successfully treated in the emergency department and discharged directly, with subsequent management on an outpatient basis.

10.6 Management (step 4): treatment of atrial tachyarrhythmias

The immediate treatment of atrial tachyarrhythmias diverges from that of junctional tachycardia in several important respects, and more closely resembles the management of acute atrial fibrillation (see Chapter 9). The key differences are as follows:

- If the patient presents more than 48–72 hours after onset, cardioversion may be associated with some risk of systemic thromboembolism (as in acute AF), and the safest approach is ventricular rate-control plus anticoagulation, usually followed by interval cardioversion as an outpatient 4–6 weeks later. Immediate cardioversion should only be considered for severe haemodynamic compromise, ideally after left atrial thrombus has been excluded by transoesophageal echocardiography, and patients should be anticoagulated afterwards to protect against the phenomenon of "atrial stunning" (see Chapter 9). If the arrhythmia is of less than 48–72 hours duration, the risk of systemic thromboembolism is low and it should be reasonably safe to undertake pharmacological or electrical cardioversion without anticoagulant pre-treatment.
- Vagal manoeuvres and adenosine will not terminate most atrial tachyarrhythmias. The exceptions are sinus node re-entrant tachycardia, rare forms of adenosine-sensitive atrial tachycardia, and occasional cases of atrial flutter which convert to sinus rhythm via transient acceleration.
- Pharmacological cardioversion is generally less successful with atrial flutter than with acute AF (see Chapter 9). Intravenous amiodarone is probably the most effective agent but converts less than 50% of cases. Class I drugs are even less effective, relatively contraindicated if there is evidence of underlying heart disease, and also associated with a risk of paradoxically accelerating the ventricular by slowing the atrial rate to the point at which 2:1 atrioventricular ratio converts to 1:1 conduction. For all of these reasons, electrical cardioversion of atrial flutter is often required. Newer class III agents such as ibutilide (already released in the USA but not yet available in the UK or Europe) appear to be much more effective at terminating atrial flutter than traditional agents and may reduce the need for DC cardioversion in the future.[7]
- Pharmacological conversion of atrial tachycardia may be attempted in patients with no definite evidence of structural heart disease or haemodynamic compromise. In

this setting, class I agents such as flecainide (2 mg/kg, maximum dose 150 mg) may restore sinus rhythm in over 70% of cases. As in atrial flutter, care needs to be taken with cases of atrial tachycardia and 2 : 1 atrioventricular conduction because of the possibility of slowing the atrial rate sufficiently to allow 1:1 conduction. DC cardioversion may be undertaken in patients for whom pharmacological therapy is unsuitable or unsuccessful.

- If patients present with atrial flutter or atrial tachycardia more than 48–72 hours after onset, i.e. too late to be candidates for immediate cardioversion, rate-control may be required to reduce the response to < 100 bpm. The most commonly used agents are digoxin, verapamil, and β-blockers. It should be noted that rate-control can be problematic in patients with atrial flutter and combination treatment (e.g. digoxin plus β-blockers) is often needed.

Most patients can be discharged directly from the emergency department if cardioversion (pharmacological or electrical) is successful. Even if the immediate management is rate-control rather than cardioversion, there is no automatic need for hospitalisation provided that the arrhythmia is well tolerated. However, arrangements should be made for all such cases to be reviewed in outpatients for further clinical assessment and echocardiography, before determining subsequent management. If an attempt at interval cardioversion is likely, it may be worth initiating full anticoagulation with warfarin.

Patients generally require admission if the atrial tachyarrhythmia is poorly tolerated, or if there is associated cardiac disease that merits further investigation and treatment on an urgent basis, for example acute myocardial infarction or decompensated congestive heart failure.

Clinical cases

Case 10.1

A previously fit 26-year-old man presented to the A&E department with a 4-hour history of rapid palpitation and mild lightheadedness. His admission ECG showed a regular narrow complex tachycardia at 200 bpm and the P waves could not be seen with certainty. Vagal manoeuvres produced no effect. Incremental bolus doses of IV adenosine were administered up to 6 mg which terminated the tachycardia. Back in sinus rhythm his ECG showed manifest pre-excitation indicating the diagnosis of Wolff–Parkinson–White (WPW) syndrome. He was started on atenolol 50 mg od and allowed to go home but was subsequently referred for intracardiac electrophysiological studies. He was found to have a left free wall pathway with a short antegrade refractory period which was successfully treated by catheter ablation.

All patients with WPW syndrome and paroxysmal SVT should be referred for specialist evaluation and possible catheter ablation as there is a risk of sudden cardiac death (approximately 0.25% per annum) due to degeneration of rapid pre-excited atrial fibrillation.

Case 10.2

A 19-year-old man was admitted with an episode of narrow complex tachycardia at 220 bpm which had persisted for 2 hours and caused severe palpitation and central chest tightness. He had had a similar attack 3 years previously which had terminated spontaneously after 40 minutes. On arrival, he was extremely anxious but haemodynamically stable, BP 90/60 with no signs of heart failure. Incremental bolus doses of adenosine were administered up to 12 mg without effect and were poorly tolerated to chest pain and dyspnoea. However, the tachycardia was terminated with IV verapamil 5 mg. His ECG in sinus rhythm was normal. He was discharged from the A&E department directly on no medication but was instructed in the use of vagal manoeuvres. No routine follow-up was organised but his GP was advised to refer him to a cardiologist if he experienced further attacks of tachycardia.

It is not uncommon for patients to require doses of IV adenosine above 12 mg (usually 18 or 24 mg) to terminate narrow complex tachycardia, but as the adenosine had been poorly tolerated verapamil was used instead. As this was only the second attack in 3 years and there was no evidence of pre-excitation or structural heart disease, it was reasonable not to initiate maintenance antiarrhythmic drug therapy. If he had suffered recurrent episodes of tachycardia, it would have been appropriate to start a β-blocker or verapamil. Referral for electrophysiological testing would only be required for patients with recurrent, troublesome symptoms despite drug therapy, or those in whom medical therapy fails due to intolerance of antiarrhythmic drugs, or who are reluctant to take drugs at all (for example, young women planning to become pregnant).

Case 10.3

A 64-year-old man was referred with a 2-week history of lassitude, worsening dyspnoea and vague palpitation. He had a past history of hypertension treated with a thiazide diuretic, but no other cardiac problems. He was found to have a resting tachycardia, BP 150/90 with cardiomegaly, S3 gallop and both clinical and radiological signs of mild pulmonary congestion. The ECG showed regular narrow complex tachycardia at 160 bpm and the admitting registrar was uncertain about the underlying P wave activity and whether the rhythm was sinus tachycardia, a junctional SVT or atrial flutter. Vagal manoeuvres had no effect but IV adenosine 18 mg produced transient AV block to reveal a "sawtooth" baseline. Thus, the diagnosis was atrial flutter with 2 : 1 block. He was admitted and initially treated with digoxin, loop diuretics and IV heparin (followed by anticoagulation with warfarin). Over the next 36 hours, the ventricular rate slowed to 100 bpm and his clinical condition stabilised. Echocardiography showed LVH with moderately impaired systolic function but no other abnormality. An ACE inhibitor was added and he was loaded with amiodarone, discharged and brought back 4 weeks later for interval DC cardioversion which was successful. At follow-up 6 weeks after that, he remained in sinus rhythm with dramatic symptomatic improvement and normalisation of LV function on echocardiography. Warfarin, digoxin and diuretics were stopped but he was maintained on amiodarone and the ACE inhibitor.

In this case adenosine provocation showed that the electro-physiological mechanism was atrial flutter, occurring on a background of hypertensive heart disease and with secondary depression of LV function due to rate-related cardiomyopathy. Had the patient presented within 48 hours of onset, immediate cardioversion could have been considered without the need for prolonged anticoagulation before and afterwards (as in acute AF, see Chapter 9). In fact he had been in atrial flutter for 2 weeks, but his condition was easily stabilised with digoxin plus diuretics and so it was no problem to defer the cardioversion for another 4 weeks. If he had been more severely affected by the tachyarrhythmia and had not responded to the initial treatment, he could have been offered early DC cardioversion provided that transoesophageal echocardiography showed no evidence of left atrial thrombus, and the cardioversion was followed by at least 1 month of anticoagulation.

Case 10.4

A 23-year-old woman presented with rapid palpitation. This had come on abruptly the previous day and had been well tolerated but she had consulted her GP after the attack had persisted through the night. Her ECG showed a regular narrow complex tachycardia at 150 bpm with apparently 1 : 1 relationship of the P waves to the QRS complexes. The P waves appeared to be inverted in the inferior leads and upright in VI and V2. She was haemodynamically stable with no abnormal findings in the cardiovascular system apart from the tachycardia. IV adenosine 12 mg produced only transient AV block revealing an underlying atrial tachycardia with discrete P waves. IV flecainide

2 mg/kg was administered and resulted in slowing and then termination of the arrhythmia. She was discharged from the A&E department on no treatment and reviewed in the cardiology clinic a few weeks later at which time echocardiography showed normal cardiac structure and function. Over the next 12 months, she had numerous further attacks of atrial tachycardia which could not be suppressed by flecainide, β-blockers or sotalol. Accordingly, she was referred for electrophysiological studies and eventually underwent successful catheter ablation of a left atrial focus near the mouth of the left inferior pulmonary vein.

Focal atrial tachycardia is a less common cause of narrow complex tachycardia in adulthood than junctional SVT but must be differentiated because both medical management and ablative therapy are quite different.

Summary

Narrow complex tachycardia is always supraventricular in origin but should, if possible, be diagnosed from a 12-lead ECG rather than a rhythm strip to avoid misrecognition of broad complex tachycardia.

Classification of narrow complex tachycardia is according to electrophysiological mechanism as: "junctional tachyarrhythmias" (AV junction is obligatory component of arrhythmic substrate); and "atrial tachyarrhythmias" (intra-atrial arrhythmic substrate not involving AV junction).

The common forms of junctional tachycardia are AV nodal re-entrant tachycardia (AVNRT) and AV re-entrant tachycardia (AVRT). AVRT also occurs as part of the Wolff-Parkinson-White syndrome. These arrhythmias are not associated with structural heart disease and the prognosis is benign except for Wolff–Parkinson–White syndrome.

Intra-atrial tachyarrhythmias include atrial flutter, atrial tachycardia and sinus node re-entrant tachycardia (SNRT). These arrhythmias may be associated with structural heart disease and a risk of systemic thromboembolism.

It may not be possible to determine the mechanism of narrow complex tachycardia from the ECG alone. Vagal manoeuvres and IV adenosine terminate junctional tachycardia, but only transiently slow, atrial tachyarrhythmias (except for SNRT).

Junctional tachycardia can invariably be terminated with IV adenosine or verapamil. Pharmacological cardioversion of atrial tachyarrhythmias is often ineffective and DC cardioversion (immediate or interval) may be required.

Junctional tachyarrhythmia may be suppressed by AV nodal blocking drugs (verapamil, digoxin, etc.) as well as β-blockers and class I agents. Atrial tachyarrhythmias can only be suppressed by drugs acting on the atria (class I agents, sotalol, amiodarone, etc.), and efficacy is generally poor.

References

1. ACC/AHA Task Force. Guidelines for intracardiac electrophysiological and catheter ablation procedures. *J Am Coll Cardiol* 1995;**26**:555–73.
2. Bar FW, Brugada P, Dassen WRM, Wellens HJJ. Differential diagnosis of tachycardia with narrow QRS complex (<0.12 second). *Am J Cardiol* 1984;**54**:555–60.
3. Rankin AC, Brooks R, Ruskin JN. Adenosine and treatment of supraventricular tachycardia. *Am J Med* 1992;**92**:655–64.
4. Mehta D, Wafa S, Ward DE, Camm AJ. Relative efficacy of various physical manoeuvres in the termination of junctional tachycardia. *Lancet* 1988;**i**:1181–5.
5. Rankin AC, Oldroyd KG, Chong E, Rae AP, Cobbe SM. Value and limitations of adenosine in the diagnosis and treatment of narrow and broad complex tachycardias. *Br Heart J* 1989;**62**:195–203.
6. DiMarco JP, Miles W, Milstein S, *et al.* Adenosine for paroxysmal SVT: dose ranging and comparison with verapamil. *Ann Intern Med* 1990;**113**:104–10.
7. Stambler BS, Wood MA, Ellenbogen KA, *et al.* Efficacy and safety of repeated intravenous doses of ibutilide for rapid conversion of atrial flutter or fibrillation. *Circulation* 1996;**94**:1613–21.

11: Broad complex tachycardia

N WEST, Y BASHIR

11.1 Introduction

Broad complex tachycardia is a common presentation in emergency medicine. The term refers to cardiac arrhythmias with ventricular rate >100 bpm and QRS duration >120 ms, and usually regular cycle lengths. The vast majority of cases are due to either monomorphic ventricular tachycardia (VT) or supraventricular tachycardia (SVT) with "aberrant" conduction (bundle branch block), although rarely the differential diagnosis may include pre-excited tachyarrhythmias in the Wolff–Parkinson–White syndrome (see below). Correct identification of VT and SVT is of considerable importance because the immediate management and prognosis of these two conditions are completely different. Unfortunately, numerous studies have shown that misdiagnosis of broad complex tachycardia occurs commonly, almost invariably, incorrect classification of VT as SVT, sometimes with disastrous consequences.[1] Moreover, the problem appears to have persisted despite publication and dissemination of various algorithms to assist diagnosis. Several factors may have contributed to this:

- Lack of awareness that VT is much more common than SVT in unselected cases of broad complex tachycardia, and overwhelmingly so among those patients with known or suspected ischaemic heart disease.[2-4]
- The erroneous perception that VT is invariably associated with haemodynamic compromise, whereas SVT is not.[5]
- Over-reliance of existing algorithms on relatively complex ECG criteria (matching QRS morphologies etc.), which less experienced or non-specialist physicians can find difficult to apply in the heat of the emergency setting.[6-8]
- The tendency to opt for the "lesser" diagnosis of SVT when there is uncertainty about the ECG criteria even though the odds are usually heavily in favour of VT (sometimes referred to as the "looks like SVT" syndrome because that is invariably the comment entered in the notes without supporting reasons!).

The correct approach is to regard VT as the default diagnosis of broad complex tachycardia if there is any degree of uncertainty,[9] whereas a diagnosis of SVT should only be made on the basis of definite evidence. On purely statistical grounds, this will yield the correct diagnosis in most cases, and occasional misclassification of SVT as VT is very unlikely to lead to adverse consequences. Evidence of antecedent ischaemic heart disease is highly predictive of VT and should be accorded greater weight than ECG criteria. Finally, the availability of adenosine has not only provided a valuable provocative test for positive identification of SVT [10,11] (difficult on ECG criteria alone), but has also largely eliminated the hazardous practice of administering intravenous verapamil to patients with broad complex tachycardia of uncertain origin.[12] Adherence to these simple principles should enable accurate diagnosis and appropriate management in the vast majority of cases.

11.2 Electrocardiographic mechanisms and differential diagnosis

The normal narrow QRS complex (duration < 110 ms) reflects rapid and simultaneous depolarisation of both ventricles via the specialised His-Purkinje network. If any part of the ventricular myocardium is activated directly, i.e. bypassing the His-Purkinje system, this will result in delayed depolarisation and QRS broadening. Thus, broad complex tachycardia may arise from one of three mechanisms.

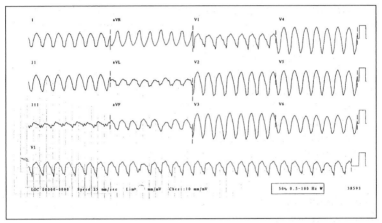

Figure 11.1 Ventricular tachycardia. ECG recording of sustained monomorphic ventricular tachycardia (see case history 1).

(1). **VT.** Activation originating within ventricular myocardium (Figure 11.1).

(2). **SVT with aberrant conduction.** Because of the bundle branch block, one ventricle is normally activated and the other by delayed depolarisation spreading directly across the interventricular septum, thereby altering QRS morphology. The bundle branch block may be pre-existing (i.e. still present in sinus rhythm), but more commonly represents a functional state of refractoriness during tachycardia. Although this is often assumed to be a purely rate-related phenomenon, in most cases the mechanism involves repetitive "concealed" excitation of the affected bundle. Thus, functional aberration may occur in young, fit patients with entirely normal conduction systems, and may be switched on and off by spontaneous ectopic beats (or programmed extrastimuli during intracardiac electrophysiology studies), resulting in abrupt transition from broad to narrow complex tachycardia or vice versa (Figure 11.2).

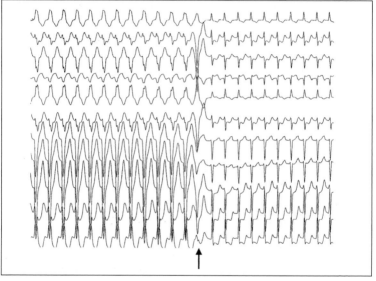

Figure 11.2 Broad complex tachycardia due to SVT with aberrant conduction. An example of broad complex tachycardia converted to narrow complex tachycardia by a single ventricular extrastimulus (marked with an arrow). This patient had atrioventricular reentrant tachycardia (AVRT) with "functional" LBBB aberration. The electrophysiological mechanism involves critically timed concealed excitation of the bundle rather than rate-related refractoriness – this explains why the bundle branch block can be abolished by a single ectopic beat.

(3). Pre-excited tachycardias. In Wolff–Parkinson–White syndrome, during sinus rhythm the QRS complex is broadened by the delta wave representing direct depolarisation of part of the ventricular myocardium via an accessory pathway (Figures 11.3(a), 11.4(a)). In the common or "orthodromic" form of atrioventricular re-

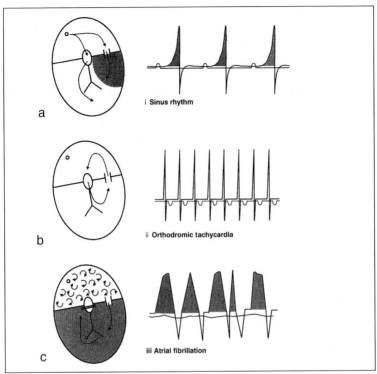

i Sinus rhythm

a

ii Orthodromic tachycardia

b

iii Atrial fibrillation

c

Figure 11.3 Wolff–Parkinson–White syndrome. Schematic diagram of the Wolff–Parkinson–White syndrome with atrial activation shown as red arrows and ventricular activation shown as black arrows. (a) During sinus rhythm, there is dual activation of the ventricles via the AV junction/His-Purkinje system and the accessory pathway; pre-excitation, i.e. direct ventricular depolarisation via the pathway (shaded) results in broadening of the QRS complexes, the so called "delta wave". (b) During orthodromic atrioventricular reentrant tachycardia (AVRT), the pathway conducts in the retrograde direction to the atria to form the reentrant circuit and the ventricles are activated exclusively via the the normal AV conduction system. Thus, the delta wave disappears and a narrow complex tachycardia is produced with retrograde (inverted) P waves after the QRS complexes (see Chapter 10). (c) During atrial fibrillation, ventricular activation via the AV junction is delayed due to the decremental conduction properties of the AV node in the face of extremely rapid, chaotic atrial depolarisations. The non-decremental properties of the accessory pathway allow "pre-excitation" and rapid depolarisation of the ventricles. Thus, ventricular activation is predominantly via the accessory pathway (shaded grey) resulting in an irregular, broad complex tachyarrhythmia. At very fast heart rates, this may simulate regular broad complex tachycardia (see Figure 11.4c).

entrant tachycardia, the pathway only conducts retrogradely (in the ventriculo-atrial (VA) direction) and activation of the ventricles is entirely via the atrioventricular (AV) node, so the delta wave disappears to produce a narrow complex tachycardia (Figures 11.3(b), 11.4(b)). In the rarer "antidromic" atrioventricular re-entrant tachycardia the ventricles are activated via the accessory pathway (in the AV direction) to produce broad complex tachycardia. Atrial fibrillation (AF) with rapid antegrade conduction via the accessory pathway also produces a broad complex tachyarrhythmia. The ventricular rate may exceed 260 bpm making it difficult to appreciate irregularity of RR intervals, and so pre-excited AF is easily mistaken for VT (Figure 11.4(c)).

In practice, pre-excited tachyarrhythmias are rare and the differential diagnosis is usually confined to VT or SVT with aberrant conduction. However, if a younger patient with no antecedent history of cardiac problems presents with an extremely rapid broad complex tachycardia at around 300 bpm, the possibility of Wolff–Parkinson–White syndrome with pre-excited AF should always be considered.

11.3 Management (step 1): initial evaluation

When approaching any patient with broad complex tachycardia, the two immediate priorities are: (i) to assess haemodynamic status; and (ii) to obtain a 12-lead ECG recording unless the patient has arrested or is otherwise in extremis.

In evaluating haemodynamic status, the absolute blood pressure is less significant than signs of critical organ hypoperfusion or other adverse clinical effects. Conscious level is the most important indicator of "haemodynamic instability": a patient who is fully alert must have reasonable cerebral perfusion irrespective of the recorded BP, whereas obtundation or unconciousness indicate circulatory collapse. Angina, pulmonary oedema, or oliguria (if urine output is

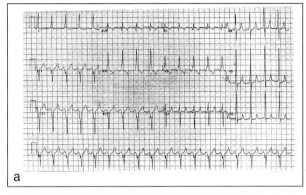

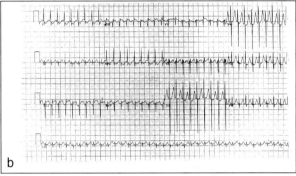

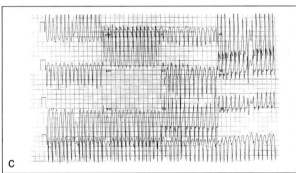

Figure 11.4 Wolff–Parkinson–White syndrome. ECG recordings from a patient with Wolff–Parkinson–White syndrome during: (a) sinus rhythm, showing a delta wave; (b) orthodromic AVRT, showing regular narrow complex tachycardia with retrograde (inverted) P waves visible particularly in leads I, III and aVL; (c) during rapid pre-excited atrial fibrillation, showing an extremely rapid (>300bpm), broad complex tachyarrhythmia with only subtle irregularity of the cycle length and QRS morphology similar to the delta waves during sinus rhythm. See text and Figure 11.3 for explanation.

being monitored) are other signs of haemodynamic compromise. Many such patients will also exhibit significant hypotension (systolic blood pressure <90 mmHg), but one should bear in mind that non-invasive BP measurements, particularly by automated sphygmomanometry, may be unreliable in this setting.

A 12-lead ECG must be recorded and scrutinised as soon as possible. Other than in a cardiac arrest situation, management should never be based on rhythm strips alone as these offer only limited diagnostic information (see below). ECG tracings of all tachyarrhythmia should be marked with the date/time and patient details, and carefully retained both for medico-legal purposes and as essential clinical records for subsequent review by senior clinicians, on which complex management decisions are often based.

11.4 Management (step 2): differentiating VT from SVT with aberrant conduction

In most cases the correct diagnosis can be rapidly made on the basis of simple clinical and ECG criteria, occasionally backed up by adenosine testing (Figure 11.13). The golden rule in applying any algorithm is that VT should be regarded as the default diagnosis of broad complex tachycardia if there is any uncertainty about the diagnosis.[9] A diagnosis of SVT with aberrant conduction should only be made on the basis of definite criteria, usually including positive adenosine provocation (see below). This approach is safe because it avoids the potential hazards of misclassifying VT as SVT, and is also the "percentage game": if you guessed VT in all cases of broad complex tachycardia, you would be correct at least 80% of the time.

11.4.1 Clinical features

An antecedent history of myocardial infarction (MI) and/or other evidence of ischaemic heart disease (angina pectoris, coronary artery bypass graft/percutaneous transluminal coronary angioplasty (CABG/PTCA), or congestive heart failure) are highly predictive of VT. In particular, several studies have shown that, among patients presenting with broad complex tachycardia and a prior MI, the likelihood of VT is close to 100%,[2-4] and so in this situation VT should be automatically regarded as the diagnosis unless there is compelling evidence of SVT (Figure 11.13).

A common misconception is that blood pressure is helpful in determining the origin of the arrhythmia, but numerous studies have refuted the simplistic notion that hypotensive patients have VT and normotensive patients have SVT.[5] Physical signs of ventriculo-atrial dissociation (variable S1 intensity and cannon waves in the jugular venous pulse), if present, indicate VT[13] but are difficult to detect in the emergency setting even for experienced clinicians and are of little practical value.

11.4.2 ECG criteria

Various algorithms have been proposed to facilitate diagnosis of broad complex tachycardia on the basis of ECG criteria,[6-8] but seem to have had little impact on the incidence of misdiagnosis in clinical practice despite impressive claims of their sensitivity, specificity, and predictive accuracy. These algorithms are difficult for junior medical staff to apply in the emergency setting and can easily result in a blinkered approach. For example, there are numerous instances of overreliance on a specific QRS morphological appearance leading to erroneous diagnosis of SVT when other ECG features and/or the clinical context are highly suggestive of VT.[1] Such difficulties are perhaps not surprising, given that the evaluation of published ECG algorithms has invariably been been based on retrospective analysis of ECG tracings by arrhythmia specialists. To date, no protocol for diagnosis of broad complex tachycardia has ever been assessed prospectively in "live" clinical settings by "non-experts."

Ventriculo-atrial (VA) dissociation

VA dissociation, as the term implies, refers to independent activation of atria and ventricles due to complete retrograde

AV nodal block during VT, resulting in P waves "marching through" with no relationship to the QRS complexes, and more QRS complexes than P waves (Figure 11.5). Occasionally this may manifest as 2:1 retrograde VA block with two QRS complexes for each conducted P wave (Figure 11.6). If the VT is relatively slow (usually < 150 bpm), a sinus node impulse may be conducted to the ventricles during diastole to produce either a "capture beat" or a "fusion beat" depending on whether the conducted impulse depolarizes the entire ventricular myocardium (normal QRS complex) or only part of it (hybrid QRS complex due to fusion with the activation front from the VT focus) (Figure 11.7). If present, electrocardiographic features of VA dissociation are highly predictive of VT[14,15] (rare exceptions are seen in SVT due to atrioventricular nodal re-entrant tachycardia). However, VA dissociation may not be apparent in more than 50% of cases of VT for a variety of reasons: in rapid VT, the P waves may be hidden amidst the QRS complexes and ST segments; there may be 1:1 retrograde VA conduction; there may be no organised P wave activity, for example if the atria are fibrillating. Absence of discernible VA dissociation in itself

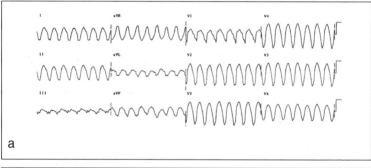

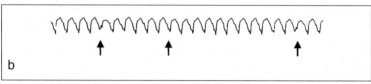

Figure 11.5 Ventricular tachycardia. Broad complex tachycardia arising in a 67 year old man with a prior history of inferior myocardial infarction. (a) The 12-lead ECG shows ventricular concordance with negative QRS complexes in leads V1–6; (b) the expanded lead V1 rhythm strip shows examples of independent P waves (marked with arrows) unrelated to the QRS complexes, indicating VA dissociation.

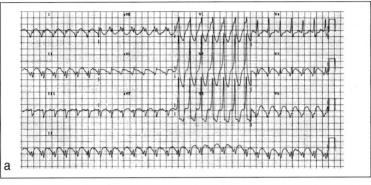

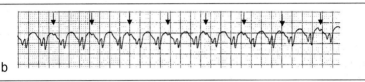

Figure 11.6 Ventricular tachycardia. Broad complex tachycardia arising in a 48 year old woman following a recent inferoposterior MI. (a) The 12-lead ECG shows an atypical RBBB morphology with extreme deviation of the frontal QRS axis (−120); (b) the expanded lead II rhythm strip shows 2:1 VA block with P waves (marked with arrows) following every second QRS complex.

does not indicate SVT. VT is still more likely, and SVT should only be diagnosed if there is additional supportive evidence. VT should likewise be the default diagnosis if you are uncertain about the presence of VA dissociation.

QRS width/axis

Total QRS width or duration >140 ms has traditionally been regarded as suggestive of VT, although recent studies have questioned the specificity of this criterion. A more stringent cut-off such as QRS duration >160 ms is usually diagnostic of VT.[14] Left axis deviation (beyond −30°) of the QRS complex in the frontal plane is another classical indicator of VT but is particularly unreliable in broad complex tachycardia of "LBBB" morphology and should not be used as the sole basis for classification.

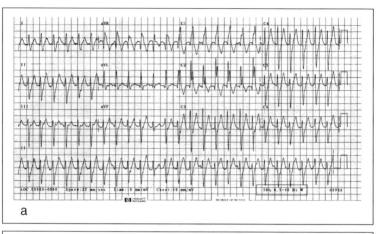

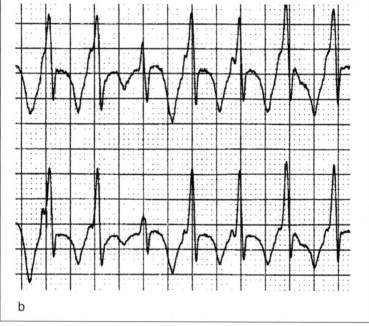

Figure 11.7 Ventricular tachycardia. Broad complex tachycardia arising in a 25 year old man with no evidence of structural heart disease. (a) The 12-lead ECG shows an atypical RBBB morphology with left axis deviation, independent P waves (not marked) and a fusion beat (marked with arrow) indicating VA dissociation; (b) expanded 2-lead rhythm strip showing the fusion beat.

QRS morphology

Analysis of the morphological characteristics of the QRS complexes in the precordial leads forms the central plank of most existing diagnostic algorithms for broad complex tachycardia. The rationale for this approach is that SVT with aberration will produce classical RBBB or LBBB patterns, so that any divergence from these is indicative of VT. Although intellectually appealing, such diagnostic schemes rely upon ECG pattern recognition and terminology which is entirely familiar to cardiologists and arrhythmia experts, but often confusing and difficult for inexperienced and non-specialist clinicians practising in the emergency setting. Junior medical staff frequently complain that the QRS morphologies displayed on wall charts in A&E departments never match the ECG in front of them, and misinterpretation of such algorithms appears to be a common cause of erroneous diagnosis, particularly the "looks like SVT" syndrome. We believe that QRS morphology is often accorded too much importance in the acute diagnosis of broad complex. tachycardia, compared to other more "user-friendly" criteria. A few cases exhibit ventricular concordance (all precordial leads negative or positive), which is diagnostic of VT[16] and can be confidently identified by all clinicians (Figure 11.5a), but most patients have one of the commoner "RBBB" or "LBBB" type tachycardias. In general, any bizarre or atypical QRS morphology will usually indicate VT and "simplified" guidelines based on the specific patterns of V1 and V6 have been proposed to assist with differentiation (Table 11.1). However, these criteria probably should not be relied upon in isolation by non-experts, particularly to make a classification of SVT. As always, if there is any uncertainty, assume that the diagnosis is VT.

Table 11.1 Classical ECG morphologies of left and right bundle branch block

	V1	V6
RBBB	rSRi	RS with R>S
LBBB	QS with no R (delay to S nadir <70 ms)	R with no Q

11.4.3 Adenosine testing

Adenosine is a purine nucleoside which produces transient blockade of AV nodal conduction following bolus intravenous administration but is rapidly metabolised (circulatory half-life approximately 10 seconds) and does not exert any negative inotropic effects. The main side-effects such as flushing, bronchoconstriction, and chest tightness are unpleasant but short-lived. Unlike verapamil, it can be safely administered to patients with broad complex tachycardia without fear of precipitating haemodynamic collapse. The rationale for the use of adenosine as a diagnostic aid in broad complex tachycardia is that it will: (i) terminate junctional forms of SVT involving the AV node as part of the re-entrant circuit (AVRT and AVNRT) (Figures 11.8, 11.12); or (ii) produce AV block and transiently slow the ventricular rate in atrial forms of SVT (atrial flutter or atrial tachycardia), revealing the underlying atrial rhythm (Figures 11.9, 11.11), but (iii) not affect VT (Figure 11.10).[17] Thus, adenosine provocation should primarily be regarded as a means to establish a positive classification of SVT. A negative result (absence of termination or slowing) must be regarded as indicative of VT.[10,11]

Table 11.2 Adenosine in the diagnosis of broad complex tachycardia

	Dose	n	Correct classification VT	Correct classification SVT
Rankin et al.[11]	2.5–25 mg	24	93%	100%
Griffith et al.[10]	0.25 mg	26	94%	100%

Published experience has shown that to achieve close to 100% sensitivity in diagnosis of SVT requires administration of intravenous bolus doses of adenosine up to 24 mg (Table 11.2), twice the maximum dose stipulated in the British National Formulary and widely used in clinical practice. Specificity is slightly less than 100% because some forms of idiopathic VT are adenosine-sensitive and may be misclassified by this approach[10] (however, such cases are extremely unusual in clinical practice and may have been overrepresented in the published series from supraregional referral centres). Confusion can also arise with rare cases of pre-excited

Figures 11.8–11.10 Adenosine provocation. Schematic diagram to illustrate the rationale of adenosine provocation in the classification of broad complex tachycardia. Atrial activation is represented in red, ventricular activation in black. The "No Entry" symbols indicate the site of AV nodal blockade by adenosine.

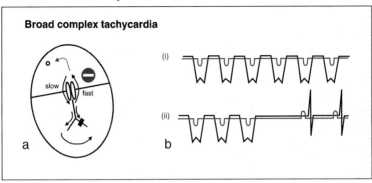

Figure 11.8 Junctional SVT. The diagram shows a broad complex tachycardia due to atrioventricular nodal reentrant tachycardia (AVNRT) with functional bundle branch block. Thus, there is a 1:1 VA relationship and the retrograde P waves coincide with the QRS complexes (a) and would probably be hidden on a 12-lead ECG. IV adenosine (b) transiently blocks AV nodal conduction and terminates the broad complex tachycardia, restoring sinus rhythm with normal QRS complexes.

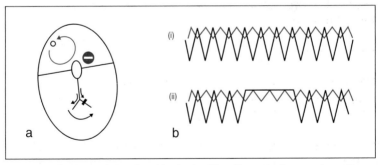

Figure 11.9 Intra-atrial tachyarrhythmia. The diagram shows a broad complex tachycardia due to atrial flutter (macroreentrant excitation of the right atrium) with 2:1 conduction to the ventricles and functional or pre-existing bundle branch block (a). The flutter waves would probably be inapparent on a 12-lead ECG due to fusion with the QRS complexes and T waves. IV adenosine (b) transiently interrupts AV nodal conduction and slows the ventricular rate of the broad complex tachycardia to expose the underlying flutter waves. However, adenosine does not terminate the flutter circuit and so the broad complex tachycardia resumes as soon as it has worn off.

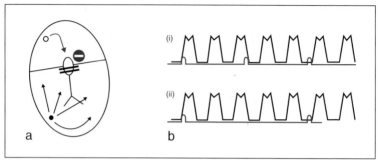

Figure 11.10 Ventricular tachycardia. The diagram shows a broad complex tachycardia due to ventricular tachycardia with retrograde VA block and independent P waves (arising from the sinus node) "marching through" the QRS complexes (a). IV adenosine (b) transiently interrupts AV nodal conduction but does not affect the broad complex tachycardia (it will cause transient sinus bradycardia but this will seldom be apparent from the surface ECG).

tachycardia in the Wolff–Parkinson–White syndrome (atrial flutter or antidromic AVRT) in which adenosine may produce transient acceleration. Despite these minor limitations, adenosine testing has revolutionised the emergency diagnosis of broad complex tachycardia. The key rules governing its application may be summarised as follows:

- Adenosine testing should only be used if a diagnosis of VT cannot been made on the basis of clinical history plus review of the 12-lead ECG. The proportion of cases in which it is required will depend on the individual clinician's level of experience: a junior doctor may have to resort to adenosine testing much more often than a cardiologist. However, any, diagnosis of SVT should usually be confirmed by adenosine provocation (Figure 11.13).
- Incremental bolus doses of adenosine up to 24 mg are required (if tolerated). The sensitivity of this technique for detection/diagnosis of SVT will be significantly reduced if testing is restricted to a maximum dose of 12 mg. A suitable schedule would be iv adenosine 12 →18 →24 mg.
- A negative result (i.e. neither termination nor transient slowing) indicates VT. Intravenous verapamil should *never* be used if adenosine proves ineffective.

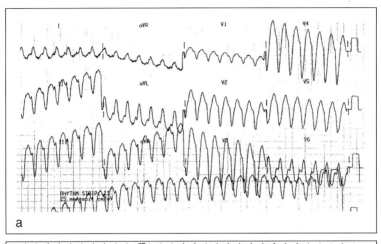

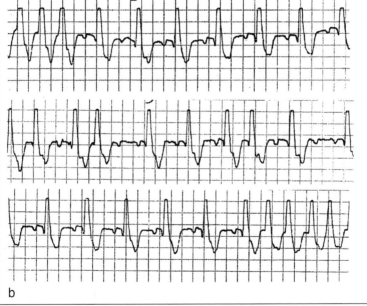

Figure 11.11 Adenosine provocation in atrial flutter. Broad complex tachycardia arising in a 65 year old woman taking flecainide for paroxysmal atrial fibrillation. (a) The 12-lead ECG shows LBBB tachycardia with unusual QRS morphology (QS waves to V5 and left axis), but (b) iv adenosine 18mg results in transient AV block (2:1 or 3:1) and slowing of the ventricular rate to reveal the underlying tachyarrhythmia. Although the appearances in this single lead recording were suggestive of atrial tachycardia, subsequent multilead recordings showed the typical sawtooth baseline of atrial flutter.

11.5 Management (step 3): immediate treatment of VT

The treatment of SVT has been addressed in Chapter 10, "Narrow complex tachycardia". This section will deal with the immediate management of patients with a definite or presumptive diagnosis of VT. The priority is always to restore sinus rhythm as soon as possible; even patients who are haemodynamically stable at presentation may progressively deteriorate if subjected to prolonged periods of tachycardia,

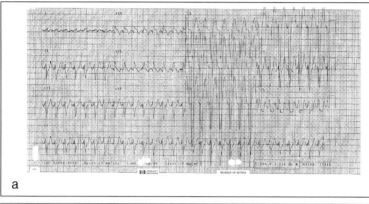

a

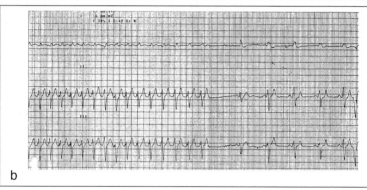

b

Figure 11.12 Adenosine provocation in junctional SVT. Broad complex tachycardia in a 60 year old woman with a long history of paroxysmal tachycardia. (a) The 12 lead ECG shows LBBB tachycardia, and (b) iv adenosine 12 mg restores sinus rhythm without any change in QRS morphology. Thus, this patient had pre-existing LBBB (as opposed to functional aberration) with a junctional SVT. Subsequent investigations showed the mechanism of her arrhythmia to be atrioventricular reentrant tachycardia (AVRT) via a left-sided accessory pathway.

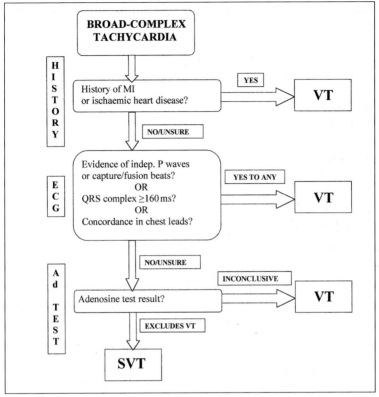

Figure 11.13 Algorithm for differentiation of VT from SVT in broad complex tachycardia. See text for details.

particularly those with impaired LV function and/or extensive coronary artery disease. The available therapeutic options are DC cardioversion, intravenous antiarrhythmic agents, and anti-tachycardia pacing. These are discussed in more detail below.

11.5.1 DC cardioversion

Synchronised DC cardioversion remains the most effective and reliable method of terminating VT.[18] In contrast to antiarrhythmic drug administration, there is no associated risk of haemodynamic depression or proarrhythmia. It is the treatment of choice if the presenting tachyarrhythmia is haemodynamically unstable or otherwise poorly tolerated. Otherwise it is used when antiarrhythmic drug therapy has failed to restore sinus rhythm. Some clinicians advocate DC cardioversion as first-line treatment for all cases of VT (irrespective of haemodynamic status) in the belief that it is safer than pharmacological conversion, but there has never been a prospective, randomised comparison.

Although availability of anaesthetists is often perceived as a barrier, the advent of transcutaneous O_2 saturation monitoring and effective reversal agents for benzodiazepines (flumazenil) and opiates (naloxone) has enabled DC cardioversion to be performed routinely and safely under neuroleptic sedation. This is almost invariably preferable to leaving a patient in extremis for prolonged periods awaiting arrival of anaesthetic support. The key points are as follows:

- Ideally DC cardioversion should be performed under general anaesthesia (most commonly propofol or etomidate). However, if an anaesthetist is not immediately available, the patient may be sedated with a short-acting benzodiazepine (e.g. iv midazolam 2.5–10 mg) ± a short-acting opiate (e.g. iv fentanyl 25–50 μg). Supplemental oxygen should be administered routinely with O_2 saturation monitoring. Availability of reversal agents and airway management equipment (oropharyngeal airways, laryngeal masks, etc.) should be ensured beforehand.
- The defibrillator must be switched to the "synchronised" mode and the markers should be synchronised with the QRS complexes.
- Higher delivered energies should be used from the outset to minimise the total number of shocks required. There is no advantage to lower energies (indeed anecdotal evidence suggests that subtherapeutic shocks may even be proarrhythmic). A suitable protocol would be 200 J →360 J → 360 J.

11.5.2 Antiarrhythmic drugs

Intravenous antiarrhythmic agents are widely used for termination of haemodynamically stable VT, when there is no mandatory indication for immediate DC cardioversion. The main advantage of the pharmacological approach is its simplicity compared to either electrical cardioversion or transvenous antitachycardia pacing. Treatment can be delivered at the bedside without delay or the need for general anaesthesia, invasive instrumentation etc. However, there is a paucity of data concerning efficacy and safety. Lidocaine (lignocaine) (1.5 mg/kg or 100–150 mg) remains the most commonly used agent and is generally promoted as the drug of choice. Following bolus intravenous administration, it rarely causes significant haemodynamic depression and is cleared within 30 minutes, affording a good safety profile for this clinical setting. Unfortunately, recent studies have consistently shown that lidocaine will only terminate spontaneously occurring VT in 10–20% of cases, although slightly higher efficacy rates of around 30% have been reported for VT induced by programmed stimulation during intracardiac electrophysiological testing (Table 11.3). By contrast, two small randomised trials have demonstrated the superior efficacy of intravenous sotalol (100 mg) and procainamide (10 mg/kg) compared to lidocaine, both agents restoring sinus rhythm in approximately 70% of cases[19,20] (Table 11.3). Adverse haemodynamic or proarrhythmic effects were rarely encountered with either drug. These results emphasise the need for more research and larger prospective studies in acute arrhythmia management.

Table 11.3 Pharmacological cardioversion of ventricular tachycardia. Efficacy of selected agents is shown as % of patients converted to sinus rhythm following intravenous administration.

	Lidocaine (lignocaine)	Sotalol	Procainamide
Griffith et al.[9]	30%	36%	
Ho et al.[20]	18%		79%**
Gorgels et al.[19]	19%	69%*	

*p < 0.01; **p < 0.005

It is likely that lidocaine will continue to be used as first-line treatment, particularly for patients exhibiting signs of mild haemodynamic embarrassment in whom early DC cardioversion would otherwise be considered. However, for patients with reasonably well tolerated VT, there is a strong case for using either procainamide or sotalol rather than lidocaine initially (Table 11.4). In general, we would advocate DC cardioversion if the first antiarrhythmic agent fails to terminate VT. There may be occasional exceptions, such as patients with well tolerated VT who have not responded to lidocaine but in whom immediate DC cardioversion under general anaesthesia may be undesirable because of an ongoing respiratory tract infection or recent consumption of a meal.

Table 11.4 Doses for drug treatment of ventricular tachycardia.

Drug	Dose (intravenous)
Lidocaine (lignocaine)	1.5 mg/kg over 2 minutes
Sotalol	1 mg/kg over 5 minutes
Procainamide	10 mg/kg at 100 mg/minute
Amiodarone	300 mg (5 mg/kg) over 30 minutes*; subsequent infusion of 600–1200 mg over 24 hours

*Into central vein.

In passing, it should be noted that intravenous amiodarone is generally unsuitable for termination of VT because of its relatively slow onset of action and negative inotropic effects resulting in a high incidence of haemodynamic depression/hypotension.[21] The major role of amiodarone is suppression of recurrent episodes of VT[21, 22] (see below).

11.5.3 Antitachycardia pacing

Antitachycardia pacing (ATP) is seldom used as the initial treatment for VT unless the patient happens to have a temporary ventricular pacemaker *in situ* (e.g. post-cardiac surgery). However, it has an invaluable role in the small minority of patients who present with frequent recurrences of VT as a simple, painless alternative to multiple cardioversions to terminate the attacks while antiarrhythmic drug therapy such as amiodarone is being introduced to suppress them. ATP is a simple, elegant technique requiring only insertion of a standard temporary transvenous pacing catheter (see Chapter 14) plus an external temporary pacemaker with a "×3 rate-function" key to deliver pacing at faster rates (typically 150–220 bpm) available on most coronary care units.[23,24]

In the vast majority of cases, sustained monomorphic VT is mediated by re-entrant excitation of a "functional" circuit involving a zone of slow myocardial conduction (usually within the border of a healed infarct). The prerequisite for perpetuation of tachycardia in such re-entrant circuits is the presence of an "excitable gap" of tissue behind the receding "tail" of electrical activation which has gone through its phase of refractoriness and recovered excitability in time to be reactivated by the advancing "head", thereby allowing the next cycle of the circuit to go ahead. Thus, the rationale of antitachycardia pacing (ATP) is to use an external, temporary pacemaker to stimulate and depolarise the excitable gap causing the VT to terminate because the advancing head of the re-entrant activation encounters refractory tissue. Although more complex algorithms are often employed during intracardiac electrophysiology studies, in the emergency setting simple overdrive pacing is the easiest method, particularly for non-cardiologists. This involves introducing a temporary transvenous pacing catheter and then using an external box with the "×3" key switched on to deliver a burst of pacing at 15–20 bpm faster than the VT rate and at a relatively high output (e.g. 5.0 V) to ensure capture. Typically, the burst is continued for 5–10 seconds with continuous ECG monitoring until the QRS complexes change morphology (indicating ventricular capture) and the pacing is switched off (Figure 11.14). This technique will terminate 80–90% of cases of VT slower than 200 bpm. However, a minority will accelerate or degenerate to polymorphic VT or VF and so ATP should only be delivered with an external defibrillator to hand. Ideally, the patient should also be sedated (e.g. with iv midazolam 2.5–5 mg) for the first attempt. The success of ATP is lower if the VT rate is above 200 bpm and conversely the chances of acceleration/degeneration are increased.

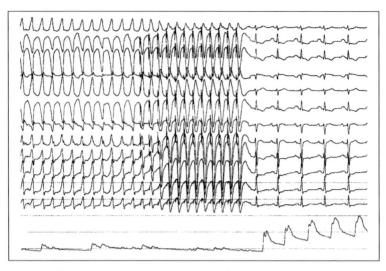

Figure 11.14 Antitachycardia pacing in VT. Recording of sustained monomorphic ventricular tachycardia at 160 bpm. Following a burst of pacing at 180 bpm via a temporary right ventricular pacing catheter, sinus rhythm is restored with dramatic improvement in arterial blood pressure (bottom tracing).

Unfortunately, generalists are becoming gradually more de-skilled in temporary cardiac pacing because the number of cases has steadily declined since the advent of thrombolytics and the availability of transcutaneous pacing. There is an understandable reluctance to undertake insertion of a temporary pacemaker and ATP in a patient with recurrent VT, but in reality this is no more challenging than pacing for bradycardia.

11.6 Management (step 4): subsequent management of VT

A detailed account of the investigation and treatment of patients with VT is beyond the scope of this book but we will briefly consider some aspects of management in the acute phase. They should all be admitted initially to the coronary care unit (CCU) for continuous monitoring, and should undergo daily 12-lead ECG recordings, measurement of renal function electrolytes (particularly serum K^+ and Mg^{2+}), and a cardiac enzyme series. Full cardiac evaluation including echocardiography (to assess LV function), coronary angiography, and possibly electrophysiological testing will be required in most cases and so the admitting medical team should liaise with their local cardiologist as soon as possible. The following general comments can be made.

- If there is clear evidence of an ongoing acute coronary syndrome, this should be treated along conventional lines. However, it should be noted that sustained monomorphic VT almost invariably arises from the scar of a healed infarct (i.e. a fixed electrical substrate) and is rarely triggered by acute myocardial ischaemia (which characteristically produces polymorphic VT or VF). Thus, monomorphic VT is usually a recurrent problem. It is very common to see modest rises in cardiac enzymes among patients admitted with monomorphic VT episodes but unless there is clinical and ECG evidence of an acute MI, this should never be dismissed as a "primary" or early ventricular arrhythmia secondary to a small infarct which is unlikely to recur (a common misconception). Most of these patients require antiarrhythmic drugs or non-pharmacological therapies (implantable cardioverter defibrillators) to protect them against recurrent arrhythmias.
- Serum K^+ should be maintained at > 4.0 mmol/l.
- Any proarrhythmic drugs should be withdrawn if possible.
- Haemodynamic function should be optimised as this contributes to arrhythmogenesis. Most patients with VT have impaired LV function and should be on an ACE inhibitor.
- If the patient presents with an isolated episode of VT which is successfully terminated, there is no automatic requirement to start maintenance antiarrhythmic drug therapy forthwith and this is often better delayed until the case can be discussed with a cardiologist (for example, the drugs may interfere with electrophysiological testing). However, if the patient experiences recurrent attacks of VT, treatment should be started without delay. In patients with underlying coronary artery disease (the majority) the drug of choice will usually be amiodarone (loading regimen 1.2 g/day for 7–10 days). Adjunctive treatment with low-

dose β-blockers has been shown to be highly effective in refractory cases and probably should be considered routinely, particularly for patients with LV dysfunction in whom there is increasing evidence of long-term prognostic benefit.

- If the attacks are occurring frequently or incessantly, amiodarone can be administered by infusion via a central venous catheter for more rapid action although this can cause haemodynamic depression with hypotension or worsening heart failure. Even if given parenterally, amiodarone can take up to 72 hours or longer in some cases to achieve therapeutic effect,[21,22] and it is important to warn the patient, family and nursing staff of the likely occurrence of frequent VT episodes during the intervening period which will have to be terminated as previously discussed (clearly antitachycardia pacing may be particularly helpful in this situation if effective). Occasionally, a piggyback infusion of lidocaine (lignocaine) may allow temporary suppression of the VT while the patient is loaded with amiodarone.

11.7 Polymorphic VT, torsade de pointes and the long QT syndromes

Polymorphic VT is a rapid ventricular tachyarrhythmia with constantly changing morphology of the QRS complexes (in contrast to monomorphic VT). The term torsade de pointes applies to polymorphic VT arising in the setting of a congenital or acquired long QT syndrome (LQTS). These are malignant arrhythmias, typically presenting with recurrent syncope and often degenerating to ventricular fibrillation. Although the ECG appearances of polymorphic VT are quite distinct from "broad complex tachycardia", this group of conditions is considered in this chapter for convenience.[25,26]

11.7.1 Polymorphic VT without QT prolongation

Polymorphic VT *not* associated with a long QT syndrome is most commonly due to myocardial ischaemia in the setting of an acute ischaemia (unstable angina, widespread ST depression, etc.), making diagnosis straightforward, but in a few cases recurrent polymorphic VT or VF may develop without symptomatic angina or striking ECG changes. Other causes of polymorphic VT without LQTS include acute myocarditis, cardiomyopathies (particularly arrhythmogenic right ventricular dysplasia/cardiomyopathy) and hereditary ion channel disorders such as Brugada syndrome (VT or VF with RBBB and precordial ST elevation). In contrast to torsade de pointes (see below), this arrhythmia is triggered by short-coupled ectopic beats without antecedent cycle length changes. Management involves urgent evaluation by echocardiography and coronary angiography and, if appropriate, anti-ischaemic therapy including β-blockers and revascularisation (emergency PTCA or CABG). For patients in whom an acute coronary syndrome has been excluded, standard antiarrhythmic agents should be used to control the polymorphic VT, including lidocaine (lignocaine), amiodarone and β-blockers. Some of these cases will eventually require implantable defibrillators (ICDs) to protect them against the risk of sudden death.

11.7.2 Long QT syndromes and torsade de pointes

These abnormalities of cardiac repolarisation have traditionally been classified into congenital and acquired forms of long QT syndrome (LQTS). Congenital LQTS includes the Romano–Ward syndrome (autosomal dominant) and Jervell–Lange–Nielsen syndrome (autosomal recessive with deafness) and comprise a heterogeneous group of inherited ion channel disorders which predispose the ventricular myocardium to catecholamine-induced arrhythmias. Typically patients present in childhood or adolescence with syncope or cardiac arrest triggered adrenergically (sudden frights, exercise, etc.) and the first-line treatment is β-blockers.

Acquired LQTS is most commonly due to drug-induced repolarisation abnormalities (Box 11.1), but may be exacerbated by bradycardia and/or hypokalaemia. In some cases a severe bradyarrhythmia, particularly complete heart block, or acute myocardial ischaemia is the sole or dominant causative mechanism. In contrast to other forms of polymorphic VT, torsade de pointes is characteristically triggered by a "short–long–short" sequence consisting of an ectopic beat followed by a compensatory pause and then another premature beat initiating the tachyarrhythmia (Figure 11.15), so called "pause-dependent" or "bradycardia-dependent" initiation. Treatment naturally involves withdrawal of the causative drug plus specific measures to suppress the tendency to torsade de pointes until ventricular repolarisation has normalised:

- Increase the heart rate by temporary cardiac pacing (VVI or AV sequential) or atropine/isoprenaline infusion. This prevents pause-dependent initiation. Usually pacing at or above 90 bpm will suffice.
- Potassium supplementation to maintain serum K > 4.0 mmol/l. Hypokalaemia dramatically exacerbates the propensity to torsade de pointes.
- Magnesium salts at pharmacological doses (e.g. magnesium sulphate 8 mmol bolus followed by 3 mmol/hr) are often highly effective at suppressing drug-related torsade de pointes, even in patients without hypomagnesaemia. The exact mechanism has not been elucidated with certainty.

Although congenital and acquired LQTS has been equated respectively with "adrenergic-dependent" and "pause-dependent" torsade de pointes, these mechanisms are not mutually exclusive. Many documented episodes of polymorphic VT in congenital LQTS are pause-dependent and may only respond to combined treatment with pacing and β-blockers. It is possible that patients who develop acquired LQTS may have subtle underlying abnormalities of ventricular repolarisation (forme fruste of congenital LQTS) which predispose them to this proarrhythmia.

> **Box 11.1 Causes of long QT syndrome and torsade de pointes.**
>
> **QT prolonging drugs**
> - Antiarrhythmic agents (quinidine, disopyramide, sotalol etc.)
> - Antimicrobials (macrolide antibiotics, ketoconazole etc.)
> - Antihistamines (astemizole, terfenadine)
> - Psychotropic drugs (phenothiazines, haloperidol, tricyclic antidepressants)

- Cholinergic agonists (cisapride, organophosphates)
Bradyarrhythmias
Electrolyte disorders
  - Hypokalaemia
  - Magnesium depletion
Congenital long QT syndromes
Acute myocardial ischaemia

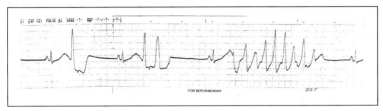

Figure 11.15 Long QT syndrome with torsade de pointes. Torsade de pointes following a "short–long–short" initiation sequence in a 67 year old woman with chronic renal impairment 24 hours after elective hip replacement. She was taking long-term sotalol 80 mg bd for paroxymal atrial fibrillation and had just completed a 7-day course of clarithromycin for a suspected chest infection. The ECG strip shows bradycardia and gross QT prolongation (> 600 ms) with a succession of triggered ventricular ectopic beats followed by compensatory pauses culminating in a short run of polymorphic VT. She degenerated to VF on two occasions but her arrhythmias were then completely suppressed by atrial pacing at 90 bpm and correction of hypokalaemia (initial serum K 2.9). Pacing was maintained for 48 hours while sotalol and clarithromycin were withdrawn.

11.7.3 Clinical approach

Both acute and long-term management of polymorphic VT require specialist input and such cases should be discussed with the local cardiologist at the earliest possible opportunity. Patients with polymorphic VT and an obvious acute coronary syndrome should be managed along conventional lines (see Chapter 4) and considered for early coronary angiography/ PTCA. Cases of acquired LQTS should be managed by withdrawal of the offending drug/drugs (if any) plus pacing or other measures to accelerate the heart rate, correction of hypokalaemia and possible magnesium salts. Patients thought to have congenital LQTS with adrenergic triggering should be immediately commenced on a β-blocker (full 24-hour coverage is required, therefore only long-acting agents such as bisoprolol or nadolol can be used once daily in this condition, whereas atenolol should be prescribed bd), and catecholamines (isoprenaline, adrenaline (epinephrine), etc.) should be strictly avoided. Patients with polymorphic VT but no evidence of LQTS or acute ischaemia require urgent evaluation by a specialist, usually including echocardiography and angiography to check for a "silent" acute coronary syndrome.

Clinical cases

Case 11.1

A 74-year-old lady presented complaining of rapid palpitation. Her past medical history included an anterior myocardial infarction 7 years previously, PTCA/stenting to the right coronary artery 6 months before admission for chronic stable angina and a diagnosis of 'paroxysmal SVT' for 5 years, currently treated with β-blockers. These infrequent attacks of tachycardia had usually been self-limiting in the past. The admission ECG showed a regular, broad complex tachycardia at 180 bpm (Figure 11.1). She was fully conscious and haemodynamically stable, BP 110/60 with no signs of acute heart failure. The presumptive diagnosis was another attack of SVT even though the arrhythmia was not altered by IV adenosine 12 mg. However, review of the history and ECG on the ward round led to the correct diagnosis of VT. It was noted that the ECG showed very broad QRS complexes (200 ms), negative concordance and independent P waves with fusion beats (best seen in the V1 rhythm strip). She then underwent DC cardioversion and was commenced on amiodarone. Retrospective analysis of the ECG tracings of 'SVT' in the past showed that these had also been incorrectly classified episodes of VT.

Broad complex tachycardia occurring in the setting of a prior myocardial infarction is always highly suggestive of VT. It is not uncommon for patients with recurrent VT to have picked up an erroneous diagnosis of 'SVT' in the past as happened here. The fact that the arrhythmia was well tolerated is not helpful in differentiating between VT and SVT. In this case, the ECG appearances were also highly suggestive of VT and adenosine testing was not strictly necessary, but there is no reason why an inexperienced clinician who is less certain about the ECG interpretation, should not resort to adenosine provocation before reaching a diagnosis – however, doses of adenosine up to 18–24 mg should have been used and the absence of effect should have led to the default diagnosis of VT.

Case 11.2

A 65-year-old man with multiple risk factors but no prior history of heart disease presented via his GP with an 8 hour history of palpitation and worsening dyspnoea. On arrival, he was tachypnoeic at rest with BP 130/85 but clinical and radiological signs of mild pulmonary congestion (O_2 saturation 90% on air). The ECG showed a regular broad complex tachycardia at 200 bpm (Figure 11.16). The admitting SHO was unsure whether the ECG showed evidence of VA dissociation and resorted to adenosine provocation. Bolus doses of IV adenosine up to 18 mg (maximum tolerated by the patient) failed to alter the tachycardia and so the default diagnosis of VT was made. IV lignocaine promptly restored sinus rhythm obviating the need for urgent DC cardioversion. Subsequent angiography and electrophysiology studies showed impaired LV function with a chronically occluded LAD and easily inducible VT.

In this case there was no prior history of ischaemic heart disease (although the patient had suffered a silent infarct in the past) but nevertheless the default diagnosis was VT throughout. A more experienced clinician may have concluded that the ECG did show VA dissociation (best seen in the fifth complex which represents a fusion beat), and that the QRS morphology was atypical for classical RBBB with marked left axis deviation, and hence been able to make a confident classification of VT without resorting to adenosine provocation. With respect to management, immediate DC cardioversion would have been the alternative strategy given that the arrhythmia was relatively poorly tolerated, but IV lignocaine had the advantage of speed and simplicity and would not have precluded cardioversion if it had proved ineffective.

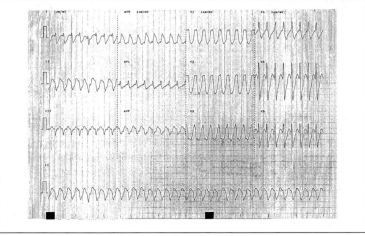

Figure 11.16 Sustained monomorphic ventricular tachycardia (see case history 11.2).

Case 11.3

A previously fit 26-year-old labourer presented to A & E with abrupt onset of a rapid heart beat accompanied by central chest tightness and tingling in his left arm. Although his blood pressure was 85/55 mmHg, he was warm, well perfused and fully alert. The admission ECG showed a regular broad complex tachycardia of classical LBBB morphology at 220 bpm. As the diagnosis was unclear, adenosine was administered at 3, 6 and 12 mg doses but without any effect on the tachycardia. Following discussion with the on-call cardiology registrar, a further bolus of IV adenosine 18 mg was administered and terminated the broad complex tachycardia. The resting ECG in sinus rhythm showed the characteristic delta wave of Wolff–Parkinson–White syndrome, and the patient was referred for further electrophysiological studies and catheter ablation.

Broad complex tachycardia of classical LBBB morphology in a young, fit patient without prior cardiac disease could well be due to SVT with aberrant conduction and this is the ideal case for adenosine provocation. However, it is not uncommon to have to use doses in excess of 12 mg. SVT should not be considered "excluded" unless a high dose (if tolerated 24 mg) has failed to slow or terminate the tachycardia.

Case 11.4

A 68-year-old man who had undergone CABG ten years previously was admitted after he had collapsed at home. His ECG showed regular broad complex tachycardia at 210 bpm with negative concordance in the chest leads. Examination revealed an obese man (> 100 kg) who appeared extremely sick. Automated sphygmomanometry measured his blood pressure at 70/50 and he was shut down and cerebrally obtunded. However, he could just open his eyes to command. The carotid and femoral pulses were palpable and transcutaneous O_2 saturation was 98% breathing oxygen at 8 l/min. Although there was no anaesthetist immediately available, it was decided to proceed directly to DC cardioversion in view of his extreme condition. He was sedated with IV midazolam 5 mg and fentanyl 25 micrograms and converted back to sinus rhythm with a single, synchronised 360 J shock. This resulted in prompt and dramatic improvement in his haemodynamic state, with the blood pressure increasing to 140/80. The sedation was reversed with flumazenil 200 micrograms. Although the patient grimaced at the time of cardioversion, he had no recollection of the event or receiving a painful shock. He was referred for further investigation and subsequently received an implantable cardioverter defibrillator (ICD).

In an ideal world, DC cardioversion would always be performed in conjunction with an anaesthetist However, immediate DC cardioversion under neuroleptic sedation may be appropriate for very sick patients if no anaesthetist is available. Access to transcutaneous oxygen saturation monitoring, simple airway management techniques and reversal agents has facilitated this approach. The amnesic properties of midazolam often result in the patient having no recollection of the event even if they appeared to experience some discomfort at the time. It is preferable to restore sinus rhythm with a single shock if possible and therefore higher delivered energies (200 or 360 J) should be used.

Case 11.5

A 62-year-old man was admitted with a 2 week history of recurrent presyncopal episodes, one of which had almost caused him to crash his car. He had suffered an uncomplicated inferior MI some 6 months previously. He arrived at the A&E department in sinus rhythm but soon afterwards went into a broad complex tachycardia at 190 bpm accompanied by profuse sweating and hypotension (75/30 mmHg). The presumptive diagnosis was VT and sinus rhythm was restored by DC cardioversion under IV propofol and he was commenced on amiodarone 400 mg tds PO. However, continuous ECG monitoring showed nonsustained bursts of VT which did not respond to IV lignocaine. Two hours later, he went into sustained VT again with hypotension and DC cardioversion was repeated. A temporary pacing catheter was inserted into the right ventricle for antitachycardia and the amiodarone was switched to an IV infusion via a central venous catheter. The patient experienced 16 further symptomatic episodes of VT over the next 72 hours, all of which were successfully terminated by overdrive pacing. The frequency of attacks steadily decreased and once he had been free of VT for 48 hours the pacing catheter was removed. Angiography and eletrophysiological studies were performed once the arrhythmia had been adequately controlled pharmacologically.

Antitachycardia pacing should be considered in any patient with frequent attacks of sustained VT, particularly if DC cardioversion has already been used on one or more occasions. The purpose of the technique is to terminate episodes of VT and so it must be complemented by pharmacological therapy to suppress the tendency to ventricular tachycardia.

Summary

In patients with broad-complex tachycardia, particularly in those with pre-existing ischaemic heart disease, VT is the most likely diagnosis.

Differentiation of VT from SVT should be straightforward if simple clinical and ECG guidelines are followed, aided by adenosine testing.

SVT should only be diagnosed if confirmed by adenosine provocation, i.e. termination of arrhythmia or transient slowing of the ventricular rate.

When differentiation of VT from SVT with aberrant conduction is not possible, **the default diagnosis should always be VT.**

The treatment aim in patients with broad complex tachycardia should be the restoration of sinus rhythm as soon as possible.

Lidocaine (lignocaine) is the first-line drug of choice owing to safety rather than cardioversion efficacy; second-line agents suitable for use include sotalol and procainamide.

If drug therapy fails to restore sinus rhythm or the patient is haemodynamically compromised, DC cardioversion should be undertaken immediately.

Most cases of broad-complex tachycardia/VT should be referred to a cardiologist.

References

1　Stewart RB, Bardy GH, Greene HL. Wide complex tachycardia: misdiagnosis and outcome after emergent therapy. *Ann Intern Med* 1986;**104**:766–71.

2　Tchou P, Young P, Mahmud R, Denker S, Jazayeri M, Akhtar M. Useful clinical criteria for the diagnosis of ventricular tachycardia. *Am J Med* 1988;**84**:53–6.

3　Akhtar M, Shenasa M, Jazayeri M, Caceres J, Tchou PJ.Wide QRS complex tachycardia. Reappraisal of a common clinical problem. *Ann Intern Med* 1988;**109**:905–12.

4　Baerman JM, Morady F, DiCarlo LA, Jr., de Buitleir M. Differentiation of ventricular tachycardia from supraventricular tachycardia with aberration: value of the clinical history. *Ann Emerg Med* 1987;**16**:40–3.

5　Morady F, Baerman JM, DiCarlo LA, Jr., DeBuitleir M, Krol RB, Wahr DW. A prevalent misconception regarding wide-complex tachycardias. *JAMA* 1985;**254**:279–2.

6　Kindwall KE, Brown J, Josephson ME. Electrocardiographic criteria for ventricular tachycardia in wide complex left bundle branch block morphology tachycardias. *Am J Cardiol* 1988;**61**:1279–83.

7　Brugada P, Brugada J, Mont L, Smeets J, Andries EW. A new approach to the differential diagnosis of a regular tachycardia with a wide QRS complex [see comments]. *Circulation* 1991;**83**:1649–59.

8　Dancy M, Ward D. Diagnosis of ventricular tachycardia: a clinical algorithm. *BMJ* 1985;**291**:1036–8.

9　Griffith MJ, Garratt CJ, Mounsey P, Camm AJ. Ventricular tachycardia as default diagnosis in broad complex tachycardia. *Lancet* 1994;**343**:386–8.

10　Griffith MJ, Linker NJ, Ward DE, Camm AJ. Adenosine in the diagnosis of broad complex tachycardia. *Lancet* 1988;**i**:672–5.

11　Rankin AC, Oldroyd KG, Chong E, Rae AP, Cobbe SM. Value and limitations of adenosine in the diagnosis and treatment of narrow and broad complex tachycardias. *Br Heart J* 1989;**62**:195–203.

12　Rankin AC, Rae AP, Cobbe SM. Misuse of intravenous verapamil in patients with ventricular tachycardia. *Lancet* 1987;**2**:472–4.

13　Garratt CJ, Griffith MJ, Young G, *et al.* Value of physical signs in the diagnosis of ventricular tachycardia. *Circulation* 1994;**90**:3103–7.

14　Wellens HJ, Bar FW, Lie KI. The value of the electrocardiogram in the differential diagnosis of a tachycardia with a widened QRS complex. *Am J Med* 1978;**64**:27–33.

15 Griffith MJ, de Belder MA, Linker NJ, Ward DE, Camm AJ. Multivariate analysis to simplify the differential diagnosis of broad complex tachycardia. *Br Heart J* 1991;**66**:166–74.

16 Wellens HJ, Brugada P. Diagnosis of ventricular tachycardia from the 12-lead electrocardiogram. *Cardiol Clin* 1987;**5**:511–25.

17 Rankin AC, Brooks R, Ruskin JN, McGovern BA. Adenosine and the treatment of supraventricular tachycardia. *Am J Med* 1992;**92**:655–64.

18 van der Watt MJ, Aboo M, Millar RN. A prospective study of electrical cardioversion for sustained tachycardias by emergency unit personnel. *S Afr Med J* 1995;**85**:508–11.

19 Gorgels AP, van den Dool A, Hofs A, *et al.* Comparison of procainamide and lidocaine in terminating sustained monomorphic ventricular tachycardia [see comments]. *Am J Cardiol* 1996;**78**:43–6.

20 Ho DS, Zecchin RP, Richards DA, Uther JB, Ross DL. Double-blind trial of lignocaine versus sotalol for acute termination of spontaneous sustained ventricular tachycardia [see comments]. *Lancet* 1994;**344**:18–23.

21 Scheinman MM, Levine JH, Cannom DS, *et al.* Dose-ranging study of intravenous amiodarone in patients with life-threatening ventricular tachyarrhythmias. The Intravenous Amiodarone Multicenter Investigators Group [see comments]. *Circulation* 1995;**92**:3264–72.

22 Levine JH, Massumi A, Scheinman MM, *et al.* Intravenous amiodarone for recurrent sustained hypotensive ventricular tachyarrhythmias. Intravenous Amiodarone Multicenter Trial Group. *J Am Coll Cardiol* 1996;**27**:67–75.

23 Camm AJ, Ward DE. Pacing for Tachycardia Control. Sydney, Australia: Telectronics.

24 Fisher JD, Johnson DR, Furman S, Waspe LE, Kim SG. Mechanisms for success and failure of pacing for termination of ventricular tachycardia: clinical and hypothetical considerations. *PACE* 1983;**6**:1094.

25 Roden DM. The long QT syndrome and torsade de pointes: basic and clinical aspects. In: El-Sherif N, Somel P, eds. *Cardiac pacing and electrophysiology*. Philadelphia: WB Saunders, 1991.

26 Viskin S, Belhassen B. Polymorphic ventricular tacharrhythmias in the absence of organic heart disease. *Prog Cardiovasc Dis* 1998;**41**:17–34.

12: Syncope, bradyarrhythmias, and temporary cardiac pacing

J FERGUSON, KM CHANNON, Y BASHIR

12.1 Introduction

This chapter deals with the acute management of bradyarrhythmias and the interrelated clinical problem of patients presenting with "syncope, ? cause". In cases of persistent bradycardia, for example a patient admitted in complete heart block, diagnosis is straightforward from a 12-lead ECG or rhythm strip. Intermittent bradyarrhythmias pose a much more difficult challenge. The patient presents in sinus rhythm and the diagnosis is suspected because of a history of one or more preceding episodes of altered consciousness (syncope or presyncope). However, syncope is a common symptom in the population, with an incidence of perhaps 20–40% in young adults and 25% or more in the elderly (over 75 years). Only a few of these cases are caused by brady- or tachyarrhythmias and the majority are due to vasodepressor mechanisms, particularly neurocardiogenic syncope (including vasovagal faints) and related disorders.[1] Similarly, syncope accounts for at least 3% of referrals to acute medical units but only a small minority turn out to have an arrhythmic basis. Nevertheless, most of these patients are admitted, and an increasing number are being subsequently referred for consideration of permanent pacemakers despite little supporting evidence, reflecting the undue concern of many hospital doctors about the possibility of bradyarrhythmias. Factors that may have contributed to this overcautious approach include:

- Traditional clinical teaching stresses the association between classical Stokes–Adams attacks and bradyarrhythmias (particularly heart block), with too little emphasis given to other (commoner) causes of syncope.
- Hospital doctors are often not familiar with the epidemiology of syncope in the community.
- Many clinicians are unaware that neurocardiogenic syncope can produce abrupt loss of consciousness without classical autonomic prodromal symptoms or triggering circumstances in some cases, especially among the elderly.

In dealing with patients who have been referred because of syncope, the priority in the acute setting is to identify those cases (the majority) who can be discharged directly and investigated on an outpatient basis. However, admission is required[2] if: the patient is considered at risk of sudden death (those with structural heart disease or other clues to ventricular tachyarrhythmias); there is evidence of bradycardia (particularly atrioventricular (AV) block) likely to require temporary or permanent cardiac pacing; the syncopal attacks are occurring frequently (daily or more often); or the patient is elderly and/or considered at risk of serious injury.

12.2 Syncope

Syncope is defined as sudden, transient loss of consciousness due to reduced cerebral blood flow. It is a very common symptom, exhibiting a biomodal distribution with peaks among adolescents/young adults and the elderly.[3] Recent research has shown that many unexplained falls or drop attacks in the elderly are also attributable to syncope with amnesia for the event itself, so that the patient denies any loss of consciousness.[4] The historic term "Stokes–Adams" attack is largely redundant in modern clinical practice and should probably be avoided. It referred to the features observed during a profound, transient bradyarrhythmia, typically abrupt loss of consciousness and associated pallor, followed by prompt recovery with minimal autonomic features.

12.2.1 Causes of syncope

The major causes of syncope are summarised in Box 12.1 and can be broadly subdivided into several categories:[5] neurocardiogenic syncope (also known as neurally mediated syncope), brady- and tachyarrhythmias, and postural hypotension. In published series,[2] neurocardiogenic syncope accounts for approximately 30% of cases, arrhythmias for 15%, and postural hypotension 10%. Although no cause could be identified in around 35% of cases, recent data suggests that most of these would also have been due to neurocardiogenic mechanisms.

Box 12.1 Causes of syncope

Neurocardiogenic or neurally mediated syncope
    Vasovagal
    Situational (micturation, coughing, swallowing, defaecation)
    Carotid sinus syncope
    Syncope associated with aortic stenosis and pulmonary hypertension

Bradyarrhythmias
    Sino-atrial disease
    Atrioventricular block

Tachyarrhythmias
    Ventricular tachycardia
    Polymorphic VT (including long QT syndromes)
    Supraventricular tachycardia (uncommon)

Postural hypotension

Miscellaneous (tamponade, atrial myxoma, massive pulmonary embolus, etc.)

Unknown

Box 12.2 Pathophysiology of neurocardiogenic syncope

The pathophysiology of neurocardiogenic syncope is not completely understood but the basic mechanisms of vasovagal syncope, carotid sinus syndrome and situational (cough, micturition, and swallow) syncope all have three common components: (i) the afferent limb; (ii) central nervous system; and (iii) the efferent limb (Figure 12.1).

The afferent signals emanate mainly from peripheral mechanical, chemical, pain, or temperature receptors but also from the central nervous system itself (the sight of blood, fear, anxiety, etc.). These stimuli transmit impulses predominantly to the nucleus solitarius in the medulla, a site closely related to the dorsal and ambiguus nuclei of the vagus nerve. In vasovagal syncope, venous pooling to the lower extremities reduces venous return to the heart. Reflex sympathetic stimulation and sinus tachycardia commonly precede the neurocardiogenic reaction. The combination of a sudden reduction in ventricular volume and forceful ventricular contraction trigger cardiopulmonary mechanoreceptors which would normally only be activated by the mechanical stretch of volume or pressure loading. After CNS processing, the efferent limb of the reflex is mediated by increased parasympathetic outflow and reduced sympathetic activity causing the bradycardia and vasodilatation that are characteristic of neurocardiogenic syncope. The bradycardia, which may be profound in some patients but only relative in others, is vagally mediated. Vasodilatation, on the other hand, depends on the interaction in sympathetic and parasympathetic tone. Release of acetylcholine from the parasympathetic system inhibits noradrenaline release from sympathetic nerve endings. Similarly, release of noradrenaline and neuropeptide Y from sympathetic nerve endings inhibits the release of acetylcholine from the parasympathetic system. As a result, the temporal sequence as well as the magnitude of sympathetic or parasympathetic responses are important in the evolution of neurocardiogenic syncope.

Although the central mechanisms contributing to this response are not clear, the role of endogenous opiates and serotonin have been studied closely and both are probably involved in the inappropriate vasodepressor response to acute haemorrhage. Studies using serotonin reuptake inhibitors, such as fluoxetine, sertraline, and paroxetine, have shown promising results in the treatment of neurocardiogenic syncope. The role of the carotid and aortic baroreceptors in neurocardiogenic syncope is likely to be important. Under normal circumstances these receptors would respond to hypotension by increasing sympathetic tone. However, for reasons that are unclear, this feedback mechanism seems to be blunted in neurocardiogenic syncope.

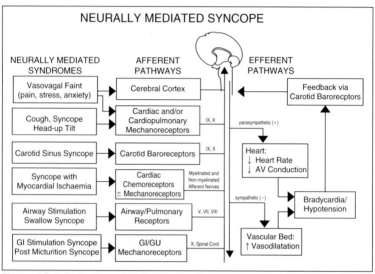

Figure 12.1 Pathogenesis of neurocardiogenic syncope. From Benditt, reproduced with permission from Futura Publishing Company, Inc.[5]

Neurocardiogenic syncope encompasses all forms of syncope due to neurally-mediated reflex vasomotor instability (Box 12.2, Figure 12.1). The group includes the common vasovagal faint, situational syncope (triggered by cough, micturition, etc.), carotid sinus syncope, and exertional syncope associated with aortic stenosis or pulmonary hypertension. Confusion may arise from some of the terminology used. "Neurocardiogenic syncope", strictly speaking, applies to the entire group but is often used loosely to refer to the common vasovagal faint. The term "malignant vasovagal syndrome" is used to describe any cases of neurocardiogenic syncope in which there is abrupt loss of consciousness without prodromal autonomic symptoms, and hence a risk of serious injury. These conditions all involve a complex interplay of neural and cardiovascular reflexes[5] organised into: (i) an afferent limb (e.g. cardiopulmonary mechanoreceptors in vasovagal syncope); (ii) central nervous system (CNS) connections and processing (predominantly within the medulla); and (iii) an efferent limb acting via the twin mechanisms of vagally-mediated bradycardia (the "cardio-inhibitory response") and vasodilatation due to withdrawal of sympathetic tone (the "vasodepressor response"). It is not generally appreciated that the vasodepressor component is usually the dominant mechanism leading to cerebral hypoperfusion[6] and loss of consciousness, often with normal heart rates or only relative bradycardia (40–60 bpm). Even in patients exhibiting severe bradycardia, there may be a major co-existent vasodepressor component, with the result that even AV sequential pacing may not prevent syncope.

The two main groups of bradyarrhythmias are sino-atrial disease (also known as sinus node disease, sick sinus syndrome, brady-tachy syndrome, etc.) which is usually a result of chronic idiopathic conduction system fibrosis, or atrioventricular conduction disease which may result from fibrosis, ischaemic heart disease, or cardiomyopathies.[7] Sino-atrial and AV conduction quite often co-exist in the same patient.

Ventricular tachyarrhythmias (VT) represent a relatively uncommon but particularly important cause of syncope, because these patients are at high risk of sudden death. Sustained monomorphic VT usually arises in the context of ischaemic heart disease and prior myocardial infarction. Polymorphic ventricular tachycardia may be a manifestation of myocardial ischaemia during an acute coronary syndrome or may arise from congenital or acquired forms of long QT syndrome (see Chapter 11). Syncope is also surprisingly common among patients with paroxysmal supraventricular tachycardia,[5] but may be primarily due to a co-existent neurocardiogenic reaction in most cases; however, the prognosis is benign.

Postural hypotension is most usually due to autonomic dysfunction or age-related physiological changes but is often exacerbated by volume depletion or medication.

An important point that emerges from all published series is that syncope occurring in the setting of structural heart disease (most commonly ischaemic heart disease) is associated with a poor prognosis,[2] compared to syncope occurring in patients with no heart disease, regardless of the mechanism. This reflects the association of life threatening arrhythmias with cardiac disease.

12.2.2 Diagnostic approach

This should always start with a careful history, physical examination, and 12-lead ECG. The account of an eyewitness is invaluable and every effort should be made to obtain this information as soon after the event as possible. The evaluation[2,8] should cover the following areas:

- Was this the patient's first ever syncopal event or is there an antecedent history of recurrent episodes?
- Circumstances leading up to syncope and any possible triggers (e.g. prolonged standing or the sight of blood in vasovagal faints)?
- Was syncope unheralded or was there a prodrome?
- Were there associated autonomic symptoms (feeling hot, nausea, sweating, tremulousness, etc.) either during the prodrome or recovery phase?
- Was syncope preceded by angina or paroxysmal tachycardia?
- Is there evidence of structural heart disease (e.g. known previous MI, aortic stenosis, pathological Q waves, etc.), or other adverse prognostic features (family history of sudden death, QT prolongation, etc.)?
- Is there significant postural hypotension (>20 mmHg fall in systolic BP within 2 minutes of standing)?

Lack of familiarity with the epidemiology, pathophysiology, and possible clinical presentations of neurocardiogenic syncope is a particular cause of diagnostic pitfalls (see Box 12.3). Following the initial assessment, three key issues arise.

Is this syncope?

Differentiating syncope from other causes of altered consciousness (epilepsy, narcolepsy, coma, etc.) is usually straightforward provided that an eyewitness account is available. The characteristic history is abrupt loss of consciousness with pallor but no ictal features. It is now accepted that many unexplained falls and drop attacks in the elderly are also due to syncope but with amnesia for the event itself, so that the patient denies losing consciousness. Occasionally, a mistaken diagnosis of epilepsy is made if syncope is followed by secondary tonic-clonic seizures due to cerebral hypoperfusion, but in such cases careful history taking will usually reveal that the fit was preceded by abrupt loss of consciousness with pallor. A more common cause of diagnostic confusion is that many syncopal episodes are associated with minor epileptiform jerks, again raising the possibility of a seizure disorder. Finally, neurocardiogenic syncope can occasionally result in prolonged loss of consciousness[9] (even up to 10–15 minutes) due to persistent vasodilatation, which is mistaken for post-ictal drowsiness.

Box 12.3 Common pitfalls in diagnosing neurocardiogenic syncope

- Vasodilatation is usually the dominant mechanism and syncope can occur without absolute bradycardia.
- The elderly often present with falls and have amnesia for the syncopal event.
- Syncope is not uncommonly associated with minor epileptiform jerks.
- Persistent vasodilatation may result in prolonged loss of consciousness (up to 15 minutes).
- There is a biomodal age distribution. Neurocardiogenic syncope occurs commonly in the elderly as well as adolescents/young adults.
- The prodrome may be abbreviated or absent ("malignant vasovagal syndrome"). However, unlike a classical "Stokes–Adams" attack due to a transient arrhythmia, neurocardiogenic syncope is invariably associated with protracted autonomic symptoms and dizziness during the recovery phase.
- Prodromal autonomic symptoms are often blunted in the elderly.
- Palpitation is commonly due to awareness of sinus tachycardia during the prodrome and/or recovery phase, and does not necessarily indicate a tachyarrhythmia.

What is the likely aetiology of the syncope?

In 40–50% of cases the cause should be apparent from the initial evaluation[2] (history, examination plus ECG) on the basis of simple pattern recognition. These will include cases of heart block or other persistent bradyarrhythmias, young patients with typical vasovagal faints, postural hypotension, and most forms of situational syncope. The remaining cases fall into the category of "syncope ? cause" and a scheme for their subsequent evaluation is summarised in Figure 12.2. In most of these patients syncope will either be due to a neurocardiogenic mechanism or an arrhythmia. The following points may help with differentiation (Box 12.4):[8]

- Patients >60 years should be assessed by carotid sinus massage (see below) to check for carotid sinus hypersensitivity.
- A longstanding history of syncopal episodes (dating back years) favours a neurocardiogenic mechanism rather than an arrhythmia.
- Associated autonomic symptoms favour a neurocardiogenic mechanism. Although prodromal symptoms may be absent in malignant vasovagal syndrome, these patients usually exhibit autonomic features during a protracted recovery phase.
- ECG conduction abnormalities (1st degree heart block, left bundle branch block (LBBB), bi- and trifascicular block) tend to favour a bradyarrhythmia.
- Evidence of structural heart disease, family history of sudden death or other ECG abnormalities (pathological Q waves, left ventricular hypertrophy (LVH), QT prolongation, etc.) also favour an arrhythmic cause.

Because of the prognostic and diagnostic importance of structural heart disease,[10] patients with unexplained syncope should be evaluated by echocardiography (supplemented by other investigations such as stress testing if appropriate). Ambulatory or Holter ECG monitoring is widely used despite poor sensitivity and diagnostic yield, especially following a single episode of syncope[11] (4% arrhythmia correlated with symptoms). Approximately 14% of recordings show an asymptomatic arrhythmia, for example prolonged sinus arrest or intermittent second degree AV block, which is then presumed to indicate the likely cause of syncope.

If ambulatory ECG recording is negative, patients with structural heart disease may be considered for invasive electrophysiological study, particularly those with prior myocardial infarction, to look for inducible ventricular tachycardia.[8] Most patients with syncope and a normal heart require no further investigation unless they are experiencing recurrent episodes. Tilt testing may confirm a diagnosis of neurocardiogenic syncope but has a relatively low diagnostic yield.[12–14] Increasingly, patients with recurrent unexplained syncope end up being offered implantable ECG loop recorders for long-term monitoring. These are activated by the patient after a syncopal episode to store the ECG data leading up to the attack for subsequent analysis.

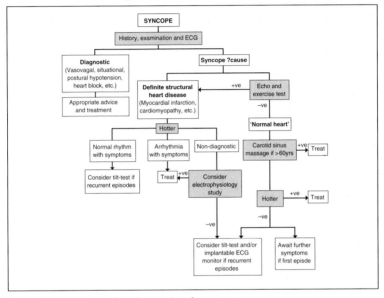

Figure 12.2 Scheme for diagnosis of syncope.

Box 12.4 Investigations in patients with syncope

12 lead ECG. First degree heart block, sinus bradycardia, and bundle branch block (including bi- and trifascicular block) may predict bradycardia as the cause of syncope, whereas old Q waves or pronounced LVH are more likely to be associated with ventricular tachyarrhythmias. Two other rare but important diagnoses are long QT syndrome (congenital or acquired) predisposing to polymorphic VT (torsade de pointes), and Brugada syndrome (right bundle branch block (RBBB)) pattern with precordial ST elevation).

Ambulatory ECG. Widely used in unexplained syncope despite a poor yield with symptom–arrhythmia correlation in only 4% and asymptomatic arrhythmias in another 14% of possible significance.

Carotid sinus massage. The patient should be positioned supine with the neck hyperextended and rotated away from the side which is being tested. The carotid pulse is located and heart rate response to very gentle initial pressure on the carotid bifurcation is assessed (profound bradycardia occurs in carotid hypersensitivity syndrome). If no bradycardia occurs after 5 seconds, more sustained pressure using the palmer aspect of the fingers should be applied for 30 seconds. The test is then repeated on the contralateral side and again with the patient standing upright. Carotid sinus baroreceptors are stimulated and the increase in vagal tone will reduce sinus rate and increase AV conduction time. Carotid sinus massage should not be performed in patients with significant carotid bruits.

Tilt-testing. Tilt-testing maintains patients in an upright posture (typically 60 degree tilt for 45 minutes) to provoke vasovagal syncope.[5-7] This leads to pooling of blood in the lower extremities with compensatory increases in heart rate and contractility. In patients prone to vasovagal syncope, forceful contraction within a relatively empty ventricle may trigger cardiopulmonary baroreceptors and initiate reflex bradycardia and hypotension. The yield of positive results may be increased by adjunctive treatment with isoprenaline infusion or sublingual glyceryl trinitrate (GTN), but at the expense of reduced specificity.[6,8,9]

Intracardiac electrophysiological study. This is only used for patients with structural heart disease (particularly prior MI) as the diagnostic yield is very low among patients with syncope and normal hearts (< 5%). Electrode catheters are introduced via the femoral vein into the right heart for measurement of conduction intervals and programmed stimulation of the atria and ventricles using extrastimuli. The most common and important finding is sustained monomorphic ventricular tachycardia (usually related to a healed infarct).

Is the patient at high risk of death or injury and do they require hospitalisation?

The majority of patients with syncope can be safely discharged from the emergency department following the initial evaluation (history, examination, and ECG) and arrangements made for further investigation (echocardiography, ambulatory ECG monitoring, etc.) and follow-up as outpatients. This applies to those with no clinical evidence of structural heart disease and a normal 12-lead ECG, particularly if the history suggests a neurocardiogenic mechanism. However, those patients in whom syncope occurred without warning prodromal symptoms or some definite trigger (for example, post-micturition) should be advised not to drive until fully evaluated, in line with current DVLA regulations.

Hospitalisation is required for the following groups of patients:[2,8]

- Those with documented and/or perisistent bradyarrhythmias likely to require temporary or permanent cardiac pacing. Patients in whom a bradyarrhythmia is strongly suspected, for example recurrent abrupt syncope with no autonomic symptoms with an ECG showing trifascicular conduction disease, should also be admitted for ECG monitoring;
- Those at high risk of sudden death, usually from ventricular tachyarrhythmias. This includes patients with adrenergically triggered syncope, family history of sudden death (hypertrophic cardiomyopathy, long QT syndrome, arrhythmogenic RV cardiomyopathy/dysplasia, Brugada syndrome), evidence of structural heart disease or significant ECG abnormalities (Box 12.5). Inpatient assessment including echocardiography and ambulatory ECG monitoring is appropriate for these "high-risk" cases. They may require invasive investigation and should ideally be seen by a cardiologist prior to discharge to formulate a plan for further management.
- Those with frequent syncopal episodes (for example, daily attacks). Clearly inpatient evaluation and ECG monitoring are likely to yield a quick diagnosis and enable appropriate management.
- Those at high risk of serious injury, particularly the elderly and possibly patients on long-term anticoagulants.

Box 12.5 Risk stratification of patients with syncope: high risk features

Adrenergic precipitation (e.g. exertion, sudden fright)

Family history of sudden death

Structural heart disease
    Ischaemic heart disease
    Chronic heart failure
    Aortic stenosis
    Hypertrophic or dilated cardiomyopathy

ECG abnormalities:
    LBBB, bifascicular or trifascicular block
    Pathological Q-waves
    AV block
    LV hypertrophy
    Prolonged QT interval
    Brugada syndrome (RBBB with praecordial ST elevation)

12.3 Bradyarrhythmias

12.3.1 Presentations

Bradyarrhythmias such as complete heart block may be well tolerated with minimal or no symptoms. However, most patients present either with cerebral symptoms (syncope or presyncope) or, if the bradycardia is persistent, lethargy and exertional dyspnoea which may progress to overt congestive cardiac failure. In the absence of a co-existent vasodilatation (as in neurocardiogenic reactions), syncope will only occur with sudden onset of profound bradycardia, for instance prolonged ventricular standstill or sinus arrest (usually for > 5 seconds).

Bradyarrhythmias encountered in the acute medical setting may represent the first presentation of chronic intrinsic dysfunction of the cardiac conduction system (for example, sino-atrial disease), or may have arisen as a consequence of transient and/or reversible conditions such as acute myocardial infarction, hypothermia, and vagotonic states (for example with abdominal pain, vomiting, ventilation on ITU). Other factors such as drugs (particularly β-blockers, digoxin and other antiarrhythmic agents) and metabolic disturbances may exacerbate minor intrinsic conduction disease to precipitate an overt bradyarrhythmia. Thus, there are two important issues for the admitting clinician:

- Although many patients will require a permanent pacemaker, it is important to identify those in whom the bradyarrhythmia will be self-limiting.
- Will temporary cardiac pacing be required, either as a bridge to permanent pacemaker implantation or until resolution of the bradyarrhythmia?

The practice of temporary transvenous cardiac pacing has evolved considerably over the past 10–15 years. The advent of thrombolysis and transcutaneous pacing have been associated with marked reductions in the total number of temporary cardiac pacing procedures, as has the introduction of permanent pacing services in most district hospitals. This has inevitably led to deskilling of junior medical staff in an invasive and potentially hazardous procedure. Accordingly, temporary pacing should only be used after careful consideration has been given to the indication, timing, and mode.

12.3.2 Classification

Sinus node dysfunction

Sinus node dysfunction[7] (also known as sino-atrial disease or sick sinus syndrome) encompasses persistent sinus bradycardia, sinus arrest, sino-atrial exit block, and combinations of atrial tachyarrhythmias with any of the above ("bradycardia–tachycardia syndrome") (Box 12.6). Intrinsic sino-atrial disease is usually due to idiopathic degenerative and fibrotic changes, but transient sinus node dysfunction is commonly encountered during acute myocardial infarction and vagotonic states such as vomiting. Most such arrhythmias can be managed conservatively and temporary cardiac pacing is seldom required. Similarly, sino-atrial disease is commonly diagnosed as an incidental finding during continuous or ambulatory ECG monitoring but the risk of sudden death is low and pacemaker therapy should only be considered if there are significant symptoms.

> **Box 12.6 ECG criteria for sinus node dysfunction**
>
> *Sinus bradycardia*
> ECG: Normal P wave axis and morphology, P wave rate < 60 bpm, constant P–R interval, unaltered QRS complex morphology
>
> Sinus bradycardia commonly occurs in young adults, particularly well-trained athletes, in whom resting heart rates at night are commonly as low as 30–35 bpm and may even be associated with sinus arrest during REM sleep. Various medical conditions, for instance vomiting or parasympathomimetic drugs may be associated with excess vagal tone and sinus bradycardia. In the vast majority of cases, sinus bradycardia does not require specific treatment.
>
> *Sinus arrest*
> ECG: Normal P wave axis and morphology, constant P wave rate except for occasional sinus arrest when the P wave falls transiently, unaltered QRS complex morphology (Figure 12.3).
>
> Failure of sinus node discharge results in loss of atrial depolarisation and ventricular asystole if escape beats from latent

pacemakers do not occur. Sinus arrest has no clinical significance if the ventricular escape rhythm can support a reasonable heart rate. Permanent pacing is generally only required for symptomatic sinus arrest with pauses >3 seconds.

Sino-atrial exit block
ECG: The criteria for normal sinus rhythm are fulfilled except during SA block. When the P-P interval is twice normal (R-R is also twice normal). The block may equal three or more normal intervals, if block occurs in consecutive cycles.

Normal sinus node impulse formation fails to depolarise the atria, or does so with delay. Permanent pacing is only required for patients with prolonged symptomatic pauses.

Bradycardia-tachycardia syndrome
ECG: Sinus bradycardia, arrest or exit block combined paroxysmal atrial tachyarrhythmias (atrial fibrillation, flutter or atrial tachycardia). Treatment often involves a combination of antibradycardia pacing and antiarrhythmic drug therapy to prevent tachyarrhythmias.

Atrioventricular conduction disease (Box 12.7)

Idiopathic conduction tissue fibrosis is also a very common cause of chronic AV conduction disorders. Patients with high-grade AV block frequently present acutely with heart failure or syncope/presyncope. Other causes include cardiomyopathy and specific heart muscles diseases (for example, sarcoidosis or amyloidosis), congenital heart block, degenerative aortic valve disease.[7] Transient, potentially reversible AV block may occur with acute myocardial infarction or other acute coronary syndromes, infective endocarditis (aortic root abscess), following open heart surgery or secondary to drugs (particularly digoxin toxicity).

The AV conduction system comprise the AV node, His bundle, plus the left and right bundles and Purkinje network (intraventricular conduction system). Delay or block developing at AV nodal level is associated with a narrower QRS escape rhythm which is relatively fast (typically ≥ 40 bpm) and stable. Conduction disease resulting in AV block below the His bundle, is associated with a slower, broad QRS escape rhythm (often < 30 bpm) which is less stable with a greater risk of ventricular standstill or degeneration to ventricular tachyarrhythmias (polymorphic VT or VF). Patients with

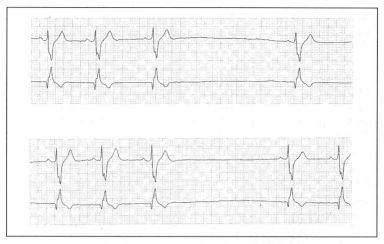

Figure 12.3 Sinus arrest. Sinus bradycardia is interrupted by a 3.5 second pause during which there are no P waves indicative of sino-atrial disease.

chronic AV block (particularly at the level of the intraventricular conduction system) are at higher risk of sudden death than those with sino-atrial disease and may be considered for permanent pacemakers even in the absence of symptoms. The role of temporary cardiac pacing is discussed below.

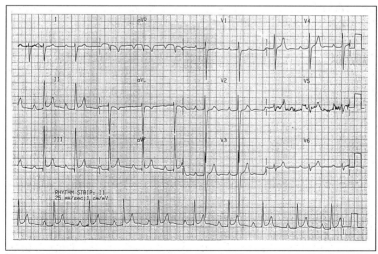

Figure 12.4 First degree heart block. Regular P waves are all followed by a QRS complex but there is a fixed PR prolongation of 280 ms.

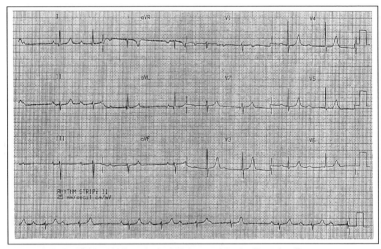

Figure 12.5 Möbitz I (Wenckebach) heart block. Regular P waves are followed by progressive PR prolongation until atrioventricular block occurs.

Box 12.7 Atrioventricular block

First degree AV block
ECG: Normal P wave axis and morphology, P–R interval is regular and > 0.20 sec, unaltered QRS complexes (Figure 12.4).

P–R intervals as long as 1.0 sec have been recorded and can occasionally exceed the P–P interval, a phenomenon known as "skipped" P waves. The site of conduction delay is most commonly the AV node but can also be His-Purkinje system, bilateral bundle branch block and, rarely, intra-atrial conduction. The block may degenerate to Type I second degree block when the atrial rate increases.

Second degree AV block
Möbitz Type I (Wenckebach)
ECG: Normal P wave axis and morphology, progressive prolongation of P–R interval until a P wave is not followed by a QRS complex (dropped beat), unaltered QRS complex morphology (Figure 12.5).

The longest P–R interval will be immediately before the dropped beat and the shortest will be associated with the first conducted P wave. There is progressive shortening of R–R interval before the dropped beat.

Möbitz Type II
ECG: Normal P wave axis and morphology, unaltered QRS complex morphology, P–R interval of conducted beats may be normal or long but remains constant prior to the non-conducted P waves (see Figure 12.6).

It is usually associated with disease within the His-Purkinje system and will often progress to complete heart block

Complete AV block
ECG: There is no consistent relationship between atrial and ventricular activity (atrioventricular dissociation), the QRS morphology may be normal but more often is abnormal, the QRS rate is usually constant (Figure 12.7), but may be prone to periods of ventricular standstill (Figure 12.8).

The atrial rhythm may be sinus or abnormal (fibrillation/flutter, tachycardia, an ectopic focus or retrograde from the ventricular escape focus). The anatomical site of the block can be determined from the escape rhythm. Block from within the node tends to have a narrow QRS and rates of 40–60 bpm compared to that arising more distally (His-Purkinje system) which tends to have a broad QRS complex with slower rates and a greater propensity to asystole.

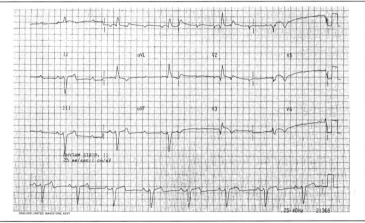

Figure 12.6 Möbitz II heart block. Regular P waves are followed by intermittent 2:1 (and occasionally 3:1) atrioventricular block without evidence of preceding PR prolongation.

12.3.3 Assessment and indications for pacing

The initial clinical assessment of patients presenting with bradyarrhythmias should address the following issues:

- Is this an acute presentation of a chronic intrinsic conduction disorder (sino-atrial disease or AV block) or is it a potentially self-limiting dysrhythmia, for example in association with acute myocardial infarction?

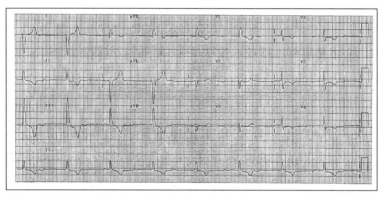

Figure 12.7 Complete heart block. Regular P wave are completely dissociated from the QRS complexes which, in this case, demonstrate a broad complex ventricular escape rhythm of 38 bpm.

- Are there other reversible factors (drugs, hypothermia, metabolic disturbance, etc.)?
- Has the patient been experiencing frequent syncope/presyncope or any life-threatening ventricular tachyarrhythmias.
- Is there evidence of pulmonary oedema or a low-output state (hypotension, oliguria, cerebral obtundation, etc.).

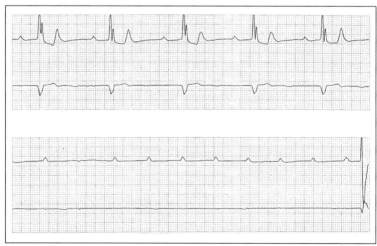

Figure 12.8 Ventricular standstill. Möbitz II heart block is followed by an 8 second run of high degree atrioventricular block where regular P waves but no ventricular activity can be seen.

Most patients with symptomatic intrinsic conduction disorders (sino-atrial disease or AV block) will require permanent pacemakers. With wider availability of specialists in district hospitals, it is preferable for such cases to proceed directly to pacemaker implantation on the next routine list, wherever possible avoiding the potential complications of temporary cardiac pacing. However, temporary pacing should be instituted in patients who have experienced recurrent syncope and/or any episodes of polymorphic VT or VF, particularly those with complete heart block and broad QRS escape rhythms because these individuals are at high risk of cardiac arrest. Patients with potentially reversible bradyarrhythmias should only require temporary cardiac pacing for recurrent cerebral symptoms, escape ventricular tachyarrhythmias or severe haemodynamic compromise. If pacing is required for haemodynamic support, ventricular-demand (VVI) pacing alone seldom helps and these patients usually require AV sequential pacing with involvement of a cardiologist. The indications for temporary and permanent pacing are summarised in Table 12.1.

Table 12.1 Indications for temporary (TP) and permanent pacing. (Recommendations for temporary and permanent pacing adapted from ACC/AHA guidelines.)

Cause of heart block	Immediate TP	TP if recurrent symptoms	Permanent pacemaker	Outpatient referral to cardiologists
AV block				
Broad complex	✓	✗	✓	✗
Narrow complex	✗	✓	✓	✗
Intermittent	✗	✓	✓	✗
Sino-atrial disease	✗	✓	✓	✗
Intraventricular conduction disease (bifascicular and trifascicular)	✗	✗	✗	✓
Carotid sinus hypersensitivity	✗	✓	✓	✗

Temporary cardiac pacing technique

This is discussed in Chapter 14.

12.4 Bradyarrhythmias and temporary cardiac pacing in acute myocardial infarction

Complete heart block (CHB) may develop in 6–14% of patients who present with acute myocardial infarction (MI) and predicts an increased in-hospital mortality. This increased mortality relates more to infarct size than the conduction disturbance itself and the role of pacing remains controversial. In the past, temporary cardiac pacing was extensively used in acute MI both for patients with established AV block or other bradyarrhythmias, and for those deemed at high risk of progressing to high-grade AV block (for example anterior MI with bifascicular or trifascicular block). The widespread use of thrombolysis has probably reduced the incidence of AV conduction disorders during the acute phase and increased the risk of invasive instrumentation, while the introduction of transcutaneous pacing has allayed fears about sudden progression to complete AV block with ventricular standstill. Thus, the modern approach to temporary pacing during acute myocardial infarction is much more conservative than in the past.

Transient sinus node dysfunction and AV block are common following inferior infarction, usually related to reflex vagal activation as well as occlusion of the AV nodal artery, a branch of the right coronary. Often such cases will respond to IV atropine. Conduction is affected at the level of the AV node resulting in a relatively stable, narrow QRS escape rhythm. Even if patients develop persistent high-grade AV block, it is usually well tolerated and almost invariably resolves within 7–10 days. Temporary cardiac pacing is rarely needed for symptomatic bradycardia (prolonged pauses with syncope) and permanent pacing is only indicated if AV block persists for 10–14 days. An important exception is complete heart block accompanying major right ventricular infarction which can lead to major haemodynamic compromise with cardiogenic shock. The noncompliant right ventricle is particularly dependent on atrial filling in this setting and AV sequential pacing offers significant advantages over VVI pacing alone.[20, 21]

Complete heart block following anterior MI is caused by large infarcts with significant septal necrosis involving the intraventricular conduction tissue. Thus, the escape rhythm is relatively unstable with broad QRS complexes and a tendency to ventricular standstill. Almost all such patients develop pulmonary oedema and/or shock. Simple ventricular demand (VVI) pacing will protect against asystole but seldom improves haemodynamic function alone, for which AV sequential pacing may be required. However, the prognosis of these patients is very poor irrespective of pacing mode.

The presence of complete heart block at presentation of acute MI is frequently cited as a cause of unnecessary delay to thrombolytic therapy to allow for instrumentation of a central vein. It is our practise not to withhold thrombolysis in patients with AV conduction disorders who are haemodynamically stable, while those who are shocked or in pulmonary oedema should receive thrombolysis as soon as central venous access has been secured.

Clinical cases

Case 12.1

A 9-year-old school boy presented with an episode of collapse during his school assembly. It had been a warm summer's day and he had been late for school and missed breakfast. He described a brief premonition of feeling faint and nauseated before collapsing to the ground. A teacher had seen him turn extremely pale before collapsing to the ground. He was rouseable within seconds of collapsing but remained pale and nauseated and felt weak and unable to stand. He described one similar episode 3 years previously while standing in church. On clinical assessment he had a normal cardiovascular examination and ECG. He was diagnosed as having a vasovagal episode, reassured and discharged home.

Case 12.2

A 75-year-old woman presented to the emergency department with her third episode of loss of consciousness within 5 years. She had been standing at the bus stop when she collapsed to the ground unconscious without any warning. A bystander had seen her fall and noticed that she was extremely pale. He had been unable to rouse her for 5 minutes after which she gradually regained consciousness. She remained pale and was sweating profusely. On clinical assessment she had recovered fully, had a normal cardiovascular examination, normal ECG and negative carotid sinus massage. She was discharged home 2 hours later. A 24-hour ECG and echocardiogram performed 2 weeks later were normal. She was diagnosed as having probable neurocardiogenic syncope but no further action was advised unless the attacks recurred.

Case 12.3

A 60-year-old man presented to the emergency department with his second episode of syncope within 48 hours. He described palpitation and diziness followed by loss of consciousness and collapse. He had abruptly regained consciousness with no particular after effects. During the second episode he had fallen against the coffee table and lacerated his forehead. He reported a history of anterior myocardial infarction 2 years previously and was currently taking an ACE inhibitor, statin, and aspirin. He was admitted for further investigation. ECG showed sinus rhythm with anterior Q waves. Echocardiogram demonstrated discrete anterior wall akinesia with moderately impaired LV systolic function. An exercise tolerance test was terminated prematurely because of dyspnoea and 2 mm ST segment depression in the inferior leads. Coronary angiography showed an occluded left anterior descending artery without any other flow limiting lesions. Ventricular stimulation studies showed inducible monomorphic VT with hypotension and he was loaded with amiodarone and β-blockers. VT remained inducible after 7 days despite antiarrhythmic therapy and he proceeded to have an ICD implanted. Three months later he presented after a defibrillator shock. Interrogation of the device showed two further episodes of VT, one successfully terminated with overdrive pacing but a second had degenerated to VF requiring shock therapy.

Case 12.4

A 52-year-old man presented with an acute inferior infarct but was not thrombolysed as he had presented more than 18 hours after the onset of symptoms. He was found to be in complete heart block on admission but was haemodynamically stable without pulmonary oedema. He was carefully monitored in the CCU and no temporary wire was inserted. The heart block resolved after 3 days and no permanent pacemaker was required.

Case 12.5

A 79-year-old man presented with a two day history of progressive dyspnoea. Clinical examination revealed a pulse rate of 48 bpm, mild congestive cardiac failure and cardiomegaly on chest radiograph. The ECG showed complete heart block with a narrow complex QRS morphology and echocardiogram showed normal LV systolic function and moderate LV hypertrophy. He was treated with diuretics but no temporary pacing was required. A permanent DDD pacemaker was implanted 3 days later.

Case 12.6

An 84-year-old woman presented with a three day history of multiple episodes of syncope and presyncope. ECG showed complete heart block, a broad-complex ventricular escape rate of 30 bpm and evidence of a left ventricular hypertrophy. Shortly after presentation she developed ventricular standstill, loss of consciousness, and a self-limiting run of torsade de pointes was recorded. A temporary pacing wire was inserted and she had no further symptoms or arrhythmias. A VVIR pacemaker was inserted 4 days later.

Summary

Syncope

Syncope is a common presentation in acute medicine. Bradyarrhythmias are often suspected but most cases are due to neurocardiogenic mechanisms.

Differentiation of syncope from other causes of altered consciousness primarily depends upon obtaining an eyewitness account.

Neurocardiogenic syncope is classically associated with automatic symptoms, but may occur with an abbreviated or absent prodrome ("malignant vasovagal syndrome"), especially in elderly patients. Vasodilatation is usually the dominant mechanism and often causes syncope in the absence of significant bradycardia.

Presence of structural heart disease, particularly impaired LV function, in patients with syncope is associated with an adverse prognosis, partly due to a high incidence of ventricular tachyarrhythmias.

Most cases of syncope can be investigated on an outpatient basis, but hospitalisation is required for those with persistent bradyarrhythmias and/or at high risk of sudden death or injury.

Bradyarrhythmias and temporary cardiac pacing

Bradyarrhythmias usually present with either cerebral symptoms (syncope/presyncope) or a lower output state.

Both sinus node dysfunction and atrioventricular block are commonly due to degenerative changes affecting the conduction system, but it is important to consider transient or reversible factors (drugs, ischaemia, etc.) before committing patients to permanent pacing.

The advent of thrombolysis plus availability of transcutaneous pacing have significantly reduced the use of temporary transvenous cardiac pacing following acute MI. Many cases of AV block complicating inferior MI will resolve with conservative management. AV block complicating anterior MI is usually associated with a massive infarct, often going on to cardiogenic shock and death.

With more widespread availability of permanent pacing, early implantation of a permanent pacemaker is preferable to temporary pacing in many cases if there is no reversible cause of bradycardia.

Temporary dual chamber pacing may be required in patients with bradyarrhythmias and haemodynamic compromise.

References

1 Savage DD, Corwin L, McGee DL, Kannel WB, Wolf PA. Epidemiologic features of isolated syncope: the Framingham Study. *Stroke* 1985;**16**:626–9.
2 Linzer M, Yang EH, Estes NA III, Wang P, Vorperian VR, Kapoor WN. Diagnosing syncope. Part 1: Value of history, physical examination, and electrocardiography. Clinical Efficacy Assessment Project of the American College of Physicians. *Ann Intern Med* 1997;**126**:989–96.
3 Abboud FM. Neurocardiogenic syncope [editorial; comment]. *N Engl J Med* 1993;**328**:1117–20.
4 Kenny RA, Ingram A, Bayliss J, Sutton R. Head-up tilt: a useful test for investigating unexplained syncope. *Lancet* 1986;**i**:1352–5.
5 Benditt DG. Neurally mediated syncopal syndromes: pathophysiological concepts and clinical evaluation. *Pacing Clin Electrophysiol* 1997;**20**:572–84.
6 Grubb BP, Kosinski D. Current trends in etiology, diagnosis, and management of neurocardiogenic syncope. *Curr Opin Cardiol* 1996;**11**:32–41.
7 Mangrum JM, DiMarco JP. The evaluation and management of bradycardia. *N Engl J Med* 2000;**342**:703–9.
8 Linzer M, Yang EH, Estes NA III, Wang P, Vorperian VR, Kapoor WN. Diagnosing syncope. Part 2: Unexplained syncope. Clinical Efficacy Assessment Project of the American College of Physicians. *Ann Intern Med* 1997;**127**:76–86.
9 Grubb BP. Pathophysiology and differential diagnosis of neurocardiogenic syncope. *Am J Cardiol* 1999;**84**:3Q–9Q.
10 Middlekauff HR, Stevenson WG, Stevenson LW, Saxon LA. Syncope in advanced heart failure: high risk of sudden death regardless of origin of syncope. *J Am Coll Cardiol* 1993;**21**:110–16.

11 Gibson TC, Heitzman MR. Diagnostic efficacy of 24-hour electrocardiographic monitoring for syncope. *Am J Cardiol* 1984;**53**:l013–17.

12 Benditt DG, Remole S, Bailin S, Dunnigan A, Asso A, Milstein S. Tilt table testing for evaluation of neurally-mediated (cardioneurogenic) syncope: rationale and proposed protocols. *Pacing Clin Electrophysiol* 1991;**14**:1528–37.

13 Kapoor WN, Smith MA, Miller NL. Upright tilt testing in evaluating syncope: a comprehensive literature review. *Am J Med* 1994;**97**:78–88.

14 Fitzpatrick AP, Theodorakis G, Vardas P, Sutton R. Methodology of head-up tilt testing in patients with unexplained syncope. *J Am Coll Cardiol* 1991;**17**:125–30.

15 Murphy JJ. Current practise and complications of temporary transvenous pacing. *BMJ* 1996;**312**:1134.

16 Bartecchi CE, Mann DE. *Temporary Cardiac Pacing*. Chicago: Precept Press, 1990.

17 Fitzpatrick A, Sutton R. A guide to temporary pacing. *BMJ* 1992;**304**:365–9.

18 Bocka JJ. External transcutaneous pacemakers. *Ann Emerg Med* 1989;**18**:1280–6.

19 Ferguson JD, Banning AP, Bashir Y. Randomised trial of temporary cardiac pacing with semirigid and balloon-flotation electrode catheters. *Lancet* 1997;**349**:1883.

20 Matangi MF. Temporary physiologic pacing in inferior wall acute myocardial infarction with right ventricular damage. *Am J Cardiol* 1987;**59**:1207–8.

21 Topol EJ, Goldschlager N, Ports TA. Haemodynamic benefits of atrial pacing in right ventricular myocardial infarction. *Ann Intern Med* 1982;**96**:594–7.

13: Cardiac arrest

CH DAVIES, M HUNT

13.1 Introduction

The large scale trials which have transformed many aspects of acute cardiology have had less impact on the management of cardiac arrest. Randomised trials have been difficult to organise, partly due to a lack of commercial incentive, and those that have been undertaken frequently produce negative results. As a result, the available evidence base is thin, and much of the animal work of questionable relevance. Within these limitations, didactic advanced cardiac life support (ACLS) guidelines have streamlined arrest management and everyone involved in resuscitation is strongly advised to attend an appropriate course. This chapter is based upon the 1998 European guidelines[1,2] with some additional information from the 2000 American Heart Association protocols;[3,4] paediatric resuscitation is not discussed.

13.2 Basic life support

The mechanics of basic life support are well covered in ACLS publications[2] and only commonly encountered problems are discussed here.

13.2.1 Management of specific problems

- Rate of chest compressions: the current recommendation is for 100/min with equal amounts of time for compression and release.
- Ratio of chest compressions to ventilation is 5:1 for two rescuers and 15:2 for single rescuers.
- The use of simultaneous CPR and ventilation is no longer recommended.
- Despite some recent encouraging studies[5] the universal applicability of active compression/decompression remains the subject of controversy.[6]
- Automatic chest compression devices are worth considering in those situations where prolonged resuscitation is appropriate (see below).[7]
- Remember that even with ideal CPR, cardiac output is only 30% of normal: CPR is not even a holding manoeuvre, one is simply sliding backwards more slowly.

13.3 Advanced life support

13.3.1 Using the universal algorithm

It is only worth giving a praecordial thump for a witnessed arrest in an unmonitored patient. Following ECG connection the universal algorithm splits into two (Figure 13.1).[1] If there is genuine uncertainty about whether VF is present, the VT/VF algorithm should be followed.

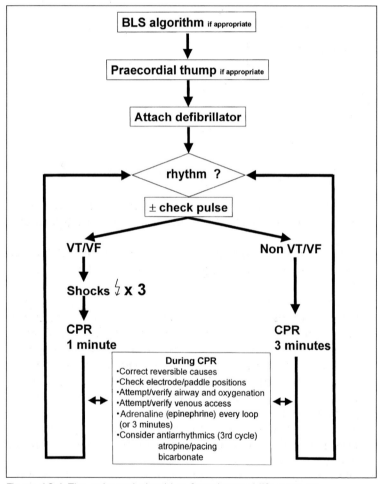

Figure 13.1 The universal algorithm for advanced life support. Reproduced from the 1998 European Resuscitation Council guidelines.[1]

13.3.2 VT/VF rhythms

(1) Defibrillate with ⚡ 200 J① then
⚡ 200 J② followed by
⚡ 360 J③.

(2) Start CPR.

(3) There is now a maximum window of 2 minutes for tracheal intubation, achieving iv access, and administering drugs.

(4) If VF persists give adrenaline (epinephrine) 1 mg iv.

(5) Defibrillate with ⚡ 360 J④ then
⚡ 360 J⑤ followed by
⚡ 360 J⑥.

(6) If still in VF, repeat sequence from 2 onwards.

(7) Antiarrhythmics can be considered at this point (i.e. the start of the third cycle).

Notes on VT/VF management

- The pulse needs only to be checked following a shock if the monitor rhythm changes to one compatible with a cardiac output.
- Push the charge button as soon as the shock is delivered: look at the monitor screen whilst the defibrillator is charging.
- The "stacked shocks" sequence should not be interrupted for CPR unless there is a flat line ECG for > one screen sweep following a shock, in which case give CPR for 1 minute (without adrenaline (epinephrine)) and reassess.
- Remember that VF is the most frequent initial rhythm in cardiac arrest, the only effective treatment is defibrillation, that VF tends to become asystolic with time and thus the probability of success diminishes rapidly.
- Shocks, not drugs, are the key to success in VF and excessive delays between shocks (which tend to occur between shocks ③ and ④) are detrimental.
- 80% of those in whom defibrillation is successful will have achieved this by shock ③.
- Patients who are successfully converted to sinus rhythm

(SR) following a 200 J shock but then have further episodes of VT/VF should be re-shocked at 200 J. Using the higher energy makes them no more likely to stay in SR and may increase the risk of myocardial damage. This is more difficult with an automatic defibrillator and it is probably not worth restarting the sequence.

- These defibrillator energies are for standard monophasic waveforms. In the near future biphasic waveform defibrillation will be available for which energy requirements (and the potential for myocardial damage) are lower.[8] Follow the instructions on the defibrillator.
- There is no benefit from attempting antero-posterior paddle positions if the standard antero-apical approach is unsuccessful.[8]

13.3.3 Non-VT/VF algorithms

(1) Administer atropine 3 mg iv and adrenaline (epine-phrine) 1 mg iv (the adrenaline is repeated on subsequent loops but the atropine is not).
(2) 3 minutes of CPR, during which iv access should be established and advanced airway management undertaken.

Notes on non VT/VF management

- This group is a composite of the previous electromechanical dissociation and asystole groups. Patients in "electromechanical dissociation" frequently demonstrate mechanical activity on echo and the term "pulseless electrical activity" (PEA) is preferable.
- Survival in this group is only 10–15% of that achieved with VT/VF and these scaled down recommendations reflect our relative inability to alter outcome in the majority of these patients.
- Always check to see that the monitor baseline moves in response to CPR in a systolic patients. If it does not, suspect lead disconnection or that the defibrillator is monitoring the paddles not the leads (since VF is much more treatable than non VT/VF it is important not to miss it).
- The only realistic hope lies in detecting a secondary cause and a rapid checklist (5H's and 4T's) should be undertaken (several of these also present as refractory VF) (Box 13.1).

Box 13.1 Potentially reversible causes

Hypoxia
Hypovolaemia
Heart block
Hyper/hypokalaemia
Hypothermia
Tension pneumothorax
Tamponade
Toxic/drugs
Thromboembolic/mechanical obstruction

- In PEA, differentiation should be made between relatively organised narrow complex ECGs which suggest a preserved myocardium struggling with a mechanical problem (hypovolaemia, obstruction, tamponade) and the broad disorganised activity of a dying myocardium. Aggressive efforts to identify a secondary problem are justified in the former group but rarely succeed in the latter.
- Precise timing of adrenaline (epinephrine) administration in isolation from the algorithm loop only complicates matters, it should simply be administered once per loop. For VT/VF this works out at every 2–3 minutes (the time for 3 shocks and 2 minutes of CPR) and for non-VT/VF every 3 minutes (by definition).
- With peripheral venous administration of drugs, a 20 ml flush of 0.9% saline (not dextrose) is required as a flush. The decision to insert a central line will depend upon the skill of the personnel involved but it is vital that they do not disrupt basic CPR, the shock sequence, or airway management.
- Administration of drugs via the ET tube remains a second line approach and only adrenaline (epinephrine), lidocaine (lignocaine), and atropine can be administered. Doses should be at least double, diluted to 10 ml in 0.9% saline and followed by five ventilations.
- Whilst tracheal intubation remains the ideal, laryngeal mask airways are becoming increasingly popular. The suggested tidal volume has been reduced to 400–600 ml/min in an attempt to reduce gastric insufflation if a bag and mask is used.

13.4 Specific clinical problems in cardiac arrest management

13.4.1 Role of antiarrhythmics

Studies of antiarrhythmics in the context of cardiac arrest (many in animal models) have produced conflicting results and there is little evidence of consistent benefit.[9,10] Matters are further complicated by the fact that antiarrhythmic action in animal models is dependent on the shock waveform (monophasic Vs biphasic).[11]

There is some evidence to support the use of bretylium in refractory VF from a small study of 36 patients.[12] However, bretylium is difficult to use as the therapeutic effect develops over 20 minutes and is frequently associated with marked hypotension.

Recent evidence suggests a small increase in survival to hospital admission following amiodarone 300 mg iv for VTNF in out of hospital arrest when administered after shock ③.[13] Hospital discharge rates were unchanged whilst both hypotension and bradycardia were more common in those receiving amiodarone. When 1.2 g amiodarone and bretylium have been compared directly in the more heterogeneous setting of haemodynamically unstable VT and VF, they appeared to be equally efficacious,[14] but hypotension was more troublesome in the bretylium group.

On the basis of current evidence, antiarrhythmics should not be used routinely during cardiac arrest in the absence of specific indications (such as a patient who manifests a monomorphic tachycardia between periods of VF). In patients with refractory VF where an antiarrhythmic is felt to be appropriate, the evidence is most convincing for amiodarone, with bretylium relegated to second place by the high incidence of hypotension and the imminent exhaustion of world supplies.

13.4.2 Use of buffers

Bicarbonate administration is now only recommended if arterial pH < 7.1 and base excess > −10 or under specific circumstances (hyperkalemia, tricyclic overdose).[15] The starting dose is 50 ml of an 8.4% solution.

13.4.3 Adrenaline (epinephrine) dose

Despite initial enthusiasm there was no increase in the hospital discharge rate with high dose adrenaline in five large studies;[15] indeed whether adrenaline is of any benefit is far from certain.[10,15,16] Adrenaline doses should be reduced or even omitted in patients whose arrest is associated with solvent abuse, cocaine, and other sympathomimetic agents. Current interest centres on vasopressin in the hope that this will possess the beneficial effects of adrenaline on perfusion pressure without the potential for increasing myocardial oxygen demand and arrhythmogenesis.[15] Current US guidelines suggest 40 U IV vasopressin in VF, reverting to the traditional adrenaline (epinephrine) regimen after 10 minutes.

13.4.4 When to pace

Only complete heart block responds to pacing, and pacing of asystole in general is of no value.[17] Confusingly, this presents as both asystole (with visible non-conducted P waves) and as VF (as an escape rhythm). An output can occasionally be generated in arrest secondary to heart block by cardiac percussion at 100/min whilst transcutaneous pacing (TCP) is attached. Though TCP is a useful holding manoeuvre this is painful and frightening for many patients and sedation is recommended. An isopresenraline infusion should be started (5 mg in 500 ml 5% dextrose = 10 μg/ml) infused at 1 ml/min titrated against response. Excessive administration can provoke ventricular arrhythmias but these respond rapidly to a reduction in the infusion rate. Meanwhile preparations should be underway for insertion of a temporary pacing wire (see Chapter 12).

13.4.5 Cardiac tamponade

Tamponade should be suspected in clinical situations where pulseless electrical activity presents following cardiac surgery, radiofrequency ablation or late in the hospital course of myocardial infarction (myocardial rupture). If available, the diagnosis on echo is so straightforward that it can be made with very little interruption of the CPR cycle. Failing this, blind pericardiocentisis should be undertaken (see Chapter 14). In the absence of a predisposing clinical scenario the success of this manoeuvre in restoring cardiac output in PEA as a whole is extremely low and pericardiocentisis "just in case" in all cases of PEA is not justified.

13.4.6 Tension pneumothorax

Like tamponade this usually occurs in the context of a predisposing clinical scenario (central line insertion, trauma, mechanical ventilation). It should be considered as a potential cause of PEA occurring later on in the course of a complex arrest where central lines have been inserted (although a non-contracting myocardium is more likely).

13.4.7 Thromboembolic/mechanical obstruction

This tends to be suggested by the preceding clinical scenario: most commonly PEA in a post-operative patient, but also in patients with malignancy. No pulse will be felt with CPR and the neck veins will be distended. Vigorous CPR has traditionally been advised in the hope of breaking up the clot. Despite anecdotal reports of thrombolysis during cardiac arrest, in reality there is little that can be done if cardiac output does not return. It is however important to make the diagnosis if output does return in order to proceed urgently to pulmonary angiography and thrombolysis or to surgical embolectomy.

13.4.8 Metabolic

Plasma K+ should be checked as soon as practicable in all protracted arrests and this is vital in refractory VT/VF. The preceding clinical scenario may include renal failure, dialysis (look for fistulae on the arms) or diabetic ketoacidosis. Treatment is with:

- Calcium gluconate 10 ml of a 10% solution iv (not in a line with bicarbonate) injected over 2–5 minutes.
- Dextrose/insulin: 50 g dextrose and 10 U soluble insulin over 15–30 minutes.
- Sodium bicarbonate 50 mmol over 5 minutes.
- Dialysis (peritoneal dialysis has been successfully performed during resuscitation).

13.4.9 Hypothermia

This represents one of the indications for prolonged resuscitation attempts. If the initial three-shock sequence is unsuccessful, further defibrillation and drugs should be postponed until core temperature is >30°C. This should be achieved by ventilating with warmed oxygen, warmed iv fluids at 40°C via a central line at 1.5 l/hr and potassium free peritoneal lavage at 43°C. Additional lavage via a chest drain or a urinary catheter have also been advocated. Extracorporeal bypass has also been successful in this situation. It is important to consider co-existing drug or alcohol intoxication.

13.4.10 Near drowning

Successful outcomes have been achieved following prolonged immersion in extremely cold water and prolonged resuscitation can be justified. Attempts to remove excess water from the airways are not necessary. Those who have inhaled water may have severe electrolyte derrangements.

13.4.11 When to consider opening the chest

Despite its haemodynamic superiority there is no evidence of benefit when open chest CPR is initiated >15 mins into an arrest. The role of open chest massage is currently limited to two situations. The first is within 36 hours of cardiac surgery,[18] when it is easily performed by a cardiothoracic surgeon who can rapidly cut the sternal sutures. The commonest problem here is tamponade secondary to haemorrhage and an echo should be performed to confirm this. Occasionally the problem is one of acute ischaemia secondary to graft failure and repeat CABG can be successful. The second indication is following chest trauma (particularly penetrating trauma) where emergency thoracotomy permits relief of tamponade and control of intrathoracic haemorrhage.

13.4.12 Cardiac arrest associated with trauma

Survival is best for younger patients with penetrating injuries, it is poor for patients who degenerate into asystole during transfer to hospital and for patients with multiple trauma who have exsanguinated. A high index of suspicion for the presence of tension pneumothorax or tamponade is essential and aggressive volume loading often required.

13.4.13 Cardiac arrest associated with pregnancy

To reduce the inferior vena caval (IVC) compression from the gravid uterus (supine hypotensive syndrome), a wedge should be placed beneath the right abdominal flank or the uterus should be displaced manually during resuscitation. Intubation is notoriously difficult in these patients and particular care should be taken to ensure correct placement of the endotracheal (ET) tube. The differential diagnoses include:

- Pulmonary embolism/amniotic fluid embolism.
- Peripartum haemorrhage and abruption.
- Uterine rupture.
- Myocardial infarction.
- Aortic dissection.

If initial resuscitation is unsuccessful, and there is potential fetal viability, summon paediatric and obstetric teams as a caesarean section should be performed within 5 minutes of the onset of cardiac arrest.[19]

13.4.14 Electrocution

With alternating current the initial rhythm is usually VF and the high potential for survival justifies intensive resuscitation. Airway management may be complicated by facial burns and rhabdomyolyis may require fluid loading and urinary alkalinisation.

13.4.15 Drug overdose

Tricyclic antidepressant toxicity is due to a combination of catecholamine elevation, anticholinergic effects, quinidine-like actions and α-blockade. Cardiac arrest occurs either due to VF-, PEA- or torsade-like arrhythmias. The patient should be rapidly alkalinised with sodium bicarbonate 1 mmol/kg, followed by hyperventilation aiming for a pH of 7.45–7.55. Torsade like arrhythmias require iv magnesium 2 g over 5 mins and overdrive pacing suppression should be considered. The administration of adrenaline (epinephrine) should be minimised. Post-arrest hypotension due to α-blockade requires a fluid challenge of 500–1000 ml.

Digoxin toxicity responds to digoxin specific antibody fragments ("Digibind"). Correction of plasma K^+ is important and magnesium infusion may be a useful temporising measure.

Calcium antagonists present as PEA or complete heart block and should receive 5–10 ml of calcium chloride iv to a maximum of 4 g. Hypotension may be partially responsive to volume loading, whilst heart block refractory to calcium should be paced.

CNS drugs: administer naloxone (2 mg) if there is any suspicion of narcotic overdose and be aware of clues such as needle tracks. Consider flumazenil (0.25 mg iv followed by a second 0.25 mg) if there is a possibility of benzodiazepine dose.

Cocaine: the adrenaline dose interval should be extended to every 5–10 minutes, with iv metoprolol 5–10 mg for refractory VF. Once the circulation returns then an α-blocker may be required for hypertension.

13.4.16 Patients with pacemakers and implantable defibrillators

In patients with implantable defibrillators (AICDs) it is usually best to let the machine follow its algorithm if it is acting appropriately. If the patient is receiving inappropriate shocks (i.e. shocks when the patient is not in VT or VF) a pacing magnet should be placed over the device. Expert advice should be sought from the implanting centre (all patients carry a card with details of their device and their implanting centre).

For patients with pacemakers, care should be taken to avoid delivering a shock within 10 cm of the pulse generator. Shocks can raise pacing thresholds and disable pulse generators leaving the patient without bradycardiac support. A magnet placed over the pacemaker will temporarily reset the pacemaker to an asynchronous mode (DOO or VOO: fixed pacing irrespective of the underlying rhythm) at maximum output. If this fails, isoprenaline and temporary pacing will be required.

13.4.17 When is prolonged resuscitation appropriate?

The guidelines state that resuscitation should continue for 20–30 minutes unless there are compelling reasons to believe that it is futile. As noted above, there are some situations where prolonged resuscitation is appropriate (Box 13.2), but these are rare. If a protracted attempt at resuscitation is appropriate, do not worry excessively about long term neurological impairment. Efforts to judge cortical perfusion during resuscitation are unreliable and experience shows that the majority of patients with severe neurological injury do not survive long term (severe impairment occurs in only 2% of survivors).

Box 13.2 Situations where prolonged resuscitation may be appropriate

Hypothermia

Near drowning (particularly if combined with hypothermia)

Electrocution

Drugs/poisoning

Hyperkalaemia

13.4.18 Knowing when to stop

Deciding when to stop is a much harder decision than the mechanics of following the universal algorithm. It is traditional to ask if there is dissent among the team before stopping and this practice is strongly recommended. Since restarting resuscitation after stopping is not a good option the rule must be that if in doubt, continue. If possible seek a senior opinion at this point. Experience shows that the senior opinion always suggests that efforts be discontinued.

Refractory asystole is not a problem as the outlook is clearly hopeless. It is much more difficult to abandon a patient in VF, particularly a repetitive cycle of VF→shock→sinus rhythm→VF. If this happens it is worth stepping back, letting someone else take over chest compressions and re-evaluating the situation. Go over the checklist of secondary causes again, particularly the plasma K^+ and gases, the possibility of poisoning or hypothermia and scrutinise the patient's drug chart. Examine the patient's notes, trying to answer two questions: why have they arrested now and what was their prior quality of life.

There are then several points to be borne in mind at this point:

- Remember the 80% rule (80% of people in whom resuscitation is successful achieve sinus rhythm within the first 3 shocks).

- Patients who were critically unwell and in whom things were not going well prior to their arrest are unlikely to do better post arrest.
- Two groups of patients do well after cardiac arrest: primary cardiac problems (particularly post MI) and those immediately following surgery (especially cardiac). The third group consists of patients with severe illnesses who were not responding to treatment or in whom the diagnosis was not certain, these people do very badly (whatever you do).
- Patients who have had extensive out of hospital resuscitation by competent paramedics and already been through multiple loops of the algorithm without success almost never survive.

The question of futility often hinges on whether an attempt at resuscitation was appropriate in the first place. For many hospital inpatients it becomes all too obvious during the arrest that resuscitation is unlikely to be in the patient's interests. Failure to make a decision as to the appropriateness of resuscitation by the team looking after the patient often means that the same decision must be made in the middle of the night in an arrest situation by someone who has never met the patient. An explicit comment in the notes of all patients concerning the appropriateness of resuscitation should be the norm. In practice, discussing these issues with patients is not as impossible as it may at first seem.

13.4.19 Return of spontaneous circulation after cessation of resuscitation

Occasionally spontaneous circulation returns immediately after it has been decided that further attempts at resuscitation are futile.[20] This does nothing for the self confidence of the clinician in charge, but matters are usually resolved by a short period of observation with appropriate supportive care: again, in reality these patients rarely survive.

13.5 Post-arrest care

With the return of a spontaneous cardiac output, patients should be examined, and a manual BP taken. Blood should be taken for electrolytes, Mg^{2+} and a full blood count whilst an ECG is obtained and a chest *x* ray ordered. At this point patients divide into two groups. Those whose arrest was precipitated by an arrhythmia are characterised by a rapid return of consciousness and haemodynamic stability. The question here is whether the arrhythmia will recur and if so whether this can be prevented. The second group remain critically unwell. This latter group consists predominantly of those patients who were profoundly unwell before the arrest (and in whom the arrest was probably part of the process of dying) with a contribution from the primary arrhythmia group whose arrest was protracted and who have developed secondary organ dysfunction.

13.5.1 Management strategy in those who recover rapidly

The first step is to identify the clinical scenario preceding the arrest (Figure 13.2). This is usually obvious as the majority of shortlived and successfully resolved arrests occur in the context of an acute myocardial infarction and the 12-lead ECG will show ST elevation. It is important to differentiate this from the established Q waves of a prior infarction or the residual ST elevation caused by ventricular aneurysm. Defibrillation itself can produce ST elevation without underlying ischaemic heart disease but this is rare, particularly with biphasic shocks. Though commonly taken at this point cardiac enzymes are uninterpretable due to damage to the chest wall muscles (although troponins may prove to be of more value). Retrospective analysis of cardiac enzymes on any sample taken before the arrest should be obtained.

The point to emphasise is that, although a patient who is successfully resuscitated from VF within the first 24 hours of infarction has a slightly worse overall prognosis than an apparently similar patient who did not experience VF, the arrhythmia is unlikely to recur in the longer term. No additional investigations (angiography, VT stimulation tests, etc.) are required before discharge and long term anti-arrhythmic medication is not required. There is no evidence of benefit (and some suspicion of potential harm) from the routine administration of iv anti-arrhythmics to these patients immediately following the arrest. The occurrence of VF is modulated by catecholamine tone and there are compelling theoretical reasons to ensure that patients are adequately β-blocked at this point and that β-blockers have not been incorrectly withheld.

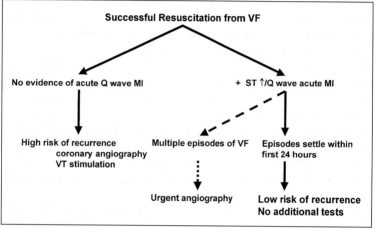

Figure 13.2 Management strategy for cases who recover rapidly from cardiac arrest.

It is also important to ensure normalisation of the plasma K+ to > 4.0 mmol/l and, unlike the routine management of K+ in patients with myocardial infarction (see Chapter 3), this should be aggressively treated. Peripheral infusions of K+ are poorly tolerated and require large volumes of fluid: a central line should be inserted and 20–60 mmol K+ infused in 100 ml of 0.9% saline at < 20 mmol/hr. Ensuring that the central line is inserted by someone with experience is also important as thrombolysis may still be indicated.

The high sympathetic tone of the arrest situation produces a transient intracellular K+ shift and whilst this should not delay replacement, plasma K+ should be rechecked 45 min post arrest. Similarly low plasma Mg^{2+} requires treatment.

If the ECG is consistent with acute infarction then reperfusion therapy should now be considered. Defibrillation and short lived (5 minutes) CPR are not contraindications to thrombolysis, but thrombolysis should not be administered without a corroborating clinical history or in an unconscious/confused patient. In patients who are unable to give a clear history but who are haemodynamically stable, then reperfusion therapy should be limited to aspirin (rectally if needed); however, if there are signs of haemodynamic decompensation then primary angioplasty should be considered as the question of whether or not this is an acute infarction can be settled at angiography.

Other situations characterised by rapid recovery are also precipitated by acute ischaemia, either following percutaneous transluminal coronary angioplasty (PTCA) or coronary artery bypass surgery (CABG) or secondary to critical ischaemia not associated with infarction. VF following PTCA or CABG usually implies infarction due to abrupt vessel closure and should prompt consideration of a return to the catheter lab or theatre.

Patients who present with unexplained VF and do not subsequently develop evolving ECG changes consistent with an ST elevation/Q wave MI require further investigation. In contrast to those developing VF in the peri-infarct period, the risk of recurrence is high and the management of these patients is discussed in Chapter 11. Patients who make an initially good recovery but subsequently experience multiple episodes of VF or polymorphic VT over the course of a few hours are candidates for urgent angiography, as this can be a manifestation of critical ischaemia; this is discussed further in Chapter 11.

13.5.2 Management strategy in the critically unwell

Patients who remain critically unwell despite the return of a spontaneous cardiac output present complex management challenges, many outside the scope of this book. Clinical examination may seem out of place among the clutter of high technology equipment, but should not be neglected. Check for rib fractures, pneumothorax, correct ET tube placement, bleeding from unsuccessful central line insertions, and the presence of abdominal distension. Pupillary dilatation should be noted but is notoriously unreliable at predicting long term functional recovery.

A period of transient stability may provide an opportunity to re-assess whether further intensive management is appropriate. Once confronted with cardiac arrest, the hopelessness of the situation becomes apparent and it becomes clear that further efforts are inappropriate. This is not a particularly rational approach and a decision that resuscitation was inappropriate prior to the arrest might have been preferable. Nevertheless once this decision has been made and after consultation with the patient's own team, management is straightforward.

In those patients in whom continued intensive efforts are felt to be appropriate, the following specific problems may be encountered.

Management of ventilation

Unless patients rapidly regain consciousness, a period of elective ventilation is strongly recommended. Restless patients should be paralysed and sedated if necessary. The evidence for hyperventilation reducing post-ischaemic cerebral damage is not as convincing as once thought and this is no longer recommended. A nasogastric tube should be inserted if there is evidence of abdominal distension secondary to gastric insulfation during resuscitation. A urinary catheter should be inserted and central venous access obtained.

Hypotension

Rapid normalisation of cerebral perfusion pressure may reduce secondary ischaemic damage. Treatment will depend on the clinical scenario preceding the arrest, however, hypotension usually represents myocardial dysfunction and requires inotropes. Aliquots of 0.25–1 mg of adrenaline (epinephrine) given as boluses may be required to hold the situation whilst infusions are made up. Again, the choice of inotrope will depend upon the clinical situation (see management of shock in Chapter 6) but dobutamine is a reasonable first choice.

Hypotension in a patient who appears salvageable is an indication for echocardiography.

Role of echocardiography (Table 13.1)

This can provide valuable information as to the cause of the arrest (i.e. segmental wall motion abnormalities suggesting ischaemic heart disease) and provide insights into the mechanisms underlying continuing haemodynamic instability. However, subtle abnormalities of left ventricular function can be difficult to detect in the presence of sinus tachycardia, atrial fibrillation and the high catecholamine levels. In particular, patients receiving high doses of inotropes and maintaining their blood pressure within the normal range may appear to have deceptively good left ventricular function. For this reason an initial scan immediately following the arrest to exclude major intracardiac pathology may need to be followed by a more detailed study once the patient has stabilised.

Table 13.1 Quick checklist for echocardiography in the post-arrest period

	Characteristic	Potential significance
LV wall motion	Overall function	Overall prognosis, though this can be very misleading
	Segmental dysfunction Segmental thinning	Coronary disease
LV cavity	Underfilled	Haemorrhage, sepsis
	Dilated with scarred segments	Substrate for VT
RV cavity	Dilated with LV cavity underfilled	Pulmonary embolus
Pericardial fluid	Tamponade	Post MI rupture, aortic dissection
Aortic valve	Doppler signal	Aortic stenosis

If the mechanism of hypotension remains unclear after clinical examination and echocardiography or if guidance is required with fluid therapy in the presence of significant disparity between LV and RV function, then a Swan-Ganz catheter should be inserted (see Chapter 14)

Hypertension

Transient hypertension can occur secondary to disturbed autoregulation of cerebral blood flow and usually settles without treatment.

Arrhythmias

Assuming that they do not cause marked haemodynamic compromise, one should actively try to avoid treating the majority of rhythm disturbances in the post-arrest period. Atrial arrhythmias and ventricular ectopics should not be treated, neither should short bursts of non-sustained VT as these often settle spontaneously as the high catecholamine levels, hypoxia, and acid–base disturbances resolve.

Sustained VT should be treated with lidocaine (lignocaine) 1 mg/kg or amiodarone 300 mg iv. Cardioversion may be also be required prior to these if the systolic BP is <90 mmHg. There is no indication for prophylactic use of lignocaine in all patients post-arrest. Further management is described in Chapters 10 and 11 (broad and narrow complex tachycardias).

Cerebral protection measures

Seizures require treatment with iv phenytoin but there is no evidence of benefit from prophylactic anticonvulsant treatment or from the use of glucorticoids or calcium antagonists.

Glycaemic control

Both hypo- and hyper-glycaemia may produce secondary cerebral damage and both should be actively treated in the post-arrest period. Do not rely solely on finger prick samples as impaired peripheral perfusion may produce unreliable results.

13.6 Psychological care

Cardiac arrest can be a terrifying experience for patients. Paradoxically those most at risk are those with primary arrhythmias who recovery rapidly after resuscitation and are often agitated and disorientated. Calm straightforward reassurance that matters are now under control is appropriate at this point, as is ensuring that someone is detailed to stay adjacent to the patient's head and continue to provide reassurance. Assuming that ventilation is satisfactory, we routinely supplement this with iv midazolam in 2.5 mg aliquots in an attempt to induce retrograde amnesia. When patients are fully recovered it is important to provide more detailed information about what has happened. In those patients in whom the arrest occurred in the context of an acute MI then reassurance about the low risk of recurrence is gratefully received. A small proportion of patients experience an out of body hallucination, they do not usually volunteer information about this unless asked tactfully and directly, yet they are often relieved at the opportunity to discuss this further.[21]

There has been much debate on whether relatives should be present during resuscitation.[22,23] Whatever the merits of this approach, attempts to simultaneously direct the arrest and cater for the psychological needs of the relatives run the risk of failing to perform either task adequately.

Most resuscitation is unsuccessful (14% survival in hospital inpatients[24]) and the focus then switches from the high technology of the arrest situation to one of caring for the patient's family. The potential damage inflicted by insensitive handling of the acutely bereaved is well recognised. This subject is well covered in both the UK and US ACLS publications and will not be reiterated. However, in addition we routinely offer relatives the opportunity to see us again the following day when they collect the death certificate (most decline) and to feel free to come and discuss matters at a later date (about one third take up this offer over the coming year). As a matter of policy the clinician in charge of the arrest should be responsible for contacting the coroner's office (if appropriate), signing the death certificate, and contacting the patient's general practitioner by telephone. The prompt arrival of a brief letter or fax from the clinician in charge to the patient's general practitioner forms a helpful basis for subsequent discussion with the relatives. Confusion caused by delegation of these apparently mundane tasks can substantially increase the family's distress.

Clinical cases

Case 13.1

A 70-year-old man who had been admitted to the CCU 24 hours previously experienced five episodes of VF over a 4 hour period. Attempts to prevent these episodes with optimisation of his plasma K^+, Mg^{2+} followed by infusions of lidocaine (lignocaine) and amiodarone were unsuccessful.

Following a further episode of VF careful examination of the monitor strip preceding the onset of VF revealed complete heart block with no underlying ventricular rhythm. No further episodes occurred following insertion of a temporary VVI pacemaker. VF can be a manifestation of heart block: an important one as it is so easily treated.

Case 13.2

A 29-year-old woman's condition was stable 2 hours following uneventful radiofrequency ablation for Wolff–Parkinson–White syndrome. She complained of nausea and then collapsed with pulseless electrical activity. In the context tamponade was felt to be the likely diagnosis and this was successfully relieved with blind pericardiocentesis.

Tamponade is an important cause of electromechanical dissociation as it is so readily treatable. It is only rarely seen outside the context of predisposing clinical scenarios; be aware of these.

Summary: Ten rules of resuscitation

Ensuring the quality of basic life support is your responsibility, not ACLS in isolation.

Shocks save lives, not drugs: give them priority.

In non-VT/VF rhythms, finding a secondary cause offers the only real hope: think hard.

Be familiar with your defibrillator: never meet it for the first time at an arrest.

Differentiate primary arrhythmias from arrhythmias occurring during the process of death.

VF during the first 24 hours of a Q wave MI does not usually recur in the longer term.

VF not associated with an acute MI has a high recurrence rate and requires further investigation.

Repetitive episodes of VF may represent acute ischaemia and urgent coronary angiography is required.

Psychological care of patients and their families forms part of good arrest management.

Assessing suitability for resuscitation is an integral part of inpatient care.

Recommended reading

Hodgetts T, Castle N. *Resuscitation Rules*. London, UK: BMJ Books, 1999.

Forthright and practical commentary on some of the many difficult issues that arise during resuscitation.

References

1 The 1998 European Resuscitation Council guidelines for adult advanced life support. Advanced Life Support Working Group of the European Resuscitation Council. *BMJ* 1998;**316**:1863–9.
2 The 1998 European Resuscitation Council guidelines for adult single rescuer basic life support. Basic Life Support Working Group of the European Resuscitation Council. *BMJ* 1998;**316**:1870–6.
3 Cummins RG. *Advanced Cardiac Life Support*. American Heart Association, 1997.
4 Guidelines 2000 for Cardiopulmonary Resuscitation and Emergency Cardiac Care. *Circulation* 2000;**102**(Suppl I):I1–383.
5 Plaisance P, Lurie KG, Vicaut E, *et al*. A comparison of standard cardiopulmonary resuscitation and active compression-decompression resuscitation for out-of-hospital cardiac arrest. French Active Compression-Decompression Cardiopulmonary Resuscitation Study Group. *N Engl J Med* 1999;**341**:569–75.
6 Stiell IG, Hebert PC, Wells GA, *et al*. The Ontario trial of active compression-decompression cardiopulmonary resuscitation for in-hospital and prehospital cardiac arrest. *JAMA* 1996;**275**:1417–23.
7 Dickinson ET, Verdile VP, Schneider RM, Salluzzo RF. Effectiveness of mechanical versus manual chest compressions in out-of-hospital cardiac arrest resuscitation: a pilot study. *Am J Emerg Med* 1998;**16**:289–92.
8 Dalzell GW. Determinants of successful defibrillation. *Heart* 1998;**80**:405–7.
9 Chamberlain DA. Antiarrhythmic drugs in resuscitation. *Heart* 1998;**80**:408–11.
10 van Walraven C, Stiell IG, Wells GA, Hebert PC, Vandemheen K. Do advanced cardiac life support drugs increase resuscitation rates from in-hospital cardiac arrest? The OTAC Study Group. *Ann Emerg Med*

1998;**32**:544–53.

11 Ujhelyi MR, Schur M, Frede T, Gabel M, Markel ML. Differential effects of lidocaine on defibrillation threshold with monophasic versus biphasic shockwaveforms. *Circulation* 1995;**92**:1644–50.

12 Nowak RM, Bodnar TJ, Dronen S, Gentzkow G, Tomlanovich MC. Bretylium tosylate as initial treatment for cardiopulmonary arrest: randomized comparison with placebo. *Ann Emerg Med* 1981;**10**:404–7.

13 Kudenchuk PJ, Cobb LA, Copass MK, *et al.* Amiodarone for resuscitation after out-of-hospital cardiac arrest due to ventricular fibrillation. *N Engl J Med* 1999;**341**:871–8.

14 Kowey PR, Levine JH, Herre JM, *et al.* Randomized, double-blind comparison of intravenous amiodarone and bretylium in the treatment of patients with recurrent, hemodynamically destabilizing ventricular tachycardia or fibrillation. The Intravenous Amiodarone Multicenter Investigators Group. *Circulation* 1995;**92**:3255–63.

15 Adgey AA. Adrenaline dosage and buffers in cardiac arrest. *Heart* 1998;**80**:412–14.

16 Behringer W, Kittler H, Sterz F, *et al.* Cumulative epinephrine dose during cardiopulmonary resuscitation and neurologic outcome. *Ann Intern Med* 1998;**129**:450–6.

17 Cummins RO, Graves JR, Larsen MP, *et al.* Out-of-hospital transcutaneous pacing by emergency medical technicians in patients with a systolic cardiac arrest. *N Engl J Med* 1993;**328**:1377–82.

18 Anthi A, Tzelepis GE, Alivizatos P, Michalis A, Palatianos GM, Geroulanos S. Unexpected cardiac arrest after cardiac surgery: incidence, predisposing causes, and outcome of open chest cardiopulmonary resuscitation. *Chest* 1998;**113**:15–19.

19 Strong THJ, Lowe RA. Perimortem cesarean section. *Am J Emerg Med* 1989;**7**:489–94.

20 Maleck WH, Piper SN, Triem J, Boldt J, Zittel FU. Unexpected return of spontaneous circulation after cessation of resuscitation (Lazarus phenomenon). *Resuscitation* 1998;**39**:125–8.

21 Appleby L. Near death experience. *BMJ* 1989;**298**:976–7.

22 van der Woning M. Should relatives be invited to witness a resuscitation attempt? A review of the literature. *Accid Emerg Nurs* 1997;**5**:215–18.

23 Robinson SM, Mackenzie-Ross S, Campbell HG, Egleston CV, Prevost, AT. Psychological effect of witnessed resuscitation on bereaved relatives. *Lancet* 1998;**352**:614–17.

24 Ballew KA. Cardlopulmonary resuscation. *BMJ* 1997;**314**:1462–5.

14: Practical procedures

CH DAVIES, J FERGUSON

All of these procedures are potentially hazardous and none should be attempted without adequate training, both in the techniques themselves and in *x* ray screening (a requirement of European law). The importance of obtaining experienced help before starting cannot be over-emphasised, but perhaps more important still is the importance of seeking help if problems are unexpectedly encountered during the procedure; the worst damage tends to occur when people persist following initial failure. If circumstances permit, written consent should be obtained (with the exception of central venous access). Although they seem minor in medical terms, these procedures may be terrifying for patients: explanations prior to the procedure reinforced by what to expect during the various stages of the procedure are important.

14.1 Central venous access

Indications for central venous cannulation range from drug administration to providing access for pulmonary artery catheterisation and temporary wire insertion. All of these procedures require full aspetic technique: simply putting on sterile gloves is inadequate. Our recommendation is always to use a Seldinger wire through needle technique and that catheter through the needle techniques are only suitable for peripheral access.

14.1.1 Subclavian route

This has the advantages of providing the easiest access for the insertion of temporary wires, for pulmonary artery catheterisation, and for patient comfort following insertion. Its major disadvantage is a relatively higher incidence of pneumothorax and an inability to compress either the subclavian vein or its adjacent artery if bleeding occurs.

Subclavicular approach

(1) Position the patient either supine or in a shallow Trendelenburg position with his/her head turned in the opposite direction (placing a rolled up towel beneath the patient's spine is uncomfortable and unnecessary).

(2) Prepare a sterile field extending to the suprasternal notch and drape the upper chest and shoulder.

(3) Select a point 1 cm below the mid point of the clavicle just laterally to the point of the 'S' bend (point C on Figure 14.1). This site is very variable and may lie anywhere within the clavicle's middle third. Palpate this point: if arterial pulsations are felt the artery lies anterior to the vein and an alternative approach (jugular, etc.) should be considered.

(4) Infiltrate 1% lidocaine (lignocaine) using an orange and then a green needle, first superficially and then more deeply under the clavicular margin.

(5) Wait whilst the anaesthetic takes effect (a minimum of 3–4 minutes).

(6) Attach a saline-filled syringe to the Seldinger needle and insert this into the anaesthetised area aiming for the suprasternal notch. Depress the point of entry so that it lies parallel to the clavicle's inferior margin. Slowly advance the needle whilst applying negative pressure to the syringe. The needle track should be aimed as close as possible to the inferior surface of the clavicle to minimise the potential of entering the pleural space. Entry into the subclavian vein is confirmed by the free aspiration of dark, non-pulsatile blood.

(7) If the vein is not entered then withdraw the needle whilst maintaining negative pressure: successful cannulation may occur during withdrawal.

(8) Remove the syringe and insert the guidewire. Unless blood is oozing out of the needle then this manoeuvre needs to be completed as quickly as possible to prevent air embolism. Cover the hub with a finger if there is any delay.

(9) The guidewire must advance without resistance or discomfort; if it will not then remove it and confirm that the needle still lies within the vein by aspirating blood. A small trickle of blood is not sufficient: you are merely aspirating the haematoma from your last unsuccessful attempt.

(10) Make a 2 mm nick in the skin with a scalpel blade (commonly forgotten).

(11) Insert the dilator over the wire, whilst warning the patient to expect some discomfort as firm pressure is required.

(12) Remove the dilator and slide the catheter over the wire, being careful that the distal tip of the wire is never lost from view within the catheter.

(13) Aspirate blood from the lumen(s) and then flush with 0.9% saline.

(14) Suture in place (using the retaining clip provided to avoid line compression) and cover with a transparent dressing.

(15) Obtain a chest *x* ray to confirm the catheter position and exclude a pneumothorax.

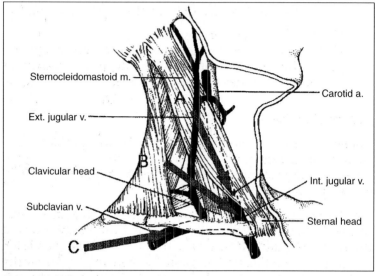

Figure 14.1 Sites of venous access for internal jugular (A), supraclavicular subclavian (B) and infraclavicular subclavian (C) central lines. (Modified from Bone.)[18]

Supraclavicular approach

This approach has the advantage of minimising problems associated with the tortuous anatomy that may occur at the subclavian/brachiocephalic junction.

(1) Positioning is identical to the subclavicular approach.

(2) The sterile field should extend above the clavicle.

(3) The local anaesthetic infiltration should be made in the triangle formed by the sternal insertion of the sternomastoid and the upper border of the clavicle (point B on Figure 14.1).

(4) The green needle should be advanced beneath the clavicle in a line joining the suprasternal notch and the contralateral nipple at an angle of 30–40° to the clavicle.

(5) It is vital to maintain an approach that is as anterior as possible (i.e. that tracks as close to the inferior aspect of the clavicle as possible). If the vein cannot be located with the exploring green needle then do not attempt to proceed further.

(6) If the vein is located, leave the green needle *in situ* as a guide, insert the Seldinger needle and proceed as described for the subclavicular approach.

Potential problems

Failure to enter the vein is the most common problem. The chances of successful puncture are maximised by head-down tilt or (if clinically appropriate) a 250 ml volume challenge using a peripheral vein.

Inability to advance the guidewire usually reflects an extravascular course. If there is any uncertainty always assume the worst at this point: withdraw the needle to the skin and start again using a slightly different angle. Occasionally there may be tortuosity at the junction of the subclavian with the brachiocephalic. It is easier to negotiate this with a J-shaped wire (which can be rotated) than a straight wire (which is not recommended). Angling the needle bevel so that the wire points towards the brachiocephalic may also be helpful. If problems persist use a supraclavicular or internal jugular approach.

Pneumothorax complicates 1% of procedures. It is important not to attempt subclavian access in patients in whom there is severe contralateral lung damage in whom pneumothorax may prove disastrous. The risk (and potential consequences) of pneumothorax are increased by mechanical ventilation, particularly PEEP. If access cannot be obtained on one side do not attempt access on the contralateral side without first obtaining a chest *x* ray to minimise the possibility of creating a bilateral pneumothorax (which may prove fatal). Perhaps surprisingly, aspirating air during needle advancement does not invariably mean that a pneumothorax has been created and conversely, pneumothorax often occurs without premonitory warning.

Haemothorax occasionally occurs and is revealed by the development of a basal pleural effusion.

Subclavian artery puncture rarely produces problems as long as its occurrence is recognised following puncture of the Seldinger needle. Attempts to introduce a dilator into the artery may produce catastrophic haemorrhage.

Excessive catheter length. The catheter tip should be situated above the junction of the inferior cava and the right atrium as more distal positioning increases the risk of arrhythmias and pneumothorax.

Chyle aspiration from puncture of the thoracic duct, usually on the left, may rarely occur: re-insert the needle at a different site and angle.

14.1.2 Internal jugular route

This has the advantage of a low incidence of pneumothorax and easy compressibility in the advent of haemorrhage, but lines are difficult to secure here and there is a suspicion of increased rates of sepsis.

(1) Positioning is identical to subclavian access, except that the head needs be rotated slightly further towards the opposite side.

(2) Prepare a sterile field extending from the clavicle to the ear and drape the patient (a turban like arrangement can be used to extend the field over the scalp). Ensure patients are able to see out from under the far side of the drapes.

(3) Ask the patient to turn their head against the resistance of your hand to demonstrate the course of the sternomastoid muscle. Locate the carotid artery by palpation.

(4) The internal jugular vein lies at the apex of a triangle formed by the two heads of the sternomastoid and the clavicle, lateral to the carotid artery (point A on Figure 14.1).

(5) Infiltrate this point with lidocaine (lignocaine) using the orange green needle technique.

(6) Using the green needle, locate the vein, usually found at a 30° angle to the skin on a line towards the right nipple, but this is very variable. Placing three fingers along the carotid pulse is a helpful guide to the vascular orientation.

(7) Leaving the green needle *in situ* as a guide, cannulate the vein with the Seldinger needle attached to a saline flIled syringe. If entry does not occur within 4 cm then withdraw the needle and re-insert with a more lateral orientation.

(8) The process of Seldinger cannulation is identical to subclavian access.

The external jugular may appear very tempting during a difficult internal jugular cannulation, but in our experience the difficulties typically encountered in negotiating its junction with the subclavian make it of little use.

Potential problems

Failure to locate the vessel is the commonest problem, followed by inadvertent carotid artery puncture. Neither of these is a problem if the rule of always locating the vessel with the green needle before inserting the Seldinger needle is followed. As with subclavian puncture, distending the vein by head down positioning is frequently helpful in hypovolaemic patients.

14.1.3 Femoral route

This is useful in an emergency but use for more than a few hours is not recommended. Pacing wires tend to be unstable and displace, whilst it is extremely difficult to navigate pulmonary artery catheters around the "S" bend between the tricuspid and pulmonary valves. In addition there are significant concerns about increased rates of sepsis and the potential for thrombus formation.

(1) Position the patient with his/her leg slightly externally rotated.

(2) Prepare a sterile field and drape from the thigh to the lower abdomen.

(3) Palpate the inguinal ligament and palpate the femoral artery.

(4) Identify an area 1 cm below the ligament and 0.5–1 cm medial to the arterial pulse and infiltrate with lidocaine (lignocaine).

(5) Connect the Seldinger needle to a saline filled syringe and insert this at an angle of 30° along a line projected towards the umbilicus, continuously aspirating during advancement.

(6) Venous cannulation is confirmed by the aspiration of dark non-pulsatile blood.

(7) If cannulation is not achieved then aspiration should be continued during withdrawal as the needle has often exited through the posterior wall of the vein.

(8) If the artery is entered then 5 minutes of firm pressure is required.

(9) Perform the rest of the Seldinger manoeuvres as described above (except that a chest x ray is not required).

Potential problems

Repeated arterial puncture may occur if the vein lies posterior to the artery, and may require the use of a subclavian or jugular approach.

Femoral nerve trauma is indicated by paraesthesiae in the leg: the needle should be inserted more medially (remember medial→lateral Vein Artery Nerve).

14.2 Temporary transvenous pacing

The indications for temporary pacing are discussed in Chapter 12. With the advent of reliable transcutaneous pacing and the decrease in the incidence of infarction-related heart block produced by the introduction of thrombolysis, there has been a sharp decline in the numbers of temporary wires inserted. As a result, experience with this technique among non-cardiologists has dwindled and there has been a noticeable increase in complications rates.[1] Before undertaking transvenous pacing, the indications for insertion should be carefully reviewed.

- Patients who are haemodynamically stable but have an indication for prophylactic pacing (particulariy following thrombolysis) should be managed with transcutaneous pacing.
- Haemodynamic compromise due to post-infarction bradycardia should be considered for temporary dual chamber pacing, not a simple single chamber system.
- Complete heart block not associated with haemodynamic compromise or syncope does not usually require temporary pacing and patients are better served by insertion of a permanent pacemaker on the next available list.[2]

Lastly, transcutaneous pacing has eliminated the misery of attempting to insert temporary wires into asystolic patients.

The fact that wires are often left *in situ* for several days and then followed by a permanent implant means that strict asepsis during insertion is particularly important. Patients requiring continued temporary pacing for more than 5 days should have a new lead inserted using a fresh site.

14.2.1 Preparation

As noted above, the subclavian is the preferred access route. In addition it is necessary to determine where any potential permanent system will be placed and to use the opposite side for the temporary wire (thus for a right handed person use a right sided approach so that the non-dominant side is available for the permanent system).

There are many temporary pacing electrodes to choose from. Although stiffer pacing wires are easier to manipulate they are potentially more likely to perforate the right ventricle and softer 5 or 6 French plastic-coated electrodes are now commonly used. The disadvantage of these is that, when warmed by the circulation, these soften, making manipulation very difficult. This problem can be partially overcome by using a balloon-flotation electrode which facilitates crossing the tricuspid valve.[3]

14.2.2 Inserting semi-rigid pacing catheters

1. Check the pacing wire. Many semi-rigid catheters have an excessive preformed curve, whilst some have none at all. A curve of 20–30° 4–5 cm from the tip is optimal.

2. Insert the electrode into the sheath and advance it into the right atrium.

3. Rotate the wire so that it points towards the apex and then advance slowly, crossing the tricuspid valve and sliding along the floor of the right ventricle to reach the apex.

4. If there is difficulty in crossing the tricuspid valve, form a loop against the lateral wall of the atrium, then rotate counter-clockwise and gently withdraw until the tip flicks across the valve.

5. Ideally the electrode tip should be at the right ventricular apex, well left of the spine with the tip pointing inferiorly (Figure 14.2). There should be a generous loop of pacing wire within the right ventricle so that the tip does not displace with inspiration (check with screening).

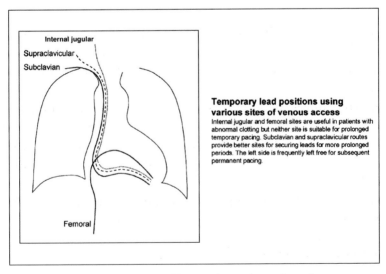

Figure 14.2 Temporary lead positions using various sites of venous access

6. Set the pacing box 10 beat/min faster than the patient's own rate and warn the patient that they will notice their heart rate accelerate as the system is tested. Setting the voltage at 3 volts the output is decreased until capture no longer occurs to define the threshold (< 1 V is ideal, < 1.5 V acceptable in an emergency).

7. Raise the output to $3 \times$ threshold and test for stability by ensuring capture during deep inspiration and forceful cough. Set the pacing rate to one appropriate for the clinical setting.

8. Carefully remove the introducer sheath whilst screening the pacing wire tip to ensure inadvertent displacement.

9. Secure the wire to the skin with 1-0 silk or equivalent.

10. Form the wire into a loop on the skin and secure this with two further sutures and cover with a sterile transparent dressing before obtaining a chest x ray.

11. Pacing thresholds should be checked daily.

14.2.3 Inserting a balloon-flotation pacing catheter

1. Check the balloon by inflating it in a small container of sterile saline.

2. Insert the electrode into the venous sheath and advance it to 15 cm before inflating the balloon.

3. Under fluoroscopic guidance, advance the balloon across the tricuspid valve.

4. The tip will tend to float up into the right ventricular outflow tract.

5. Deflate the balloon and the tip will fall to the apex and will then only require a little manipulation to optimise the position.

6. Electrical testing and lead fixation are as for semi-rigid catheters.

Potential problems

Difficulty in crossing the tricuspid valve or in obtaining a satisfactory position within the right ventricular apex are both frequent and may respond to a change in insertion technique. Balloon-flotation techniques facilitate crossing the tricuspid valve but are more difficult to position within the apex, whereas with semi-rigid catheters, problems are generally encountered crossing the valve but once this has been achieved, ventricular positioning is easier. The use of a stylet-based wire may be helpful in difficult cases as the catheter's shape can be reconfigured during insertion.

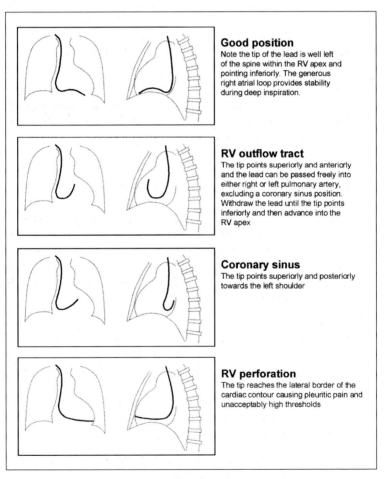

Good position
Note the tip of the lead is well left of the spine within the RV apex and pointing inferiorly. The generous right atrial loop provides stability during deep inspiration.

RV outflow tract
The tip points superiorly and anteriorly and the lead can be passed freely into either right or left pulmonary artery, excluding a coronary sinus position. Withdraw the lead until the tip points inferiorly and then advance into the RV apex

Coronary sinus
The tip points superiorly and posteriorly towards the left shoulder

RV perforation
The tip reaches the lateral border of the cardiac contour causing pleuritic pain and unacceptably high thresholds

Figure 14.3 Correct and incorrect lead positions for temporary pacing.

Inadvertent intubation of the coronary sinus will direct the electrode tip up towards the left shoulder (Figure 14.3) preventing the required inferior orientation of a position within the ventricular apex. The electrode should be withdrawn to the high right atrium prior to further attempts of positioning.

Ventricular perforation is not uncommon and particular care is required after recent inferior infarction (Figure 14.3). Patients will usually complain of pleuritic chest pain and pacing thresholds rise, although haemodynamically significant tamponade is surprisingly uncommon. The wire should be gently withdrawn and carefully repositioned. Right ventricular perforation is usually well tolerated but, urgent echocardiographic assessment should be performed.

Lead displacement is suggested by loss of capture or progressive threshold elevation and is confirmed by chest *x* ray. Microdisplacement (rise in threshold without radiographic displacement) can usually be managed by increasing the voltage but repositioning is occasionally required.

14.2.4 Temporary transvenous pacing – atrial

Temporary trial pacing in isolation is rarely appropriate due to the high rate of lead displacement. However it is increasingly employed in patients with heart block who require restoration of atrioventricular synchrony to optimise their haemodynamic status. Temporary atrial leads are usually supplied with preformed "J" curves.

(1) Obtain central venous access.

(2) Insert the wire to mid atrial level.

(3) Rotate the wire until the tip is on the left of the atrium and pointing cranially.

(4) Gradually withdraw the wire until the tip catches on the right atrial appendage (Figure 14.4): at this point further withdrawal of the wire will cause the "J" loop to open up.

(5) At this point the wire tip should make a "figure of eight" or "windscreen wiper" motion.

(6) Establish electrical parameters (< 1.5 V is acceptable), test stability, and secure the lead.

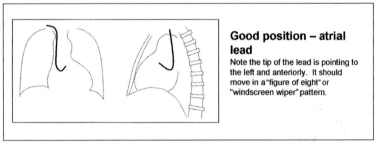

Good position – atrial lead
Note the tip of the lead is pointing to the left and anteriorly. It should move in a "figure of eight" or "windscreen wiper" pattern.

Figure 14.4 Correct position of temporary atrial leads.

14.3 Pulmonary artery catheterisation

The indications for insertion of a Swan-Ganz catheter are discussed in the relevant chapters but can be summarised as:

• Shock of unknown aetiology.
• Fluid management in right ventricular infarction.
• Differential diagnosis of pulmonary oedema.

There is something intuitively attractive and reassuring about the generation of apparently objective data in acutely ill patients and, as a result, Swan-Ganz catheters have undoubtedly been over-utilised in the USA. Subsequent concerns about safety[4] have sparked a fierce debate and have initiated calls for a moratorium in their use.[5] This debate has less relevance to UK cardiology where pulmonary artery catheterisation has always been less prevalent. However, the fact remains that the data generated is often less clear cut than anticipated and must always be viewed in the context of the overall clinical picture. In addition, the majority of useful information accrues within the first 24 hours after insertion and we strongly favour a policy of removing catheters at this point unless there are compelling reasons to continue monitoring. Subsequent reinsertion of a second catheter may be preferable to prolonged monitoring. Whilst catheters are frequently inserted successfully without the use of screening, this is not recommended, particularly in patients with cardiac disease. The practical aspects of pulmonary artery (PA) catheter placement are considered under the headings of preparation, insertion, and interpretation.

14.3.1 Preparation

(1) Zero the transducers by opening the line to the atmosphere at mid-chest level whilst depressing the "zero" option on the monitor.

(2) Prepare a sterile field and liberally drape the patient's upper extermity: the catheter is unwieldy and frequently needs to be laid on a sterile surface during insertion.

(3) Obtain central venous access: subclavian is preferable, jugular is possible, and femoral is not recommended.

(4) Unpack the catheter, attach three-way taps to the lines leading to the proximal (right atrial) and distal (pulmonary artery) ports and flush each line with saline.

(5) Inflate the balloon with air using the syringe included in the pack and then place this in a small container of sterile saline to check for leaks.

(6) Remember to thread the catheter through the mandril which will permit subsequent manoeuvre of the catheter without loss of sterility.

(7) Connect the catheter to the pressure transducer and flush.

14.3.2 Insertion

(1) Insert the catheter into the venous sheath.

(2) Inflate the balloon between the first and second 10 cm marks (when the balloon is outside the insertion sheath).

(3) Feed the catheter across the tricuspid valve: the systolic pressure rises, the balloon oscillates from right to left on screening and the ECG demonstrates ventricular ectopics. This usually occurs between the 25–35 cm marks. Failure

of these signs to appear indicates that the catheter has not crossed the valve and is merely curling round in an enlarged right atrium: deflate the balloon and start again.

(4) The balloon should now "turn the corner" and face cranially: pausing for a few seconds may facilitate this, as may asking the patient to take a deep breath.

(5) Advancing the catheter will result in the balloon crossing the pulmonary valve signalled by an increase in diastolic pressure, usually around the 40 cm mark.

(6) Feed the catheter forward into the pulmonary artery (it usually lodges on the right side and at around 40–50 cm).

(7) The catheter should migrate distally into the wedged position. This can be confirmed by the characteristic forward motion of the catheter tip when the balloon is inflated and the bifid pressure trace. Deflation of the balloon should be followed by movement of the balloon backwards into the pulmonary artery, the restoration of pulsatile motion and the re-appearance of the characteristic arterial pressure tracing (Figure 14.5).

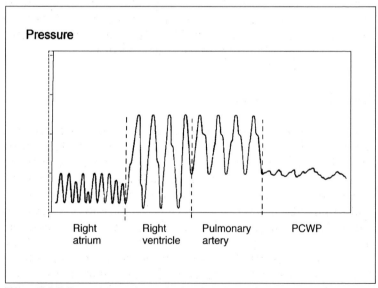

Figure 14.5 Pressure tracings obtained during pulmonary artery catheterisation.

The three most important rules in PA catheter placement are:

- Never leave the catheter with balloon wedged for longer than it takes to make a PCWP measurement (< 40 seconds).
- Never pull the catheter back with the balloon still inflated.
- Always inflate the balloon slowly and monitor the pressure tracing during inflation.

PCWP readings only represent left atrial pressure if the pulmonary capillary wedge pressure (PCWP) value is less than alveoiar pressure.[6] This condition is only satisfied for the basal one-third of the lungs (so called zone 3). This region is readily identified in erect patients where a useful rule is to ensure that the catheter tip is always below the level of the left atrium. However, in a supine patient this region can only be identified with a lateral chest x ray and this is unacceptably cumbersome for routine use. As the majority of catheters spontaneously lodge in zone 3 (due to its higher flow), a suggested compromise is to resort to a lateral chest x ray if the PCWP data do not fit into the overall clinical picture.

As the catheter is manufactured from PVC, it becomes progressively less rigid following insertion. Thus it is important to attempt to cross the tricuspid valve and to negotiate the curve of the RV (the two most difficult manoeuvres) as soon as possible after insertion.

14.3.3 Interpretation

The commonly encountered haemodynamic patterns are listed in Table 14.1. The normal range of the right heart pressures are given in Table 14.2. It is important to appreciate that the accuracy of the pressure data is limited and should be viewed in terms of a series of bands (low: 0–13, mid 14–23, and high >24 mmHg) as opposed to absolute values. In particular, a change in pressure in response to fluid loading, diuresis, etc. is more significant than isolated values. Importantly, the relationship between pressure and volume (i.e. the degree of pressure change one would expect for a given change in volume) is non-linear and varies with time due to changes in circulatory capacitance. Formulae for the derived variables are listed in Box 14.1, however, these all depend on thermodilution derived cardiac output, which is frequently inaccurate. For the majority of cardiac patients, calculation of these values adds little to patient management and use of a non-thermodilution catheter is satisfactory. In patients with obstructive airways disease, pulmonary fibrosis, mechanical ventilation, mitral stenosis, or following cardiopulmonary bypass, PCWP values tend to be higher than LV filling pressures. Conversely, aortic regurgitation, pneumonectomy and pulmonary embolus are all associated with PCWP readings in excess of true LV filling pressures.

Table 14.1 Haemodynamic patterns in shock.

Condition	RA	PA	PCWP	CI	PVR	SVR
LV infarction	↔ or ↑	↔	↑↑	↓	↓	↑
RV infarction	↑	↓ <1.5 × RA	↓	↓	↓	↑
Ventricular septal defect	↔ or ↑	↑	↑	↑	↑	↑
Papillary muscle rupture	↔ or ↑	↑	↑↑	↓	↑	↑
Massive pulmonary embolus	↑	↑	↓	↓	↑↑	↑
Tamponade	↑↑	↓	= to RA	↓	↔	↑
Early septicaemia	↓	↓	↓	↑	↓	↓
Late septicaemia	↔ or ↑	↔ or ↑	↑	↓	↑	↑
Hypovolaemia	↓	↓	↓	↓	↔	↑

RA: right atrium, PA: pulmonary artery; PCWP: pulmonary capillary wedge pressure; CI: cardiac index; PVR: pulmonary vascular resistance; SVR: systemic vascular resistance.

Notes

These represent general trends, to which there are many exceptions (for example pulmonary artery resistance and pressure may both rise in septicaemic shock, whilst both RA and PCWP may be normal despite marked hypovolaemia).

Large "V" waves may be present in the PCWP tracing of patients with both ventricular septal defects and acute mitral regurgitation.

The thermodilution cardiac index in patients with VSDs will reflect *pulmonary* flow and will therefore br higher than expected.

Saturation measurements in patients with VSDs will demonstrate the characteristic "step-up" between the RA and RV samples.

Table 14.2 Normal ranges of right heart pressures

Site	Pressure/mmHg
Right atrium (RA)	
range	0–5
Right ventricle (RV)	
systolic	15–30
diastolic	0–6
Pulmonary artery (PA)	
systolic	15–30
diastolic	5–13
range	10–18
Pulmonary wedge (PCWP)	
range	2–12

Box 14.1 Derived data formulae

Systemic vascular resistance $= \dfrac{80\,(\text{MAP}-\text{CVP})}{\text{CO}}$ $\quad$ 1000–1500 dynes/s/cm^{-5}

Pulmonary vascular resistance $= \dfrac{80\,(\text{MPAP}-\text{PCWP})}{\text{CO}}$ $\quad$ 120–250 dynes/s/cm^{-5}

Cardiac index $= \dfrac{\text{CO}}{\text{body surface area}}$ $\quad$ 2.5–4.5 l/min/m^2

CO=cardiac output, MPAP=mean pulmonary artery pressure, CVP=central venous pressure, PCWP=pulmonary capillary wedge pressure

14.3.4 Potential problems

Failure to wedge is usually due to the balloon failing to migrate distally enough. Deflate the balloon and attempt to manoeuvre it into another lung segment. If the catheter will not wedge despite this then the pulmonary artery diastolic pressure may be used as a substitute for PCWP.

Damped traces respond to flushing the system or slight withdrawal of the catheter.

Effects of mechanical ventilation and PEEP may be minimised by taking all recordings at end expiration.

Right bundle branch block occurs in 5% of patients due to the balloon coming into contact with the exposed section of the right bundle (moderator band) as it tracks across the right ventricular floor. This may produce complete heart block in patients with pre-existing left bundle branch block in whom a prophylactic temporary wire is required.

Pulmonary artery rupture, presenting as haemoptysis, may occur when the balloon is inflated too rapidly in a small peripheral branch: this emphasises the importance of slow and gentle balloon inflation.

Catheter knotting is a risk if screening is not used and the distances for the appearance of the various changes in waveform are exceeded. Once knotted it may prove impossible to withdraw the catheter into the sheath and a surgical venotomy may be needed.

14.4 DC cardioversion

The degree of preparation appropriate will depend on the urgency of the situation.[7,8] Prior to performing DC cardioversion, check the plasma potassium and correct this if time permits, though bear in mind that two oral potassium tablets will have little effect on total body potassium levels. Similarly, for elective conversion of atrial fibrillation or flutter with durations > 48 hours adequate anticoagulation (INR > 2.5 in general, but 3.5–4 with mechanical valves) both at the present time and over the preceding month should be confirmed. An alternative is to perform a transoesophageal echo to confirm the absence of intracardiac thrombi and then perform cardioversion with acute heparin. In conscious patients adequate sedation is essential and this is best obtained with general anaesthesia. Light sedation for cardioversion, other than in extreme emergencies, is unacceptable. Deep sedation using iv midazolam combined with flumazenil recovery is an alternative only in experienced hands and requires the presence of a second doctor to administer. Digoxin need not be withheld prior to cardioversion, but caution should be exercised in patients in whom digoxin toxicity is suspected.

(1) Connect the patient to the defibrillator.

(2) Switch lead orientations until a QRS of adequate amplitude is obtained.

(3) Change the defibrillator to synchronous shock mode and check that the sensing algorithm marks each R wave with a sensing artifact.

(4) Place the paddles or self adhesive pads either anterolaterally (apex and right praecordium) or anteroposteriorly (apex and posterior).

(5) Charge to the appropriate energy (see below).

(6) Check that everyone is clear, issue the "everyone clear" warning and depress the discharge button: there is a disconcerting pause of approximately 1–2 seconds (depending on heart rate) before discharge.

(7) If cardioversion is successful then a 12-lead ECG should be obtained. If unsuccessful then the energy level should be increased and/or an anteroposterior position attempted.

- Patients who transiently convert to sinus rhythm (SR) but then degenerate back to their initial arrhythmia will not remain in SR any longer despite higher energy shocks.
- Optimum results are obtained from anteroposterior paddle positions[9] (best achieved with self adhesive pads) and end expiration. It is important to appreciate that firm pressure is still required even when pads are used.
- Previous recommendations for the initial energy settings started at inappropriately low levels and the recent demonstration that myocardial damage does not occur during routine cardioversion has encouraged the use of higher initial energy levels.[10,11] For atrial fibrillation, we currently use a starting energy of 200 J followed by 360 J,[12] whilst for atrial flutter, a minimum energy of 100 J is recommended.[13] The position is less clear for ventricular tachycardia, but we currently recommend 200 J.
- Unlike troponins,[10,11] "cardiac" enzymes (including creatinine kinase MB fraction (CKMB)) are elevated following cardioversion due to skeletal muscle damage, and blood for these should be obtained taken prior to the procedure (from the sample used to check the K^+).

- There is preliminary evidence to suggest an increased rate of successful conversion following the administration of 1 mg atropine in patients with atrial fibrillation who do not successfully convert to SR.[14]
- Patients require one month of anticoagulation following successful cardioversion of atrial fibrillation (restoration of mechanical activity lags behind the electrical function by several weeks).

Potential problems

Ventricular fibrillation occasionally follows cardioversion (even with correct synchronisation). Before a defibrillating shock can be administered it is essential to switch to asynchronous mode without which no shock will be delivered despite frantic depression of the discharge buttons (the defibrillator cannot synchronise on VF).

Fulminant pulmonary oedema may complicate successful cardioversion.

Peripheral embolisation occurs in 1–2% of cases.

Permanent pacemakers may be disabled by shocks delivered < 10 cm of the pulse generator, resulting in profound bradycardia following cardioversion. A pacing magnet will revert the system to asynchronous mode (VOO/DOO) and overcome this.

Skin burns are more common with higher energy levels (both total and cumulative[15]) and are traditionally treated with 1% hydrocortisone cream.

14.5 Pericardiocentesis

14.5.1 Clinical presentation of cardiac tamponade

The classical features, encompassing Beck's triad, are of a falling blood pressure, rising venous pressure and quiet heart sounds. Added to this are pulsus paradoxus, a rise in central venous pressure with inspiration and occasionally the presence of a pericardial friction rub. Unfortunately, the possibility of tamponade is often not considered and treatment is frequently delayed.[16]

14.5.2 Investigations

The ECG may demonstrate small voltage QRS complexes (a subjective observation of little practical use). The cardiac silhouette appears globular on chest x ray. Echocardiography will demonstrate the presence of a pericaridal effusion. Unfortunately, confusion exists between the anatomical demonstration of pericardial fluid and the physiological diagnosis of tamponade. The degree of compression, and thus the restriction to cardiac filling, exerted by pericardial fluid depends upon the rate of its accumulation and the degree of pericardial distensibility. Thus the rapid accumulation of small volumes (<1 cm effusion) of fluid into a rigid pericardium may produce acute tamponade whilst the gradual accumulation of much larger amounts may not. Echo and Doppler features to determine the haemodynamic consequences of pericardial fluid do exist (Box 14.2) but the more sophisticated of these are rarely performed. In addition, it is important to appreciate that inexperienced echocardiographers may mistake pleural fluid for a pericardial effusion.

Box 14.2 Echo/Doppler quantification of haemodynamic consequences of pericardial fluid

Right ventricular collapse with inspiration

> 20% change in mitral or 40% change in tricuspid velocities with respiration (mitral flow ↓ with inspiration, tricuspid flow ↑)

For these reasons the primary determinant of the need for emergency (as opposed to diagnostic) pericardiocentisis must be made on the basis of the degree of haemodynamic compromise (hypotension with > 20 mmHg paradox) and not simply the presence of pericardial fluid per se. Failure to appreciate this may lead to severe complications from a procedure that was never likely to have benefitted the patient in the first place.

14.5.3 Blind pericardiocentesis

The traditional procedure should now only be used as a last resort: actual or impending cardiac arrest due to pulseless electrical activity (PEA). Connecting an ECG lead to the needle makes it no less barbaric and only wastes time.

(1) Attach a 16 gauge needle to a 25 ml syringe: use either a spinal needle or one taken from a central line set.

(2) Palpate just beneath the xiphisternum.

(3) Angle the needle 45° downwards and 45° to the left (aiming for the left shoulder)

(4) Advance the needle with continuous negative pressure, stopping the moment blood is aspirated.

(5) Place the aspirated blood into a plain glass test tube: ventricular blood clots, but pericardial fluid does not.

14.5.4 Echo-guided pericardiocentesis

This is now the procedure of choice, but is still hazardous and should only be performed by those with experience. If time permits, a clotting screen and platelet count should be checked.

(1) Scan the patient to determine the region with the optimum combination of fluid width and accessability, mark the skin at the proposed point of entry.

(2) Prepare a sterile field and consider the use of light sedation.

(3) Infiltrate both the superficial and deep layers with local anaesthetic.

(4) Make a small nick in the skin at the marked entry site.

(5) Open a sterile glove and ask an assistant to place echo gel and the echo transducer into this to provide a sterile transducer. Re-scan from the point of skin incision to the point of proposed pericardial penetration, noting the depth in centimetres from the display.

(6) Gradually advance the pericardiocentisis needle parallel

to the echo probe an appropriate distance to puncture the pericardium (the needle itself is often poorly visualised on the scan).

(7) Aspirate fluid. If there is uncertainty about the needle's position, gently re-inject a small volume of the fluid: echo contrast will appear within the cardiac chambers if ventricular perforation has occurred.

(8) Remove the syringe and advance the guidewire into the pericardium before removing the needle.

(9) Advance the dilator over the wire and then remove it.

(10) Advance the pericardial drainage pigtail catheter over the wire.

(11) Aspirate fluid whilst intermittently confirming that the effusion is indeed decreasing, send samples for cytology and culture as appropriate.

(12) When no further fluid can be aspirated (a small posterior collection often remains), re-insert the guidewire and remove the pigtail. Failure to re-insert the guidewire may result in the curled up end of the pigtail catheter lacerating the coronary veins. Leaving a drain in the pericardium should be avoided if possible: if recurrent fluid accumulation occurs then a pericardial window should be considered.

(13) A chest x ray should be obtained following the procedure, as pneumothorax is a potential complication.

14.5.5 Potential problems

Perforation of the cardiac chamber (usually the right ventricle) is the most common problem. The chances of this occurring are minimised by echo guidance and by avoiding drainage of effusions of < 1 cm depth at the proposed entry site. As noted above, the appearance of an echo contrast effect within the heart, when a small volume of the aspirate is injected, is diagnostic. Injection of radiocontrast and screening is an alternative. If only the needle has perforated the myocardium, matters may resolve spontaneously once it has been removed (although the effusion will enlarge); if the dilator has been advanced over the wire then emergency cardiac surgery will be required. Problems of myocardial perforation may only become apparent when the drainage catheter is removed and patients should be observed carefully at this point.

14.6 Intra-aortic balloon pump management

Balloon pump use continues to increase and the range of potential indications has enlarged significantly in recent years (Box 14.3). Although the insertion of intra-aortic balloon pumps (IABP) is not technically demanding, it calls for proficiency in skills which can only be acquired with regular experience in a cardiac catheter lab and is beyond the scope of this book. However, it is not uncommon to be involved in the care of a patient who has had an IABP inserted and some familiarity with the indications for insertion and the potential problems is useful. IABPs work by inflating to force blood back down the coronaries (when the majority of coronary perfusion occurs) then deflating during systole to present the ventricle with a reduced afterload (Figure 14.6).

Balloon pump insertion is contraindicated in patients with significant aortic regurgitation, ongoing sepsis and in whom severe peripheral vascular disease precludes insertion.

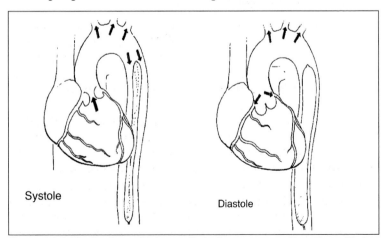

Systole

Diastole

Figure 14.6 Mechanism of intra-aortic balloon pump action. From Shah PK. Complications of acute myocardial infarction. In: Parmley W (Ed.). *Cardiology.* Philadelphia: Lippincott, 1987.

Box 14.3 Indications for intra-aortic balloon pump insertion

Cardiogenic shock: prior to revascularisation
prior to surgery for VSD or mitral regurgitation

Refractory unstable angina

Support during high risk angioplasty

Stabilisation of refractory ventricular tachycardia

Myocardial support following cardiac surgery

Severe heart failure awaiting cardiac transplantation

Balloon assisted thrombolysis in cardiogenic shock?

14.6.1 Potential problems

Mechanical problems tend to centre on vascular access and bleeding from the insertion site[17] (patients are usually anticoagulated following insertion). Sheathless insertion is increasingly used and this is more comfortable for the patient although bleeding is initially more common. Manual pressure over the entry site, followed by the use of prolonged low pressure from a sandbag or, failing this, a "Femostop" device may be required. Distal leg ischaemia is less common with the current small calibre devices than previously but foot perfusion should be checked daily.

Timing problems relate to the need to inflate the balloon just after the dichrotic notch so that the ejecting ventricle is never faced with the high outflow resistance created by an inflated balloon (Figure 14.7). Deflation should be timed to coincide with the nadir of arterial pressure prior to the next ejection. Most devices have a facility which marks the portion of the aortic pressure tracing during which the balloon is inflated to facilitate these adjustments. If there is doubt over timing, it may be helpful to switch to augmenting every other beat (1 : 2 augmentation) as this enables comparison of native and augmented beats. Unless there are compelling reasons to do otherwise, synchronisation should be set to ECG as opposed to pressure. Older devices have difficulty in tachycardic patients and all devices have difficulty with atrial fibrillation.

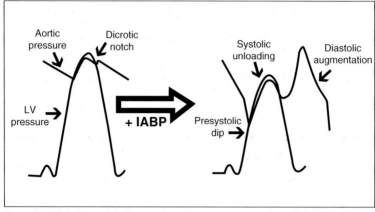

Figure 14.7 Left ventricular and aortic pressure tracings following intra-aortic balloon pump augmentation.

Weaning is usually accomplished by a combination of decreasing the ratio of augmented beats (1:1 → 1:2 → 1:3, etc.) or by reducing the amount of augmentation provided to each beat. For patients that are difficult to wean a combination of both may be helpful.

Removal is frequently painful as the local anaesthetic used at insertion will have long worn off. To minimise this we routinely infiltrate the insertion site with lidocaine (lignocaine) prior to removal and frequently administer a small dose of opiate. Twenty minutes of firm manual pressure is required following removal.

Clinical cases

Case 14.1

A 40-year-old man presented to his local hospital with a history of fatigue. He was noted to have been in renal failure and he was transferred to the regional renal unit. Prior to dialysis he was found to be hypotensive and echocardiography was requested. On examination his BP was 95/50 with 30 mmHg paradox, quiet heart sounds and positive Kussmaul's sign. Echocardiography confirmed the presence of a 2 cm pericardial effusion. Echo-guided pericardiocentesis via the apical approach revealed purulent material. Although there was a transient improvement in his condition, within 10 minutes there was an abrupt deterioration with worsening hypotension. A chest x ray revealed a new left sided pleural effusion. Despite antibiotics and fluids he suffered a cardiac arrest (pulseless electrical activity) 30 minutes later. His cardiac output returned with further volume loading accompanied by boluses and an infusion of adrenaline (epinephrine). Emergency thoracotomy revealed purulent pericarditis and laceration of an intercostal artery at the time of pericardiocentisis. The patient made a complete recovery.

Even in experienced hands, and using echo guidance, pericardiocentisis remains a hazardous procedure. Purulent pericarditis may occur secondary to pharangeal sepsis or, as in this case, be idiopathic.

Case 14.2

A 55-year-old man who was receiving low dose aspirin treatment for coronary disease was noted to be in complete heart block by his general practitioner. He was referred to his local hospital by which time he was in sinus rhythm. Insertion of a temporary pacemaker was attempted. Multiple attempts at securing subclavian access were unsuccessful and an internal jugular approach was attempted. Again, several attempts at cannulation were unsuccessful and a large haematoma developed. Following the last attempt at insertion the patient experienced a period of pulseless electrical activity which resolved with volume replacement.

On transfer, the patient was hypotensive but with no clinical evidence of tamponade. Chest x ray followed by CT scanning revealed a large haematoma arising at the junction of the subclavian and carotid arteries, tracking into the mediastinum and associated with a 1 cm pericardial effusion. Clinical examination and subsequent echocardiography failed to demonstrate evidence of significant tamponade physiology.

His condition improved following volume replacement. The haematoma (presumably caused by inadvertent arterial cannulation) gradually resolved spontaneously as did the pericardial effusion. A permanent pacemaker was implanted uneventfully one week following admission.

Patients with heart block not associated with syncope or haemodynamic compromise do not require temporary pacing. If central venous cannulation is unsuccessful then it is important to seek help rather than persist. Not all pericardial effusions produce tamponade and not all need to be tapped.

References

1 Cooper JP, Swanton RH. Complications of transvenous temporary pacemaker insertion. *Br J Hosp Med* 1995;**53**:155–61.

2 Hildick-Smith DJR, Petch MC. Temporary pacing before permanent pacing should be avoided unless essential. *BMJ* 1998;**317**:79–80.

3 Ferguson JD, Banning AP, Bashir Y. Randomised trial of temporary cardiac pacing with semirigid and balloon-flotation electrode catheters. *Lancet* 1997;**349**:1883.

4 Connors AFJ, Speroff T, Dawson NV, *et al*. The effectiveness of right heart catheterization in the initial care of critically ill patients. SUPPORT Investigators. *JAMA* 1996;**276**:889–97.

5 Dalen JE, Bone RC. Is it time to pull the pulmonary artery catheter? *JAMA* 1996;**276**:916–18.

6 Brandstetter RD, Grant GR, Estilo M, Rahim F, Singh K, Gitler B. Swan-Ganz catheter: misconceptions, pitfalls, and incomplete user knowledge – an identified trilogy in need of correction. *Heart Lung* 1998;**27**:218–22.

7 Ewy GA. The optimal technique for electrical cardioversion of atrial fibrillation. [Review]. *Clin Cardiol* 1994;**17**:79–84.

8 Yurchak PM, Williams SV, Achord JL, *et al*. Clinical competence in elective direct current (DC) cardioversion. A statement for physicians from the AHA/ACC/ACP Task Force on Clinical Privileges in Cardiology. *Circulation* 1993;**88**:342–5.

9 Botto GL, Politi A, Bonini W, Broffoni T, Bonatti R. External cardioversion of atrial fibrillation: role of paddle position on technical efficacy and energy requirements. *Heart* 1999;**82**:726–30.

10 Rao AC, Naeem N, John C, Collinson PO, Canepa-Anson R, Joseph SP. Direct current cardioversion does not cause cardiac damage: evidence from cardiac troponin T estimation. *Heart* 1998;**80**:229–30.

11 Greaves K, Crake T. Cardiac troponin T does not increase after electrical cardioversion for atrial fibrillation or atrial flutter. *Heart* 1998;**80**:226–8.

12 Joglar JA, Hamdan MH, Ramaswamy K, *et al*. Initial energy for elective external cardioversion of persistent atrial fibrillation. *Am J Cardiol* 2000;**86**:348–50.

13 Pinski SL, Sgarbossa EB, Ching E, Trohman RG. A comparison of 50-J versus 100-J shocks for direct-current cardioversion of atrial flutter. *Am Heart J* 1999;**137**:439–42.

14 Sutton AG, Khurana C, Hall JA, Davies A, de Belder MA. The use of atropine for facilitation of direct current cardioversion from atrial fibrillation – results of a pilot study. *Clin Cardiol* 1999;**22**:712–14.

15 Pagan-Carlo LA, Stone MS, Kerber RE. Nature and determinants of skin "burns" after transthoracic cardioversion. *Am J Cardiol* 1997;**79**:689–91.

16 Larose E, Ducharme A, Mercier LA, Pelletier G, Harei F, Tardif JC. Prolonged distress and clinical deterioration before pericardial drainage in patients with cardiac tamponade. *Canad J Cardiol* 2000;**16**:331–6.

17 Cook L, Pillar B, McCord G, Josephson R. Intra-aortic balloon pump complications: a five-year retrospective study of 283 patients. *Heart Lung* 1999;**28**:195–202.

18 Bone RG. *Acute respiratory failure*. New York: Churchill Livingstone, 1987:356.

Appendix: CCU drug protocols

CCU Staff. John Radcliffe Hospital, Oxford

Accelerated TPA (Alteplase)

Administration:

Route   Any IV access.

Infusion   100 mg dissolved in 100 ml water for injections.
               Bolus of 15 mg given over two minutes, followed
               by infusion of 0.75 mg/kg over 30 minutes,
               followed by infusion of 0.5 mg/kg over one hour.
               Weight-adjusted only up to maximum 65 kg.
               Heparin should be administered concurrently
               with TPA (bolus 5000 units followed by infusion
               at 1000 units/hr.) Heparin infusion is adjusted to
               achieve an APTT of 1.5–2.5 times control value).

	Weight			
	50 kg	55 kg	60 kg	65 kg+
Bolus over 2 minutes	15 mg	15 mg	15 mg	15 mg
Infusion over 30 minutes	37.5 mg	41.25 mg	45 mg	50 mg
Infusion over 1 hour	25 mg	27.5 mg	30 mg	35 mg

Adrenaline (epinephrine)

Administration:

Route   Should be given centrally.
Infusion 2 mg in 50 ml N saline or 5% dextrose.
Range   2–50 ml/hr

kg	Infusion rate in ml/hr								
	2	4	6	8	10	15	20	30	50
50	0.026	0.05	0.078	0.104	0.13	0.2	0.26	0.4	0.66
60	0.022	0.044	0.066	0.088	0.11	0.16	0.22	0.33	0.55
70	0.019	0.038	0.057	0.076	0.095	0.142	0.19	0.28	0.476
80	0.016	0.03	0.05	0.06	0.083	0.125	0.166	0.25	0.416
90	0.014	0.029	0.044	0.059	0.074	0.11	0.148	0.232	0.37
100	0.013	0.028	0.04	0.053	0.066	0.1	0.13	0.2	0.33

(Figures in table are expressed in micrograms/kg/min.)

Amiodarone

Administration:

Route   Should be given centrally.

Bolus   300 mg in 20–50 ml of dextrose 5% over 1 hour.

Infusion 450 mg in 48 ml dextrose 5% over 12 hours=4 ml/hour. Repeat once therefore total infusion of 900 mg following bolus. Maximum dose in 24 hours=1.2 g.

Atenolol

Administration:

Route   Any IV access.

Bolus   2.5 mg at a rate of 1 mg/min. Repeat every 5 minutes to total of 10 mg.

Bretylium

Administration:

Route   Any IV access.

Bolus   5 mg/kg (undiluted). If no response after 5 minutes, increase to 10 mg/kg. Maximum dose 40 mg/kg.
or
500 mg plus 40 ml 5% dextrose or 0.9% N saline (stable for up to 24 hours). Infuse over 8–30 minutes up to a total dose of 5–10 mg/kg.

Infusion   1–2 mg/min
or
5–10 mg/kg over 15–30 minutes every 6 hours.

Dalteparin (in acute coronary syndromes)

Administration:

Route   Subcutaneous.

Dose   120 units/kg bd for ≥ 5 days.

Weight (kg)	Dosage (units twice a day)
50–53	6000
54–57	6500
58–62	7000
63–66	7500
67–69	8000
70–74	8500
75–79	9000
80–83	9500
>83	10 000

Dobutamine

Administration:

Route Any IV access – ideally should be given centrally.

Infusion 250 mg in 50 ml 5% dextrose.
Usual range = 2.5–10 micrograms/kg/min.

Weight (kg)	Dose (micrograms/kg/min)														
	2	3	4	5	6	7	8	9	10	12	14	16	18	20	25
50	1.2	1.8	2.4	3.0	3.6	4.2	4.8	5.4	6.0	7.2	8.4	9.6	10.8	12	15
60	1.4	2.2	2.9	3.6	4.3	5.0	5.8	6.5	7.2	8.6	10.1	11.5	13.0	14.4	18
70	1.7	2.5	3.4	4.2	5.0	5.9	6.7	7.6	8.4	10.1	11.8	13.4	15.1	16.8	21
80	1.9	2.9	3.8	4.8	5.8	6.7	7.7	8.6	9.6	11.5	13.4	15.4	17.3	19.2	24
90	2.2	3.2	4.3	5.4	6.5	7.6	8.6	9.7	10.8	13.0	15.1	17.3	19.4	21.6	27
100	2.4	3.6	4.8	6.0	7.2	8.4	9.6	10.8	12.0	14.4	16.8	19.2	21.6	24.0	30

(Figures within the table are expressed in ml/hr)

Dopamine

Administration:

Route   Should be given centrally.

Infusion   200 mg in 50 ml 5% dextrose. Usual range 2.5–5 μg/kg/min (renal dose).

Weight (kg)	Dose (micrograms/kg/min)														
	1	1.5	2	2.5	3	3.5	4	5	6	7	8	9	10	15	20
50	0.8	1.1	1.5	1.9	2.3	2.6	3.0	3.8	4.5	5.3	6.0	6.8	7.5	11.3	15
60	0.9	1.4	1.8	2.3	2.7	3.2	3.6	4.5	5.4	6.3	7.2	8.1	9.0	13.5	18
70	1.1	1.6	2.1	2.6	3.2	3.7	4.2	5.3	6.3	7.4	8.4	9.5	10.5	15.8	21
80	1.2	1.8	2.4	3.0	3.6	4.2	4.8	6.0	7.2	8.4	9.6	10.8	12.0	18.0	24
90	1.4	2.0	2.7	3.4	4.1	4.7	5.4	6.8	8.1	9.5	10.8	12.2	13.5	20.3	27
100	1.5	2.3	3.0	3.8	4.5	5.3	6.0	7.5	9.0	10.5	12.0	13.5	15.0	22.5	30

(Figures within the table are expressed in ml/hr)

Heparin (unfractionated)

Administration:

Route   IV

Infusion   Heparin 20 000 units added to
                                  500 ml 5% dextrose

Initial bolus   5000 units

Maintenance infusion   Start at 33 ml/h ($=$1300 units/hr)

APPT	Rate change (ml/hr)	Additional action	Next APPT
<45	+6	Repeat bolus of 5000 units	4–6 hr
45–54	+3	None	4–6 hr
55–85	0	None	Next morning*
86–110	−3	Stop infusion for 1 hour	4–6 hr after restart
>110	+6	Stop infusion for 1 hour	4–6 hr after restart

* Monitor at least every 6 hours for first 24 hours.
Modified from Hyers TM *et al. Chest* 1992;**102**:408S–25S.

Insulin

Insulin infusion protocol from DIGAMI study: 500 ml 5% dextrose with 80 IU actrapid insulin ($\cong$ 1 IU/6 ml)

- Start at 30 ml/hr.

- Check blood glucose after 1 hour.

- Adjust rate according to the protocol and aim for a blood glucose 7–10 mmol/l.

- Blood glucose should be checked after 1 hour if infusion rate has been changed, otherwise every 2 hours.

- If the initial decrease in blood glucose exceeds 30%, the infusion rate should be left unchanged if blood glucose is >11 mmol/litre or reduced by 6 ml/hr if blood glucose is within the targeted range of 7–10 mmol/litre.

- If blood glucose is stable and < 10.9 mmol/litre after 10 pm, reduce infusion rate by 50% during the night.

> 15 mmol/litre	Give 8 IU of insulin as an IV bolus and increase infusion by 6 ml/hr
11–14.9 mmol/litre	Increase infusion rate by 3 ml/hr
7–10.9 mmol/litre	Leave infusion rate unchanged
4–6.9 mmol/litre	Decrease infusion rate by 6 ml/hr
< 4 mmol/litre	Stop infusion for 15 minutes. Then test blood glucose and continue testing every 15 minutes until blood glucose is ≥ 7 mmol/litre. In the presence of symptoms of hypoglycaemia, administer 12 ml 50% glucose intravenously. The infusion is restarted with an infusion rate decreased by 6 ml/hr when blood glucose is ≥ 7 mmol/litre.

Labetolol

Administration:

Route   Any IV access.

Bolus   If BP to be reduced quickly. 50 mg in 10 ml over 1 minute. If necessary repeat at 5 minute intervals.

Infusion 500 mg (100 ml) in 500 ml 5% dextrose. Commence infusion at 120 mg/hr. Titrate to keep systolic BP at approximately 100 mmHg.

Lidocaine (lignocaine)

Administration:

Route   Any IV access by slow injection – too rapid may cause fitting.

Bolus   Usually 50–100 mg. A further 50–l00 mg can be given.

Infusion Lidocaine (lignocaine) 1 g in 250 ml 5% dextrose (0.4% solution).
4 mg/min for 112 hr=60 ml/hr
3 mg/min for 1 hr=45 ml/hr
2 mg/min for 2 hr= 30 ml/hr
1 mg/min for up to 44 hr=15 ml/hr.

Metoprolol

Administration:

Route   IV peripheral/central.

Bolus   5 mg every 2 minutes to a maximum of 15 mg followed by oral administration.

Noradrenaline (norepinephrine)

Administration:

Route   Should be given centrally.

Bolus   4 mg in 50 ml 5% dextrose.

Weight (kg)	micrograms/kg/min									
	0.05	0.1	0.15	0.2	0.25	0.3	0.35	0.4	0.45	0.5
50	1.9	3.8	5.7	7.5	9.5	11.0	13.2	15.0	17.0	19.0
60	2.3	4.5	6.8	9.0	11.0	13.5	16.0	18.0	20.0	22.5
70	2.6	5.0	7.9	10.5	13.2	15.8	18.5	21.0	23.0	26.5
80	3.0	6.0	9.0	12.0	15.0	18.0	21.0	23.5	27.0	30.0
90	3.4	6.8	10.0	13.5	16.9	20.5	23.0	27.0	30.0	34.0
100	3.8	7.5	11.0	15.0	18.8	22.5	26.5	30.0	34.0	37.5

(Figures within table are expressed in ml/hr)

Streptokinase

Administration:

Route   Any IV access.

Bolus   1 500 000 units in 50 ml N saline given over 1 hour.

Sodium nitroprusside

Administration: Dissolve the 50 mg powder in 2 ml 5% dextrose. Make up the solution as 50 mg in 50 ml 5% dextrose or 0.9% sodium chloride (i.e. 1000 micrograms/ml). Protect the solution from light during administration using foil. Sodium nitroprusside degrades in light forming toxic products. Amber syringes do not provide adequate protection from light. Use an opaque giving set. Discard the solution after 24 hours. Titrate the dose given to the blood pressure. Wean off over 10–30 minutes to avoid a rebound increase in blood pressure

Weight (kg)	micrograms/kg/min						
	0.5	1	2	3	4	5	6
50	1.5	3.0	6.0	9.0	12.0	15.0	18.0
60	1.8	3.6	7.2	10.8	14.4	18.0	21.6
70	2.1	4.2	8.4	12.6	16.8	21.0	25.2
80	2.4	4.8	9.6	14.4	19.2	24.0	28.8
90	2.7	5.4	10.8	16.2	21.6	27.0	32.4
100	3.0	6.0	12.0	18.0	24.0	30.0	36.0

(Figures within table are expressed in ml/hr)

Tirofiban

Administration:

Route: IV

Infusion: Rmove 50 ml from a 250 ml container of 0.9% saline or 5% dextrose and replace with 50ml tirofiban concentrate (=50 micrograms/ml)

Weight (kg)	Infusion (ml/hr) 30-min loading	Maintenance
50	20	5
55	22	6
60	24	6
65	26	7
70	28	7
75	30	8
80	32	8
85	34	9
90	36	9
95	38	10
100	40	10

The dose of both the loading and maintenance infusions should be reduced by 50% in patients with renal failure (GFR < 30 ml/min).

Tirofiban should be administered at the same time as unfractionated heparin with KCCT titrated to 2×control. Unless contraindicated aspirin should also be administered.

Minimum recommended duration of infusion is 48 hours.

Index

Page numbers in **bold** type refer to figures; those in *italic* refer to tables or boxed material. Where material appears on the same page in more than one format, only one reference is given.